Dental Practice Transition

T0176879

Dental Practice Transition
A Practical Guide to Management

Second Edition

Edited by

David G. Dunning, Ph.D.,
Professor of Practice Management
Department of Oral Biology
University of Nebraska
Medical Center College of Dentistry
Lincoln, NE

And

Brian M. Lange, Ph.D.,
Professor of Behavioral Science
Department of Oral Biology
University of Nebraska
Medical Center College of Dentistry
Lincoln, NE

WILEY Blackwell

Editorial offices: 1606 Golden Aspen Drive, Suites 103 and 104, Ames, Iowa 50010, USA
The Atrium, Southern Gate, Chichester, West Sussex, PO19 8SQ, UK
9600 Garsington Road, Oxford, OX4 2DQ, UK

For details of our global editorial offices, for customer services, and for information about how to apply
for permission to reuse the copyright material in this book, please see our website at www.wiley.com/
wiley-blackwell.

Library of Congress Cataloging-in-Publication Data

Names: Dunning, David G., 1958- editor. | Lange, Brian Mark, editor.
Title: Dental practice transition : a practical guide to management / edited
    by David G. Dunning and Brian M. Lange.
Description: Second edition. | Ames, Iowa : John Wiley & Sons, Inc., 2016. |
    Includes bibliographical references and index.
Identifiers: LCCN 2016016542 (print) | LCCN 2016017184 (ebook) | ISBN
    9781119119456 (pbk.) | ISBN 9781119119463 (pdf) | ISBN 9781119119470 (epub)
Subjects: | MESH: Practice Management, Dental | Economics, Dental | Practice
    Valuation and Purchase | Dentistry
Classification: LCC RK58 (print) | LCC RK58 (ebook) | NLM WU 77 | DDC
    617.60068–dc23
LC record available at https://lccn.loc.gov/2016016542

A catalogue record for this book is available from the British Library.

2   2017

Table of Contents

Contributor List

Alderman, Bradley, D.D.S., Dental Practice Owner, Lincoln, NE

Anderson, Ronda, Hu-Friedy, Iowa/Nebraska Regional Account Manager, Louisville, NE

Boartfield, Rebecca, Human Resource Consultant, Bent Ericksen & Associates, Eugene, OR

Callan, Richard, D.M.D., Ed.S., Associate Professor and Department Chair, General Dentistry, College of Dental Medicine, Georgia Regents University, Augusta, GA

Crist, Ross L., D.D.S., M.A., M.S., Dental Practice Owner (orthodontics), Sioux Falls, SD

Cumby, Dunn, D.D.S., M.P.H., Chair, Division of Community Dentistry and Dental Services Administration, University of Oklahoma, College of Dentistry, Oklahoma City, OK

Dunning, David G., Ph.D., Professor of Practice Management, Department of Oral Biology, University of Nebraska Medical Center College of Dentistry, Lincoln, NE

Harris, David, M.B.A., C.P.A., C.M.A., C.F.E., C.F.F., Chief Executive Officer and Embezzlement "Guru," Prosperident, Halifax, Nova Scotia, Canada

Heller, Eugene, W. D.D.S., Vice President, Henry Schein, Inc.; Vice President, Professional Practice Transitions Division, Woodstock, GA

Itaya Lisa, E., D.D.S., Associate Professor and Group Practice Leader, Department of Dental Practice, University of the Pacific Arthur A. Dugoni School of Dentistry, San Francisco, CA

Kirsch, Amy, R.D.H., Founder and President of Amy Kirsch & Associates, Centennial, CO; Member of the Academy of Dental Management Consultants; Formerly a Senior Dental Consultant with the Pride Institute

Lange, Brian M., Ph.D., Professor of Behavioral Science, Department of Oral Biology, University of Nebraska Medical Center College of Dentistry, Lincoln, NE

Lyon, Lucinda J., R.D.H, D.D.S., Ed.D., Associate Professor and Chair, Department of Dental Practice, University of the Pacific Arthur A. Dugoni School of Dentistry, San Francisco, CA

Madden, Robert, D.D.S., M.B.A., Dental Practice Owner, Littleton, CO

Nadershahi, Nader A., D.D.S., M.B.A., Ed.D., Interim Dean, University of the Pacific Arthur A. Dugoni School of Dentistry, San Francisco, CA

Neumeister, David, D.D.S., Dental Private Owner, Brattleboro, VT

Opp, Darold, D.D.S., Dental Practice Owner, Aberdeen, SD

Shea, Gavin, Senior Director Sales and Marketing, Wells Fargo Practice Finance, Pleasanton, CA

Smith, Tyler, D.D.S., Dental Practice Owner, Omaha, NE

Spitsen, Jim, Insurance Broker and Consultant, Harold Diers & Company, Lincoln, NE

Strasheim, Kristen, R.D.H., Amertias Group Customer Connections and Operations, Manager Dental Consultant Review, Lincoln, NE

Terronez, Thomas, Chief Executive Officer, Medix Dental, Bettendorf, IA.

Twigg, Tim, Owner and President, Bent Ericksen & Associates, Eugene, OR; Board Member, Academy of Dental Management Consultants

Wacker, Mike, Equipment Specialist, Benco, Omaha, NE

Webb, William "Dana", Co-Founder and Financial Advisor, Fortress Wealth Advisors, Omaha, NE

Wiederman, Arthur S., C.P.A, C.F.P, Wiederman & Associates, Tustin, CA

Willis, David O., D.M.D., M.B.A., Professor Emeritus, Practice Administration and Health Policy Research, University of Louisville, School of Dentistry, Louisville, KY

Wolff, Steven C., D.D.S., Owner of ADS MidAmerica Dental Practice Sales, Raytown, MO

Workman, Rick, D.M.D., Founder and Chief Executive Officer, Heartland Dental, Effingham, IL

Preface

As anyone who has ever edited or written a book fully knows, this project could not have been completed without the untiring support of several vital people. Our lead department office staff member, Debbie Merritt, provided indispensable and timely support on many occasions. Key team members at Wiley, especially Teri Jensen and Catriona Cooper, also provided timely support throughout the project.

This book is designed so that each chapter "stands" in essence on its own. This means that the chapters are complementary and may even cover in a few cases the same or similar content in varying degrees of depth. Still, each chapter is intended to address a topic in ample fashion without relying on other chapters. Readers will certainly and intentionally glean much more from the book by reading chapters with augmenting content. Still, instructors in practice management may assign chapters individually or in combination, and readers may review individual chapters based on their needs and interests.

Profound market differences in dentistry and in cost of living typify the United States. For example, the value of dental practices may vary from 30–50% of average annual collections (or less) in sparse rural areas to well over 100% in highly competitive cities. Similarly, personal budgets vary greatly by region, especially owing to rent/mortgage expense. Internet sources may help understand some of the cost of living differences in various locations (for example, www.bestplaces.net—Sperling's best places—and city-data.com).

We are very grateful to all the chapter authors, all of whom have very busy schedules and thus basically participated in chapter writing "above and beyond the call" in normally hectic schedules.

We are also *very* appreciative of our chapter reviewers who invested significant time providing feedback while continuing their considerable regular work responsibilities:

Dr. Bradley Alderman
Ms. Ronda Anderson
Ms. Rebecca Boartfield
Dr. Richard Callan
Dr. Ross Crist
Dr. Dunn Cumby
Dr. David Dunning
Mr. David Harris
Mr. Drew Hinrichs
Ms. Amy Kirsch

Dr. Brian Lange
Dr. Lucinda J. Lyon
Dr. Robert Madden
Dr. Nader Nadershahi
Dr. David Neumeister
Dr. Darold Opp
Mr. Gavin Shea
Dr. Tyler Smith
Mr. Jim Spitsen
Ms. Kristen Strasheim
Mr. Tom Torronez
Mr. Tim Twigg
Mr. Mike Wacker
Dr. David O. Willis
Dr. Steven Wolff
Dr. Rick Workman

These individuals donated their time, literally, in order to provide valuable input to improve the already solid book chapters. Inasmuch as possible, writers were granted freedom of expression in writing style. Consequently, the reader will note variability in writing style from chapter to chapter. This is purposeful on our part as editors.

This book is not intended to, nor does it provide, legal, financial, investment or accounting advice. Readers are strongly encouraged to obtain the counsel of qualified attorneys, financial planners, accountants, and consultants for professional services.

Without God's grace, guidance and blessing, this project would not have been started or completed. Without support and encouragement from our families, especially our wives Kathy and Anne, this project would not have been accomplished.

About the Companion Website

This book is accompanied by a companion website:

www.wiley.com/go/dunning/transition

The website includes:

- Sample worksheets and lists
- All figures from the book
- Video of a dental health morning huddle

How to access the website:

1. The password is the first word of Chapter 14.
2. Go to **www.wiley.com/go/dunning/transition** to enter the password and access the site.

Part 1
An Introduction to Practice Transition, Dental Practice Financial Statements and Practice Financial Analysis

Chapter 1
Introduction and Overview
David G. Dunning and Brian M. Lange

This book is aimed at providing you with necessary concepts and perspectives for making practice transition decisions. The emphasis is on presenting sound ideas in a fair and balanced manner inasmuch as that is possible. We are not trying to sell you anything other than good information for decision making.

Assembling all that is necessary for practice transition in a single volume is a daunting task. More detail treatments are available for many of the topics addressed here (for example, see a partial list of American Dental Association [ADA] publications at the end of this chapter). Still, this book provides essential information not typically available in one book.

Career Choices

> The future you see is the future you get.
>
> Robert G. Allen

The major career question has already been answered. You are in dental school or have already graduated. For those still in dental college, questions often center on what area of dentistry: private general practice, private specialty practice, public health, military service, dental education, or are you one of the few that will join one or more of your relatives in "your" family practice? Our purpose here is not to duplicate an entire American Dental Association publication on career options, *Roadmap to Dental Practice: The Guide to the Rest of Your Career After Dental School and Licensure. Rather, we encourage you to take a couple of cleansing breaths or deep sighs, and* to take a step back and reflect on the process of making a career choice and some of the key issues in that process.

Most dental students in their first and second years are asking, now that I am in dental school, what is next? Questions begin to race through your mind. Where do I want to live? Or if married, where do we want to live? If I specialize, how does that affect where I can live? Do I want a metropolitan lifestyle, rural lifestyle, or something that allows a little of both? If you have or are planning a family, you find yourself asking about the best educational and social opportunities for your children. What values do you want your children exposed to day by day? For those who follow a faith-based

Dental Practice Transition: A Practical Guide to Management, Second Edition.
Edited by David G. Dunning and Brian M. Lange.
© 2016 John Wiley & Sons, Inc. Published 2016 by John Wiley & Sons, Inc.
Companion Website: www.wiley.com/go/dunning/transition

lifestyle, where does God want me to be? Can I get student loans repaid, and should this, based on interest rates, be a slow or a quick repayment process?

The questions listed above are by no means an exhaustive list. They are meant to get you thinking about the relationships among you, your family, the location of your practice, and the type of practice (general, specialty, etc.). The matrix in Table 1.1 is meant to give you a *starting point* for your decision-making process. You can list across the top all the issues you need to consider in making a decision about the type of dentistry you want to practice and then see which area of dental practice best meets most or all of your criteria. Approach the matrix (decision-making process) with the following in mind:

- Gather input from the people closest to you who will be affected by your decision.
- What seems like a good idea in your second year of dental school may not seem like a good idea in your third year of dental school. Be flexible; at times, life can take a sharp turn.
- It is called a decision-making process for a reason. Decisions, especially of the nature you are considering, require sound data and input, and take time. Be patient.

This question often arises when working with people making important decisions: what if I do all the right things, and I am comfortable with my decision. However, after being in the practice or another career path, I realize I do not like it? This is a challenging and multidimensional question with both a simple and a complex answer. The simple answer is that you can always move, although this may take some time depending on your situation. There is a demand for dentistry in many places. The complex answer is based on a series of questions:

- What do you not like about the practice/career path?
- What do you not like about the community?
- Can anything be changed that would make you more at ease?
- How does what you are experiencing differ from what you expected?
- What would you do differently in choosing another practice/career path?

If you invest the time to go through the series of questions with family, and if you are in a position of working for (associateship) or with (partnership or buyout) another dentist, you may find out that you can eventually resolve the issues causing your discontent. However, if you are not able to resolve the issues causing your discontent by answering the questions above, you will be better prepared to decide on what you will do next.

Some points to remember when making decisions, adapted from McDaniels et al. (1995):

- Decisions are tentative; you can change your mind.
- There is usually no one right choice.
- Deciding is a process, not a static one-time event. We are constantly reevaluating in light of new information.
- When it comes to a career decision, remember you are not choosing for a lifetime. Choose for now and do not worry whether you will still enjoy it in 20 years. Life is fluid and change occurs.
- There is a big difference between decision and outcome. You can make a good decision based on the information at hand and still have a bad outcome. The

Table 1.1 Decision matrix.

	Lifestyle We Want (e.g., Rural Area)	Values We Want	Loan Repayment	Educational Opportunities for Children	Close to Family	Housing We Want and Can Afford	List Other Important Considerations
General Dentistry							
Specialty Practice							
Military							
Public Health							
Dental Education							
Dental Service							
Management Organization							
Institutional Practice (Hospital)							

decision is within your control, the outcome is not. All decisions have an element of risk.
- Think of the worst outcome. Could you live with that? If you could live with the worst, then anything else does not seem that bad.
- Try to avoid either/or thinking: usually there are more than two options.

The Current Market and Its Implications for You

The dental market in its 21st century "adolescence to early adulthood" stage of life presents some unique opportunities and challenges for dentists and patients alike. These exigencies have profound implications for you. Let us consider the current age of dentistry and the present market as representing both the best of times and the worst of times as a background for this book.

The Platinum Age: Now Tarnished

The term "platinum age of dentistry" seems to have first been used as early as the spring of 2000 (Takacs 2000). So, why *did* people describe dentistry as being in the platinum age at that time? Much of the rationale hinges on the numbers, most of which you have probably already heard and so we will only point out the most critical ones.

Our population is living longer and is more likely than a generation or two ago to have had relatively good oral health. With fewer missing teeth and more teeth and supporting structures to be maintained and restored, there is, plainly speaking, more work to be done assuming patients have the means to pay for it and access to care to get the treatment done. In addition, research suggests that dentists now make more money per hour than physicians, although physicians make more annual income because of longer work hours (Seabury, Jena, and Chandra 2012). Finally, *U.S. News and World Report* ranked dentists as the No. 1 career in 2015 (http://money.usnews.com/money/careers/slideshows/the-25-best-jobs-of-2015/2), with vital practice team members, dental hygienists, not far behind at No. 5.

While these and other reasons may have justified dentistry being anointed as a "platinum age" for dentists for a time, we would remiss if we failed to mention that such is not the case for certain groups of patients. Patients lacking dental insurance, patients in some rural areas, and patients with lower incomes are all less likely to receive the care they need. So while dentistry may have enjoyed a platinum age for providers, it may have been more of an iron age for certain patient groups. Since you will be receiving much, we hope you will consider giving back much in whatever manner you are led to help close the gap in access to care. Options are many but include state Medicaid programs, nonprofit clinics, Missions of Mercy (volunteer weekends for providing care for the poor), and even providing free or discounted care or negotiated care based on bartering.

So, why now depict the platinum age as being tarnished? Several key variables are diminishing the "platinum age of dentistry," even in light of dentists being named the No. 1 career. There are probably many variables at play here, but four in particular stand out.

First, the expenditures ($) for dental services appear to have flattened and may not rebound amidst the ebb and flow of economic conditions. Meanwhile, utilization (those going to the dentist for services) has increased for children and dropped for adults (Wall, Vujicic, and Nasseh 2012; Vujicic 2013). Further, and brace yourself for some sobering statistics, The total number of dental care visits in the United States, across all settings, decreased by 7% between 2006 and 2012. There were approximately 271 million dental care visits nationwide in 2006 compared with 252 million in 2012 (this means 19 million fewer dental visits in 2012 versus 2006). Over this same time frame, the US population increased by 5.3%, and the number of practicing dentists increased by 9.4%. As a result, average dental care visits per capita and per dentist decreased substantially. Even though more people now seem to have dental coverage of some kind—Medicaid, preferred-provider, and so on (see McGill 2014), patients still struggle to access care and still need some expendable income for any deductibles or co-pays.

Second, dental student debt has skyrocketed, prompting studies about its influence on recruiting students and impact on career decisions. As of this writing, average debt hovers around the $247,000+ area and is rising precipitously, with lower averages for public college graduates and higher for private college graduates (http://www.asdanet .org/debt.aspx). A debt of $225,000 at a blended 6.5% rate over 10 years results in a monthly payment of $2,555, without factoring in rather severe limits on the tax deductibility of student loan interest and income taxes owed on gross income. A recent graduate would need to earn on average $30,660 in annual income just to make a $2,555 monthly payment ($2,555 × 12). This indebtedness redefines the economic landscape for associateship positions and for obtaining practice purchase loans (study the related chapters on these topics—especially Chapters 3, 20, and 21).

Third, new dental colleges have been and are being created, and this may eventually saturate the market with an excess number of providers, especially in some markets (see Solomon 2015a, 2015b).

Fourth, decreased reimbursement schemes from some dental insurance companies are putting increased pressure on practice profit margins, presenting an ongoing challenge to dentists (McGill 2014). Summarizing an aggregate data set, Boechler asserts that "although the dentists and hygienists are working more hours on average each month, their net production per hour and per patient represents a smaller percentage of the gross. This is due to the increased use of insurance as payment, leading to more adjustments and a smaller percentage of net production. Unfortunately, for dentists, with the ACA [Affordable Care Act] . . . this trend is likely to continue into the future." In other words, *dentists can expect to work longer hours and realize increasing pressure on profit margins*. Peruse several related chapters in this book, especially Chapters 3, 12, and 13, for insights about practice profitability, dental fees, and dental insurance/benefits.

The Best of Times, the Worst of Times?

A particularly astute and famous quotation from Charles Dickens's *A Tale of Two Cities* accurately describes the current transition opportunities for the general practice of dentistry: "It was the best of times, it was the worst of times, it was the age of wisdom, it was the age of foolishness, it was the epoch of belief, it was the epoch of incredulity." How do these literary observations relate to transitioning into private practice?

In so many ways, it is indeed the best of times. In spite of the "tarnishing" impact of the variables described earlier (such as debt and lower utilization levels), it is certainly not by accident that dentistry was ranked in 2015 as the No. 1 profession as already mentioned. The return on investment remains good at least for the foreseeable short-term future (Dunning 2015).

However, it is also, ironically, the worst of times in a sense. Why? Because blazing a career path is becoming increasingly complicated with unpredictable demand for dental services and the need to make student loan payments. There is a need, among other skills, to be able to objectively evaluate the options that are available in order to make an informed decision. Further, the word has now been widely broadcast: dental students will likely become wealthy in their lifetimes. This means that many individuals and corporations are, metaphorically speaking, circling above the heads of dental students, not waiting for them to die, but waiting for them to live out their careers and to share in the revenue stream! The need to be watchful regarding personal and business insurance, regarding practice transition concepts and processes, and regarding investing has never been greater. Refer to the chapters addressing these issues, including Chapters 25 and 26 on personal/business insurance and personal finance/investing.

Amidst this best of times and worst of times, a plethora of transition arrangements and models have emerged. We are, frankly, surprised at the way that some associate-ship arrangements and practice purchases are structured, particularly in view of student indebtedness. Still, there apparently is room in the competitive market for contracts that seem to be heavily biased in some ways for the owner-dentist. Some very competitive market conditions give the owner-dentist incredible negotiating positions that, in such a context, may warrant many fewer advantages for an associate position and much higher prices for practices. Some consulting firms market and implement their business models of transitioning practices across incredibly variable market conditions, causing others to scratch their heads and wonder how these models can work in such diverse markets.

One of the main purposes of this book is to provide for you some perspective of wisdom based on historically proven concepts so that you can sort your way through this best of times and worst of times, through this fog of a somewhat tarnished platinum age of dentistry. In the end, there may not be any absolutely and indisputably "right" way to structure an associateship experience or to purchase a practice. Nevertheless, there certainly are reasonable ranges within which these endeavors can be structured, and some of these will be more or less favorable to you. This, then, calls for you to be a very wise consumer with business acumen.

The "Bermuda Triangle" of Practice Transition

Transitioning from dental school or early career paths (military or public health) into private practice represents a tenuous activity in which opportunities can readily disappear into oblivion. Hence, the reference in the heading to the infamous "Bermuda Triangle," where, according to folklore and myth, ships and planes have disappeared without a trace (see Figure 1.1). Regardless of the veracity of the Bermuda Triangle in history, as a metaphor the name helps us to focus on the particularly tender and easily tipped process through which recent dental graduates enter the business world by trying to start, buy, buy into, or become associates of dental practices.

The three-dimensional triangle in the practice transition model includes these parties/sides: the dental student/graduate, the owner-dentist(s), and the advisors for both parties (see the model itself). Inside the model are the particular dynamics and characteristics of the practice that, depending on how they "load" with each party, can also readily sink the deal. For example, suppose a prospective buyer understood that the staff in a given practice would be staying after the purchase, only to discover that all the team members are leaving. Such information could easily sink the deal, as could discoveries related to the opinions of area dentists, overhead percentages, and so forth.

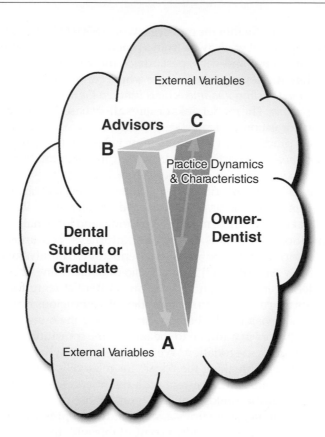

Figure 1.1. The "Bermuda Triangle" of practice transition.

Outside the model are the external variables influencing the practice, including the wider economic conditions such as unemployment, inflation, and interest rates.

Three specific principles undergird this model; principles that, admittedly, are themselves subject to debate.

Principle #1: *No single party in the transition process should retain all of the power or control.* We believe this principle is an equitable one. The dentist-owner, obviously, enjoys more "position power" than a prospective associate or buyer. Still, the interests of the latter cannot simply be ignored. Some sense of balance and mutual interest must be preserved for a successful transition to occur.

Principle #2: *Each party has competing interests, and thus this process requires some degree of negotiation, ranging from making minor adjustments to standardized employment agreements to developing unique contracts.* Sometimes individuals have interests that seem somewhat odd. These may arise from personal history. Occasionally, for example, an associateship contract will contain some very specific provision regarding a rather obscure circumstance that presented itself in a previous associate's employment (for example, thou shalt not approve the purchase of any dental supplies).

Principle #3: *This process of negotiation can easily/readily "tip" or fall (sink into the ocean) if any party maintains an unreasonable bargaining position or an unreasonable stance.* We are of the opinion that practice transitioning needs to major in majors rather than get tipped by relatively minor issues. It seems unwise to walk away from an associateship contract because of a dispute about who pays for malpractice insurance for 1 year or because of a disagreement about whether the practice is worth $500,000 instead of $530,000. It is our opinion that you do not walk away from a practice sale for $30,000 (though maybe you should certainly pause and get expert advice for $100,000!).

Let us explore the nexus of the triangle where competing interests meet. *At juncture "A" reside the relationships and interactions between the dental student (or recent graduate) and the dentist-owner.* The model sinks or stays afloat based on the relationships between the person in transition and practice owner(s). How do the personalities mesh the philosophies of practice, the values governing behavior, the type of dental services to be provided? Do these two parties agree on some fundamental concepts and principles to structure an associateship or a practice purchase?

At juncture "B" emerge the dynamics of relationships and interactions of the dental student or dentist in transition with his/her advisors and the advisors of the dentist-owner. Importantly, note that advisors here may be both formal and informal. Formal advisors could include transition consultants/companies, attorneys, accountants, lenders, faculty, and so on. Informal advisors include parents, other family members, friends, and classmates. How well (if at all) are the basic understandings negotiated between the student or dentist in transition and the owner-dentist communicated to the formal advisors? Does the consulting firm offer a flexible, efficacious business model to handle the transition as envisioned by both the student and the owner? May the student hire independent advisors in addition to the ones in the transition firm? Do spouses assert proper influence in the negotiation? We have seen cases where spouses exert incredible influence, potentially breaking the "deal" for relatively minor issues or by applying general business models inconsistent with the nuances of the dental market. Does a student agree with the philosophy/business model of the transition firm if one is involved? For example, some firms assert that they represent both parties (known as "dual representation"), is the student comfortable with this? Should a student have to pay an up-front fee to look at practices or an "earnest" payment to hold the final purchase until after graduation? Will the lender offer the money needed for the practice—and, if so, are there any liens against the practice?

The relationships and interactions of the dentist-owner with his/her formal and informal advisors and the student's advisors develop at juncture "C." Does the owner-dentist communicate clearly to transition consultants the previously agreed-to basic understandings negotiated with the student? Unfortunately, the answer is often "no." In other words, it is fairly common in transitions for the communication between the owner-dentist and his/her advisors to fail to include what the student and owner thought had been negotiated through several extensive conversations. This is often because the owner's advisor failed to edit a standardized employment agreement or utilizes a possibly inflexible approach to transition. Do the student's advisors offer what is perceived to be reasonable positions with respect to practice valuations or associateship contracts?

Inside the Triangle

Every dental practice has unique characteristics that make up the inside of the triangle. Some of the key "inside" variables include practice location, patient base (and its historical, current, and future dental needs), unique staff, the practice's office design (which can make life much easier or more difficult for the practitioner), technology, number of active patients, and financial information (see Chapters 2 and 3 on dentistry financial statements and key quality performance indicators for an excellent overview by Dr. David Willis). This inside picture of the practice needs to be understood, especially by associates intending to buy and by potential buyers. This is all part of due diligence. For example, a practice showing production of $510,000 and collections of $450,000 for the previous year creates a "due diligence opportunity" for you. Is this uncollected revenue and/or dental insurance adjustments"

Outside the Triangle

Outside the triangle are the external variables unique to the neighborhood, town/city, county, and state. Is the neighborhood older and established, deteriorating, or growing? What is the general population of the city/county, and how many general dentists are in practice? This information can be researched through a variety of sources as well as purchased from certain firms. Is the dental market highly competitive for patients? If so, practices will likely sell for much higher prices, comparatively. Two states may be separated by a mile-wide river. Yet this may be a great divide representing two distinct markets: one essentially saturated with third-party payers; the other, primarily fee-for-service patients. In addition, the wider economy, interest rates, unemployment, and inflation have incredible influences on any dental practice. In total, these external variables cannot be overemphasized.

Broadly speaking, the continued growth of group practices represents a fundamentally profound and ongoing shift in the national dental market and dental economy. This growing trend includes not only groups of dentists operating within the same building(s) with variously defined legal/business corporate relationships but also dental service organizations (a.k.a. "corporate dentistry"). Chapters 10 and 21 discuss, respectively, business entities and dental care organizations.

Some Common Pitfalls Causing the Triangle to Sink

In associateships:

- Compensation offers from owners and/or expectations of would-be associates below and/or above typical norms.
- Form of relationship: employee versus independent contractor. The IRS has a rigorous test for dentist-workers to qualify as independent contractors (search www.irs.gov). As you probably know, an independent contractor must pay his/her own share of social security tax AND that of the employer (just over 15% as of this writing).
- Assignment of patients: is this fair and balanced? Does this match the compensation provisions of the contract to cover base pay or the "draw"? Patient assignment becomes particularly critical in practices with significant managed-care/third-party payers with resultant "adjustments" (reductions) in collections.
- Buy-in provisions/process (timing, procedures, etc.).
- Influence of third-party carriers on associate's compensation and on practice overhead and profitability.
- Insufficient practice revenue for adding another dentist? Some argue that a single-dentist practice should have ~$800,000 or more in collections before an associate should be hired.
- Allocation of dental hygiene income: does the associate receive any income for supervising dental hygiene?
- Restrictive covenant terms viewed as unreasonable.
- An associate demonstrating weak interpersonal communication skills or marginal technical skills (Halley et al. 2008)

Dr. Eugene Heller (1999) also astutely details ten specific reasons for associateships failing; refer to his article listed in the references.

In purchases:

- Practice value unknown or viewed as unreasonably high by associate and/or advisors.
- Practice allocation of value seen as inaccurate (for example, a value of $10,000 for all equipment and supplies and a value of $375,000 for the goodwill or blue sky).
- Can the buyer secure enough financing? Some lenders may cap the lending limit of new graduates.
- Major change in the practice during the process of purchase (disability of owner, departure of staff, divorce of owner, etc.).
- Practice projections that appear too good to be true from a transition consulting firm.
- Undue and inappropriate influence of a key advisor (formal or informal).

Some Suggestions to Avoid Tipping the Deal

- Study the dental market in the specific area. What do associates tend to earn in salary and benefits? What methods are used to evaluate practices? What is the extent of third-party involvement and reimbursement in the area? What are typical overhead/profit ranges? What are some ballpark figures for which practices typically sell in terms of percentages of revenue? Chapter 4 covers the basics of practice valuation.
- Identify your "nonnegotiables," if any, in an employment arrangement and in a practice purchase. Are you willing to do prophies? What is your "bottom line" for income and benefits based on a detailed personal/family budget? How soon do you want to purchase the practice, and is this process in writing? What is the most you would be willing to pay for the practice?
- Identify your negotiable positions: compensation level beyond minimums, practice value within a certain range, how the transfer will proceed with respect to patients, staff, and so forth.
- Utilize a variety of advisors and weigh their input based on their expertise. Solomon advised, "Refuse good advice and watch your plans fail; take good counsel and watch them succeed" (Proverbs 15:22).
- Make sure all items of importance are specifically documented in contracts and agreements.
- Manage your credit rating; the higher your rating, the better. And while the "below which no loan" bottom threshold changes based on market conditions, generally speaking it is critical to maintain a credit rating higher than ~665 as of this writing.

Selecting Key Advisors

Before you start the process of selecting advisors to help you through the maze of decisions that end up with you practicing dentistry, you need to answer this question: which advisors do I need? The list of professionals that you need to find the best practice fit for you is rather extensive. Most certainly your choice of practice (associateship, partnership, ownership) will influence the number of advisors and type of advisors you will require. However, before we dig deep into securing the best possible advice, do not overlook the invaluable input of any family members or family friends, particularly those in business or in dentistry. Conversations about the practice of dentistry with practitioners, especially family members, are most productive if you have a list of questions that reflect your goals. It is a good idea to verify information obtained about the practice of dentistry from family and friends with the perspectives of other trusted sources.

Two of your best resources in dental school are the faculty who teach practice management and the faculty who practice in the community. For most dental schools, talking to part-time faculty who maintain a private practice is one of your best resources for issues that face a dentist in private practice.

Faculty who teach practice management should teach you about or have references that can help you decide which advisors you should contact to help you achieve your practice goals. Many schools maintain a list of practice opportunities and dental practices for sale, as well as recommended advisors such as lenders and transition firms. Most practices may be within the state and region in which the dental school is located, and many listed practices are owned by alumni of the college. Nevertheless, your college's practices list is a good place to start.

Also, do not overlook the advice you can get from dental suppliers. Dental suppliers often know about dentists interested in selling their practices before the dentist goes to a broker or lists the practice. Most dental suppliers are happy to pass on information to prospective buyers in the hope of establishing a long-term business relationship.

The number and type of advisors that you use will depend on the type of practice opportunity you are pursuing. For example, if you are pursuing an associateship without the option to purchase, your banking, accounting, and tax needs will be different than if you are pursuing a purchase of a solo private practice or a future buy-in of a multiple-owner practice.

Let us examine in alphabetical order the advisors available to assist you in obtaining the practice environment of your dreams, or at least the practice environment that matches your goals. This is a basic list, *not* an exhaustive one. For example, architects are not discussed here and yet have a pivotal role in marketing your practice and lowering your stress level via insightful office design (Figure 1.2).

Look at the list below as a menu from which you need to choose the advisors who will help you accomplish your goals:

Accountant/CPA
Attorney
Banker
Insurance broker
Investment counsel
Practice broker

There are key organizations specializing in dental services, including the Academy of Dental Practice CPAs (www.adcpa.org) and the Academy of Dental Practice Management Consultants (www.admc.net).

When looking for advisors, make sure they are skilled in working with small business/dental practices. If you use an advisor who does not deal with dental practices on a regular basis, you may end up paying to help educate the advisor and possibly pay again through lost income or legal entanglements because of outdated or inaccurate advice.

(a)

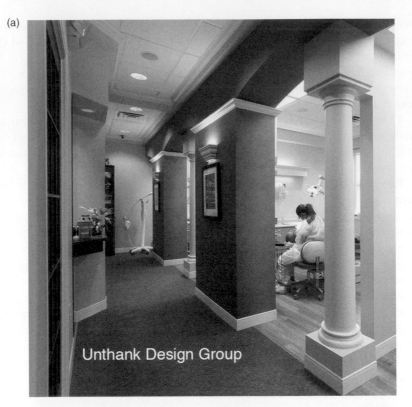

(b)

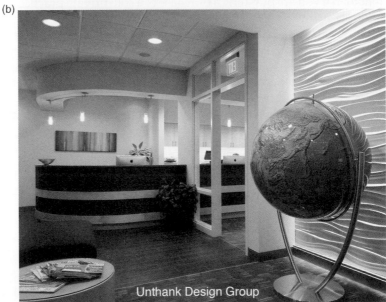

Figure 1.2.   Unthank Design Group is an award-winning planning, architecture and interior design firm providing services exclusively to the dental professions. Dr. Michael Unthank is a dentist and registered architect and has designed over 2,000 dental and specialty offices throughout the world. (a) Dr. Davila's eight chair prosthodontic office in Tampa, Florida. This view of the treatment corridor illustrates the classical nature of Dr. Davila's heritage. (b) Drs. Glenn and Katzberg's office in Lincoln, Nebraska. Based on their theme for Genesis Orthodontics, a 42″ diameter globe is center stage in this contemporary new office.

Selecting an Accountant

Consider, for example, what an accountant/CPA potentially has to offer:

- Prepare periodic financial statements and annual audit reports
- Assist you in analyzing your financial statements
- Help develop a budget and a system of monthly reporting so that you can regularly check on your financial transactions in relation to what was budgeted
- Prepare tax returns and assist with tax and retirement/estate planning
- Set up a tax calendar and a system to help you comply with all filing requirements
- Help set up your accounting system
- Assist with determining loan or capital requirements
- Act as your advisor on financial and administrative matters
- Consult with you to set and monitor key financial and quality performance targets and to maximize profitability (see Chapters 2 and 3)

The following suggestions are intended to help you find the right professional accountant, attorney, banker, CPA, practice broker, and so on. For the purpose of consistency, we will continue using an accountant in this example.

Determine the scope of work that you want an accountant to provide for your practice. Do you want someone to keep your books and prepare monthly financials? Are you looking for an annual audit? Are you looking for advice?

- Ask for referrals from other dentists in private practice.
- Set up interviews with two or three accountants so that you can see which one you are most comfortable with.
- Keep interviews focused on whether you would be comfortable with and have confidence in the accountant. Questions you ask should be general in nature. Do not ask for accounting or tax advice in the interview screening process.
- Ask accountants you interview to provide two or three references from dentists with whom they have worked for several years.

The following questions should be covered in the interview (adapted from www .smallbusinessnotes.com):

- What primary services do you provide to a dental practice?
- How will you charge for your services? Most accountants will establish a monthly retainer for recurring services like monthly or quarterly financial statements and charge by the hour for audits. Tax returns can be charged by the hour or by the form.
- What can I do to reduce your fees? Determine if you will be able to keep your accounting and business overhead costs down by using the advice provided.
- As my practice grows, how will you be able to help me? Ask them to describe services they provide to other dental practices.

You can keep your accounting costs down by the following measures:

- Finding out what you can prepare in advance to make the accountant's work easier. The easier it is for the accountant to read and understand the information you bring in, the quicker the work gets done. Modern dental practice software provides many reports helpful to you and your accountant.

- Choosing an accounting system that you can understand and that allows you or a staff member to do as much of the bookkeeping work as you have time for.
- Talking to your accountant and tax professional before making major decisions so that you will know the tax implications ahead of time. This also allows you to fill out all documents in a timely manner, thus saving the accountant time.
- Preparing and organizing for your meetings. Taking time to prepare for your visit can save money and time. Take notes so that you will not have to ask questions a second time.
- Asking for a detailed bill that specifies the billing for each type of service, including time and billing rate. This will help give you some clues about what you can do to save money.

It is good to keep in mind that contracting out services that would take you a lot of time to learn can actually save you money. You can be far more productive doing dentistry than doing your own books, billing, or tax forms. There is a lot to be said for quality of life: having time to spend with your family, enjoying your hobbies, and relaxing.

Selecting an Attorney

When selecting an attorney, it is important to determine the type of attorney you will need. If you are interested in becoming an associate or a partner in a dental practice or are considering purchasing a dental practice, you will best be served by an attorney who specializes in small business contract law, particularly with dental practice experience. If you are looking for an attorney who is also a CPA, consider a member of the American Association of Attorney-CPAs (https://www.attorney-cpa.com).

In many localities, attorneys are permitted to advertise in an area of specialization. Often the area of specialization is regulated by the American Bar Association. This association, like state dental associations, may require members to maintain a skill level that mandates the annual completion of additional study in the area of expertise under which they are listed. A primary consideration in selecting an attorney should be how comfortable you are after your interview with a prospective attorney.

The suggestion list intended to help you find an accountant can and should be modified and used to find the right attorney. For example, determine the scope of work that you want an attorney to provide. Do you want the attorney to give you examples of contracts or review a contract you have been offered? If the attorney is reviewing a contract for you, know in advance what you want in the way of compensation, benefits, and overhead expenses.

The questions you ask of a prospective attorney should include the following (adapted from https://attorneypages.com/help/ch11-attorney-interview-questions.html):

- Does the attorney specialize in the area of law in which you are interested?
- Will you be charged for your first consultation?
- How much does the attorney charge per hour?
- How many hours does the attorney think it will take to complete the task?
- Are there any government licensing or filing fees involved?
- Are there any statutory guidelines for this type of work?
- Does the attorney provide the client with a written contract or letter confirming employment? If so, ask to see an example.

- Has the attorney ever had complaints filed against him/her?
- Does the attorney refer work to other attorneys in other areas of law where he/she is not an expert?

Throughout the course of your lifetime, you will need the services of attorneys to help you with issues such as wills, trusts, and the sale of your practice when the time comes. Even if the attorney you have identified to work with cannot handle all of your needs, they can refer you to the expertise you require. As with accountants, trusted dentists in your area will likely have recommended attorneys for you to interview.

Selecting a Banker

How should you choose a bank or financial institution? The steps to choosing a bank or financial institution are very similar to choosing an accountant or attorney. Not all financial institutions are the same. Each institution establishes its own policies for the following:

- Types of products and services that are offered
- Criteria for qualifying for a loan
- Minimum balances for accounts
- Interest rates
- Charges for account services

Your banker can offer you the following:

- Assistance with cash management needs—for you and your business
- Investment products of varying maturities and varying risk (see Chapter 26)
- Advice about qualifying for the loan that best meets your needs
- Special loan programs for small businesses

Compare financial institutions in order to find the one that serves you best. Do not overlook local and regional banks. They may have more of an interest in the local community, and the majority of their resources stay in the community. Start gathering information to help you select the best financial institution and identify a banker with whom you can build a relationship with for the future:

- Approach the decision as a long-term investment.
- Ask trusted dentists, your accountant, and attorney to introduce you to bankers with whom they are familiar.
- Check with your local Chamber of Commerce to find out which banks are active in the community.
- Look for a complementary personality—someone you are comfortable with.
- Introduce yourself to the banking center manager or vice president. If looking for a loan, ask to meet the loan officer who will be assigned to you.
- Educate the banker about your business so that they can tell you what special products and services or restrictions might apply.
- Do not make a decision on costs alone, but do compare interest rates on deposit accounts and basic consumer loans. Most business loans are negotiated. Also, you may be able to negotiate charges for services. Do some comparison shopping (see www.smallbusinessnotes, for example).

It is a good idea to establish a relationship with a banker before you need money. The right banker will be someone who understands your needs and the needs of your business.

Selecting an Insurance Broker

An insurance broker or agent source (brokers) contracts for insurance on behalf of his/her customers. Basically, there are two types of insurance agents: those who work for one main insurance company, and independent brokers who work for their clients by vetting policies from many companies. Brokers who work for insurance companies can offer only the products and prices established by the company they work for. Independent insurance agents shop all insurance companies and try to offer the best coverage at the best price.

Your insurance needs will fall into the two broad categories of personal and business. Areas of your personal life that should be covered by insurance policies include but may not be limited to the following:

- Homeowner/rental
- Automobile
- Life insurance (you/spouse)
- Disability
- Umbrella liability policy
- Health (may be offered as a practice benefit)

Areas of your professional life that require insurance coverage include but may not be limited to the following:

- Malpractice
- Disability
- Health

If you are a partner in a dental practice or the owner of a solo practice, you will need to consider insurance coverage for the following:

- Building and/or equipment
- Staff members
- Liability/personal injury
- Employee life
- Business overhead (which provides coverage for practice disruption due to fire and flooding as examples)

You may need to use more than one insurance broker, depending on your insurance needs. When looking for a broker to help you with selection and coverage for your practice, you should follow the interview process as outlined for accountants, attorneys, and bankers. Importantly, as discussed in Chapter 9, a lender may require life insurance and disability insurance of a borrower in order to provide security for a loan.

Please refer to Chapter 25 on insurance needs as they apply to you and to dental practice.

Selecting an Investment Counsel

When it comes to investing your money for you and your family's future, whether children's education, a new house, or retirement, you have basically three choices. First, you can do all the investing and manage your own portfolio. A second choice is to hire someone else to manage all your investments; and your third option is you manage some of your assets and someone else manages the remainder of your assets. Unless you have been trained as Certified Financial Planner™ (CFP), an investment counselor, or have made investing a hobby over several years, going it alone can be very risky, and not all the risk is in choosing poor-performing investments. If you are obligated to the practice of dentistry 35+ hours a week and have a family, precious little time remains learn the intricacies of investing and monitoring your investments.

Turning all or most of your investments over to someone to manage should be done only after you have developed your investment goals, determined the level of risk you can tolerate, and established your investment philosophy. A financial advisor certainly may assist you in setting goals, assessing risk, and developing a philosophy of building wealth, but in the end these are your informed decisions. The process of developing your investment goals starts with the budgeting process. See Chapter 26 on personal finance/investing. Once you have established a budget and your emergency fund and maintained your budget-driven lifestyle, you will have identified money for investments. Investment goals at the top of the list for most younger couples include the following:

- Education for children/spouse
- New house/car
- Vacations
- Retirement

Once goals have been identified and the amount of money has been agreed upon, it is time to determine your tolerance for risk; this is one question that an investment counselor should ask you. Basically, risk is defined in terms of potential rate of return on your investment. Usually, the higher the rate of return, the higher the risk. Bank certificates of deposit (CDs) and savings accounts are considered to have the least risk of losing your investment. However, it is possible to essentially lose money on CDs and savings accounts. If your rate of return is 2%, and inflation is 2%, you are really making a 0% return. Still, you will be taxed on your 2% return on interest, and therefore are actually losing money. Most investment counselors will suggest a mixture of investments (diversified portfolio), with percentages of your investment money being allocated to different investments. If you are in your thirties, you may get a recommendation of 50–70% equities in the form of mutual funds and stocks, 10–20% in bonds, and the remainder in foreign equities, precious metals, or cash.

The use of more than one investment modality is referred to as an "asset allocation." For a beginner's guide to asset allocation, diversification, and rebalancing, go to investor.gov. Once on the site, go to investing basics and click on guiding principles.

Investors who can tolerate high levels of risk and volatility may invest 90–100% in stocks. Their rationale is that from 1920 to 1999, the stock market has averaged an 11% return rate. However, there have been volatile days when the market dropped and people lost significant amounts of their investments. If you have the personality to ride out the bad days—and sometimes years—and you are in the right stocks and/or mutual funds, you will see good returns.

Next, you need to decide if your investments will be active (someone manages) or passive (stocks or funds that are reviewed once or twice a year). There will be fees and investment costs for either the active or passive approach to investing. The key to choosing an investment counselor is how he/she charges you. Pick financial advisors that charge an annual management fee. People who are paid only on up-front commissions have no incentive to watch your money and make suggestions as to when adjustments are needed.

For review purposes, your investment philosophy should include the following:

- Allocation of assets
- Portfolio diversification
- Identifying and sticking with your investment style
- Active or passive management of your investments

Selecting a Practice Broker

The role of a practice broker includes these and other functions:

- Listing of practices for sale
- Recruiting associates
- Marketing-listed practices
- Showing practices to potential buyers
- Writing offers to purchase
- Serving as a practice buyer representative
- Making sure all appropriate paperwork is legally compliant and signed

Choosing a practice broker is much like choosing an accountant or attorney. In addition to using the suggestions for finding an accountant or attorney, you will need to ask if the broker represents the practice owner or both the practice owner and you as the would-be associate/buyer. The latter is called "dual agency" and includes built-in ethical challenges. Is it really possible to represent both parties equitably and equally? Dual agents may be paid by both the buyer and the seller. In an ideal world, dual agents work for the best outcome for both parties. If you are working with a broker who is a seller's agent (or with a dual-agency broker), you really should consider hiring an independent attorney or broker to represent your interests.

You will also want to ask how your earnest money will be handled. Typically, earnest money is deposited in an account and used toward the purchase price of the practice at closing. The amount of earnest money can be negotiated. Another question you will want to ask is, what is the average length of time from acceptance of offer until close? The longer the wait, the more financial resources you will need to live on before income can be earned from the practice.

There are *many* associations/organizations focused on brokering dental practices, including ADS Transitions (www.adstransitions.com) and Professional Practice Transitions (https://dentalpracticetransitions.henryschein.com).

Before closing this chapter, it should be mentioned that a growing number of leaders in organizations, including dentists, engage short- or long-term coaching consulting services. An internet search of "dental coaching" will yield many dental coaching services. Some coaches have formal training such as that offered through http://coachfederation.org.

References and Additional Resources

Abernathy, Michael. 2013. *The super general dental practice.* Available at http://summitpractice solutions.com/.

American Dental Association. Various years. A few of these titles may be out of print: *Associateships; CEO Crash Course; Dental Office Design: Creating an Office Manual; Dental Letters; Creating an Employee Office Manual; Roadmap to Dental Practice: The Guide to the Rest of Your Career After Dental School and Licensure; Smart Hiring: A Guide for the Dental Office; Terminating Employment in a Dental Office; Transitions: Navigating Sales, Associateships and Mergers in Your Dental Practice; Starting Your Dental Practice; Valuing a Practice.*

American Dental Education Association (ADEA). 2013. A report of the ADEA Presidential Task Force on the cost of higher education and student borrowing. Washington, DC.

Boehlert, Alito. 2014. *Trends in dental practice management: 2012 to 2014.* Available at dental-practicerports.com (accessed June 18).

Costes, Mark. 2013. *Pillars of Dental Success.* North Charleston, SC: CreateSpace Independent Publisher Platform.

Dunning, David. 2013. Dental student debit in the U.S.: a mountain to be scaled. *Dent Hypothec* 4(4): 112–114.

Dunning, David. 2015. Resources for practice management. *Dent Hypothec* 6(2): 1–3.

Halley, Meghan, Lalumandier, James, Walker, Jonathan, and Houston, James. 2008. A regional study of dentists' preferences for hiring a dental associate. *J Am Dent Assoc* 139(7): 973–979.

Heller, Eugene. 1999. Top ten reasons why many associateships fail to result in practice purchase. *Preview* Fall, 12–17.

———. 2005. Lecture comments. *What to Expect from a Practice Broker.* Lincoln, NE: University of Nebraska Medical Center, College of Dentistry, September.

———. 2007. The most important number—active patient count. *New Dentist,* Spring, 6–10.

McGill, John. 2014. Ramp up marketing as managed care increases. *The McGill Advisory* 29(4): 1–3.

Seabury, Seth, Jena, Anupam, and Chandra, Amitabh. 2012. Trends in the Earnings of Health Care Professionals in the United States, 1987-2010. *JAMA* 308(20): 2083–2085.

Solomon, Eric. 2015a. The future of dentistry: dental economics. *Dent Econ* 105(3) (online).

Solomon, Eric. 2015b. The future of dental practice: dental education. *Dent Econ* 105(1): (online).

Takacs, Gary. 2000. Strategies to reduce insurance dependency. *Dental Angle Online,* Magazine, Spring. Available at http://www.dentalangle.com.

Vujicic, Marko. 2013. *National Dental Expenditure Flat Since 2008 Begin to Slow in 2002.* Chicago, IL: American Dental Association, Health Policy Resources Center.

Vujicic, Marko. 2015. Where have all the dental care visits gone? *J Am Dent Assoc* 146(6): 412.

Wall, Thomas, Vujicic, Marko, and Nasseh, Kamyar. 2012. Recent trends in the utilization of dental care in the United States. *J Dent Edu* 76(8): 1020–1027.

Learning Exercises

Decision Matrix

Complete the decision matrix for the career path toward which you are leaning. Make sure that you involve your immediate family members.

Buy-In

You are just beginning your D4 year. Over your all too short summer break, you found what you think is the ideal practice to purchase. An appraisal from 3 and a half years ago from a national consulting firm placed a value of $450,000 on the practice. Dr. Smith, the current owner, said that he would sell you the practice for $400,000, in spite of increased practice revenues averaging $650,000 for the past 3 calendar tax years.

1. What can you do to facilitate this successful sale in order to make the deal mutually beneficial for you and Dr. Smith? In other words, how can you avoid "tipping" the Bermuda Triangle of practice transition?
2. What can Dr. Smith do to facilitate this successful sale in order to make the deal mutually beneficial for you and for him? How can he avoid "tipping" the Bermuda Triangle of practice transition?
3. Identify key advisors for you and for Dr. Smith, and how you would select them.
4. Identify some practice information you would need to obtain and study as you pursue this purchase.

Chapter 2
Financial Statements
David O. Willis

Financial statements are the basic language of business and finance. They take the same general form, regardless of the size or type of business. They are used for many purposes, including tax compliance, assessing practice performance, applications for borrowing, and practice valuation, among others. Understanding how to develop these statements, what each component is, and what they show is important.

Financial statements come in two styles: personal and business. The format of the forms is similar, though not exactly the same. This chapter discusses personal and business financial statements, and describes differences between them. Four types of financial statements are presented: (1) statement of financial position (balance sheet), (2) profit and loss, (3) cash flow, and (4) pro forma. You will work with your accountant to develop and utilize these forms, as the rules for the personal and business forms are different.

Types of Financial Statements

1. The *statement of financial position (balance sheet)* shows what someone owns (assets) and what they owe (liabilities) at a specific point in time. The general formula for a statement of financial position is given in Table 2.1. This statement is a "snapshot" of a financial position. It will be different tomorrow, as assets change value and loans are paid off. Bankers and financial planners like to examine changes in the balance sheet to decide how well someone is doing financially. (Total net worth should be growing.) Net worth can grow in two ways. One, assets can increase by savings or through increasing the value of an asset. Two, liabilities can decrease by paying off debt. Borrowing and then using the money to purchase an asset leaves the net worth unchanged. This happens when a new dentist buys a dental practice. He or she takes on debt but also now owns an asset of equal value. The total net worth remains unchanged. As he or she pays down the debt or the value of the practice increases, net worth becomes more positive.

    It is possible to have a negative net worth. This happens to young professionals who have significant educational debt and few assets. Their total liabilities

Dental Practice Transition: A Practical Guide to Management, Second Edition.
Edited by David G. Dunning and Brian M. Lange.
© 2016 John Wiley & Sons, Inc. Published 2016 by John Wiley & Sons, Inc.
Companion Website: www.wiley.com/go/dunning/transition

Table 2.1   Personal balance sheet formula.

Statement of Financial Position (Balance Sheet)

ASSETS – LIABILITIES = NET WORTH

ASSETS
    Cash/Cash Equivalents
    Business Assets
    Invested Assets
    Personal Use Assets

LIABILITIES
    Short-Term
    Long-Term
        Mortgages
        Notes

(educational and other debts) are more than the total of what they presently own (assets). While not an enviable position, it is frequently encountered.

The corporate balance sheet is similar to the personal in form. It shows the amount of business assets held, the amount of money owed (liabilities), and the amount of the owner's capital. (Corporations call this "Shareholder's Equity," partnerships call it "Partner's Capital," and proprietorships call it "Owner's Capital.") Note that these are business, not personal, assets and liabilities.

Bankers often require borrowers to develop both a personal balance sheet, and a balance sheet for the practice. If the practice is incorporated or has multiple owners, the practice entity will have a statement. Each of the owners also may need to develop a personal statement of financial position, depending on the needs of the lender. Banks may have specific forms to complete. These are usually their particular versions of the generic balance sheet.

An example of a personal balance sheet is shown in Table 2.2. This table shows that John and Mary Doe own assets that total $570,830 in value. These assets have been grouped according to their financial use (cash, personal, business, investment). Mary's dental practice has been valued at $300,000. John and Mary owe a total of $344,070. These debts are categorized by when they will pay them. Short-term liabilities will be paid within a year. Long-term liabilities are loans used to purchase assets that last many years, such as houses, autos, and dental practices. Mary still owes $250,300 on her dental practice, so she has just less than $50,000 of value, or equity, in the practice. The difference between what they own and what they owe is the couple's net worth, in this case $226,760. This means that if the couple sold everything they own and paid off all their loans, they would have $226,760 in cash remaining.

2. Another statement, called a *profit and loss statement*, an operating statement, or an income statement, shows business income and expenses and the resulting net income or net loss. The general formula for a proprietorship profit and loss statement is given in Table 2.3. This statement shows a summary of the taxable income and expense items over a specific period. The period may be a day, month, quarter, year, or any other period that gives meaningful information. If the income items of the practice are greater than the expense items, a profit results. If the expenses are greater, there is a loss. We find office expense items in the office checkbook. (The register, whether a

Table 2.2   Example balance sheet.

Statement of Financial Position
John and Dr. Mary Doe
As of December 31, 201X

ASSETS

Cash/Cash Equivalents			
Checking Account	3,050		
Credit Union Savings	4,000		
Money Market Account	7,500		
Life Insurance Cash Value	8,000	22,550	
Personal Use Assets			
House	135,000		
Automobiles	28,000		
Personal Property	52,000	215,000	
Business Use Assets			
Dental Practice	300,000	300,000	
Investments			
Stock Portfolio	7,800		
Mutual Funds	6,500		
SEP/IRAs	18,980	33,280	570,830

LIABILITIES

Short-Term Liabilities			
Credit Card Balance	950	950	
Long-Term Liabilities			
Auto Notes Balance	4,920		
Home Mortgage Balance	87,900		
Dental Practice	250,300	343,120	344,070

NET WORTH		226,760

Table 2.3   Profit and loss statement.

Profit and Loss (Income) Statement

REVENUE − EXPENSES = PROFIT (LOSS)

REVENUE
  Collections

EXPENSES
  Practice Costs
  Business Taxes
  Depreciation

manual or computer system, should group expenses according to type.) We find income information in the office management computer system.

Profit and loss statements may be arranged in two ways, according to their use. (Both contain the same information; they are simply organized differently.) Expenses may be listed alphabetically, which is the same as the format for the tax form Schedule C (Profit or Loss from Operating a Business). Others organize the information by categorizing items of expense. This format makes it easier to do

Table 2.4   Example proprietorship profit and loss statement (Schedule C format).

Profit and Loss (Income) Statement
Mary Doe, DDS
For the Year Ending December 31, 201X

Revenue		
Production	337,470	
Collections		327,346
Expenses		
Advertising	1,854	
Auto Expenses	1,928	
Commissions	0	
Depreciation	23,047	
Employee Benefit Program	3,640	
Insurance	2,650	
Interest Expense	12,487	
Legal and Professional	1,790	
Office Expense	3,817	
Pension/Profit Sharing Plan	3,048	
Rent or Lease	18,000	
Repairs and Maintenance	270	
Supplies (Office)	4,082	
Taxes and Licenses	10,108	
Meals, Travel, and Entertainment	139	
Utilities	10,955	
Wages	65,950	
Other Expenses		
Temporary Services	340	
Bank Charges	120	
Office Cleaning	3,055	
Dental Supplies	23,584	
Dental Lab	33,754	
Dues and Publications	2,050	
Continuing Education	3,492	
Postage	690	
Total Expenses/Costs		230,850
Profit (Loss)		96,496

financial analysis on the practice because similar costs (staff, facility, etc.) are grouped together.

Examples of both types are presented in Tables 2.4 and 2.5. Both show a summary of the income and expenses Mary Doe had in her dental practice for the year ending December 31, 201X. These statements show that Mary produced $337,470 of dentistry during the year. Her practice collected $327,346 in cash, checks, and credit card payments for the year. Her expenses are summarized by item in both forms and grouped by categories in the categorized form. The total cost of $230,850 leaves her a profit of $96,496 for the year. If she had shown a loss

Table 2.5   Example proprietorship profit and loss statement (categorized format).

Profit and Loss Statement
Mary Doe, DDS
For the Year Ending December 31, 201X

Income			
Production	337,470		
Collections			327,346
Expenses			
Staff Costs			
Commissions	0		
Employee Benefit Program	3,640		
Pension/Profit Sharing Plan	3,048		
Wages	65,950		
Temporary Services	340	72,978	
Office Space Costs			
Depreciation	23,047		
Rent or Lease	18,000		
Repairs and Maintenance	270		
Utilities	10,955		
Office Cleaning	3,055	55,327	
Office Expenses			
Insurance	2,650		
Office Expense	3,817		
Postage	690	7,157	
Marketing Expenses			
Advertising	1,854	1,854	
Bank Expenses			
Interest Expense	12,487		
Bank Charges	120	12,607	
Variable (Production) Expenses			
Dental Supplies	23,584		
Dental Lab	33,754		
Office Supplies	4,082	61,420	
Professional Expenses			
Legal and Accounting	1,790		
Taxes and Licenses	10,108	11,898	
Owner's Expenses			
Auto Expenses	1,928		
Meals, Travel, and Entertainment	139		
Dues and Publications	2,050		
Continuing Education	3,492	7,609	
Total Expenses			230,850
Profit (Loss)			96,496

for the year, expenses would have been more than income, and the number for the loss would be in parentheses.

If the income statement is from a sole proprietorship or partnership, then it does not report any salary expense for the owner(s) who work in the business. The amount that the business owner actually withdraws from the business doesn't matter. The profit or loss from the business is reported on the owner's personal income tax return. However, if the business is a corporation, then that is a separate tax paying entity. In this case, the income statement reports owner's salary as a corporate expense. (The owner pays personal income tax on salary, dividends, and bonuses.) Due to these differences, the net income from corporate and proprietorship income statements will be different. A proprietorship's profit or loss statement shows the amount that is left over after subtracting all deductible operating expenses from the practice's gross revenue. A corporate profit or loss statement includes officers' salaries (including owner-officers) as a deductible expense.

The personal income statement is similar in format to the proprietorship statement. It shows personal income and expenses over a specified period. Most people prepare a family statement, which includes income and expenses from both spouses and children. If you don't commingle money, then develop separate statements.

3. The *cash flow statement* is primarily a business statement, although we may adapt it to personal situations. The general formula for a cash flow statement is given in Table 2.6. It is similar to a profit and loss statement, with a few important differences. This statement shows the cash receipts and cash disbursements for a specific period and the resulting cash balance changes. The cash flow statement represents changes in the checkbook. The cash flow statement shows the cash changes. The income statement shows noncash accounting items. Some transactions involve tax events, but not cash. For example, the income statement lists "depreciation" as an expense. (Depreciation is the reduction in the value of an asset over its useful lifetime.) The dentist did not write a check for depreciation, although he or she claimed it as a tax expense. Some transactions involve cash transfers, but not tax events. For example, if a dentist borrows cash and puts it into a checking account, the dentist has made a cash transaction, although this is not a taxable event. (The dentist does not pay tax on borrowed money. Likewise, when he or she pays back borrowed money to a lender, the principal portion is not an expense, only the interest portion.)

Cash flow statements are often used to decide if there is enough money flowing through the practice to make recurring mortgage and other loan payments or other expense items, such as payroll or supplies. If the cash flow statement doesn't "balance," then we must cover any cash shortage from savings or borrowing. Any

Table 2.6 Cash flow statement formula.

INFLOWS − OUTFLOWS = NET CASH FLOW

CASH INFLOWS
  Collections
  Withdrawal from Savings
  Loan Proceeds

CASH OUTFLOWS
  Office Expenses
  Loan Payments
  Taxes
  Additions to Savings

excess goes to savings or cash accounts. That is to say, total cash inflows must equal total cash outflows.

An example of a projected practice cash flow statement is shown in Table 2.7. It details the projected (estimated) production, collections, and costs by month for the first year of a practice. It includes a mortgage payment each month and a draw or salary for the owner's living expenses. The line "Monthly Net Cash Flow"

Table 2.7 Example cash flow projection.

	Month 1	Month 2	Month 3	Month 4	Month 5
Doctor Production	7,621	8,764	10,079	11,590	13,329
Hygiene Production	1,732	2,078	2,494	2,993	3,591
TOTAL PRODUCTION	9,353	10,842	12,573	14,583	16,920
TOTAL COLLECTIONS (CASH RECEIPTS)	4,676	7,946	11,084	12,855	14,912
Dental Laboratory	842	976	1,132	1,312	1,523
Clinical Supplies	561	651	754	875	1,015
Office Supplies	187	217	251	292	338
TOTAL VARIABLE COSTS	1,590	1,844	2,137	2,479	2,876
Staff Wages	5,265	5,265	5,265	5,265	5,265
Employment Taxes	684	684	684	684	684
TOTAL STAFF COSTS	5,949	5,949	5,949	5,949	5,949
Office Rent/Lease	1,500	1,500	1,500	1,500	1,500
Utilities	800	800	800	800	800
Repairs	100	100	100	100	100
TOTAL OFFICE SPACE COSTS	2,400	2,400	2,400	2,400	2,400
Office Expenses	317	317	317	317	317
Insurance, Business	416	416	416	416	416
TOTAL OFFICE EXPENSES	733	733	733	733	733
Bank Charges	50	50	50	50	50
Mortgage Payment (Practice)	3,041	3,041	3,041	3,041	3,041
TOTAL BANK EXPENSES	3,091	3,091	3,091	3,091	3,091
Marketing and Promotion	583	583	583	583	583
TOTAL MARKETING EXPENSES	583	583	583	583	583
Management Consulting	0	0	0	0	0
Accounting	200	200	200	200	200
TOTAL PROFESSIONAL EXPENSES	200	200	200	200	200
Draw	4,000	4,000	4,000	4,000	4,000
Personal Insurances Paid	300	300	300	300	300
Continuing Education	50	50	50	50	50
Professional Dues and Journals	83	83	83	83	83
TOTAL OWNER'S EXPENSES	4,433	4,433	4,433	4,433	4,433
TOTAL EXPENSES	18,979	19,233	19,526	19,868	20,265
MONTHLY NET CASH FLOW	−14,303	−11,287	−8,442	−7,013	−5,353
CUMULATIVE CASH POSITION	−14,303	−25,590	−34,032	−41,045	−46,398

Table 2.7 (*Continued*)

Month 6	Month 7	Month 8	Month 9	Month 10	Month 11	Month 12	Year 1
15,328	17,627	20,271	2,312	26,809	30,830	35,455	221,015
4,310	5,172	6,206	7,447	8,937	10,724	12,869	68,553
19,638	22,799	26,477	30,759	35,746	41,554	48,324	289,568
17,304	20,086	23,322	27,088	31,473	36,580	42,531	249,857
1,767	2,052	2,383	2,768	3,217	3,740	4,349	26,061
1,178	1,368	1,589	1,846	2,145	2,493	2,899	17,374
393	456	530	615	715	831	966	5,791
3,338	3,876	4,502	5,229	6,077	7,064	8,214	49,226
5,265	5,265	5,265	5,265	5,265	5,265	5,265	63,180
684	684	684	684	684	684	684	8,208
5,949	5,949	5,949	5,949	5,949	5,949	5,949	71,388
1,500	1,500	1,500	1,500	1,500	1,500	1,500	18,000
800	800	800	800	800	800	800	9,600
100	100	100	100	100	100	100	1,200
2,400	2,400	2,400	2,400	2,400	2,400	2,400	28,800
317	317	317	317	317	317	317	3,804
416	416	416	416	416	416	416	4,992
733	733	733	733	733	733	733	8,796
50	50	50	50	50	50	50	600
3,041	3,041	3,041	3,041	3,041	3,041	3,041	36,492
3,091	3,091	3,091	3,091	3,091	3,091	3,091	37,092
583	583	583	583	583	583	583	6,996
583	583	583	583	583	583	583	6,996
0	0	0	0	0	0	0	0
200	200	200	200	200	200	200	2,400
200	200	200	200	200	200	200	2,400
4,000	6,000	6,000	6,000	6,000	6,000	6,000	60,000
300	300	300	300	300	300	300	3,600
50	50	50	50	50	50	50	600
83	83	83	83	83	83	83	996
4,433	6,433	6,433	6,433	6,433	6,433	6,433	65,196
20,727	23,265	23,891	24,618	25,466	26,453	27,603	269,894
−3,423	−3,179	−569	2,470	6,007	10,127	14,928	−20,037
−49,821	−53,000	−53,569	−51,099	−45,092	−34,965	−20,037	

shows the anticipated cash flow for the month. The line "Cumulative Cash Position" shows the running total cash excess or shortage. Since the cash inflows must equal cash outflows, this statement shows that the dentist buying into or starting this practice would need to borrow cash to pay the bills until month 9, when monthly net cash flow becomes positive. At this point, there should be enough cash coming through the practice to pay monthly expenses. The maximum amount of cash needed (as working capital) is estimated to be $53,569 in month 8, the largest negative "Monthly Net Cash Flow." After this point, estimates show the excess cash flow that can be used to pay down the accumulated cash borrowed.

4. *Pro forma statements* are projected statements for expected future outcomes. They can be any of the four types described above. The essential element of a pro forma is that it is an educated guess of what the statement will be at a given time in the future. For practice statements, this requires estimates of numbers of patient visits, average charges, numbers and pay rates of staff, and many other items of expense. Obviously, a pro forma statement is only as accurate as the educated guess about the future. Often, banks will ask borrowers to develop a pro forma cash flow (to assess whether there is adequate cash to meet expected expenses) and an income statement (to determine your expected income and tax situations).

Using Financial Statements

Financial statements have several vital uses. These include the following:

1. Meeting the needs and desires of creditors or lenders, required either by contract or to secure funds (borrowing)
2. Providing information that may be required by law, such as income tax returns (compliance)
3. Developing information to be used in control of the practice (analysis)
4. Providing information to be used in planning changes in the practice (planning)

Borrowing

Bankers are in the business of lending money. However, they want to lend to people that they believe will repay their loans in a timely manner. So the banker will gather extensive information to "qualify" a new dentist for a loan (or to decide whether he or she is a good loan risk). Borrowers should show the banker that they know what they are doing from a business perspective so that the banker will be more comfortable with the loans. Borrowers should approach the first meeting with a budget, cash flow analysis, and business plan, rather than asking what the banker needs for a loan. Bankers may have specific items (for example, tax returns from the past 3 years) that they want in addition, but being prepared at the initial contact will help to convince the banker that the borrower is worthy of a loan. Two other chapters of this book relate directly to borrowing money to purchase a practice—Chapter 4 (business planning) and Chapter 9 (financing a practice).

Compliance

Financial statements form the basis of business and personal income taxes. Depending on the form of business entity, the practitioner needs an income statement and a balance sheet, showing changes in financial position for the year. Generally, the accountant will develop these forms. The professional needs to understand that they can also be used for analysis of the practice.

The profit and loss statement is the basis for determining federal income taxes. The items placed on a business profit and loss statement are the same ones that are tax items. A sole proprietor reports tax items on the IRS's Schedule C, which is nothing but a glorified P&L statement. Other forms of business ownership have different requirements and forms, but most involve some form of a profit and loss statement and balance sheet calculations. Chapter 10 discusses various business forms or entities and some of their tax implications.

Financial Analysis

Financial statements provide the raw numbers to analyze the financial health of a dental practice. These data are used in several ways. A given practice may be compared with other similar practices to detect areas where the practice exceeds or falls short of benchmarks. The analysis can look for changes by comparing data over time (monthly, quarterly, or yearly). The practitioner may set his or her own internal standard and use data to decide how well the practice met these specific goals. Chapter 3 discusses these financial analysis in detail.

Planning

In the traditional dental practice mode, the new practitioner established or bought a practice and remained there for 30 years. The current marketplace is much different. Today's graduate may work in a network practice for several years, buy a small practice, build it, and then move to a different location in several years. They may look to establish satellite practices or joint practice ventures with other practitioners. To do these ventures requires detailed planning. One phase of this planning is financial, proposing changes and calculating the expected result. The basis of these calculations is the current financial statements of the practice(s).

   Several chapters in this book expand upon the key role of financial statements in dental practice, especially Chapter 3 (financial analysis), Chapter 4 (business planning), Chapter 7 (buying/buying into a practice), Chapter 8 (starting a practice), and Chapter 9 (financing a practice).

References and Additional Resources

Books

Finkbeiner, Betty Ladley, and Finkbeiner, Charles Allan. 2001. *Practice Management for the Dental Team*, 4th ed. Philadelphia: Mosby.

Pinson, Linda. 2001. *Keeping the Books: Basic Recordkeeping and Accounting for the Successful Small Business*, 5th ed. Chicago: Dearborn Trade Publishing.

Rattan, Raj. 1996. *Making Sense of Dental Practice Management: The Business Side of General Dental Practice*. Abingdon, UK: Radcliffe Medical Press.

Willis, David O. 2007. *The dental practice: a management simulation.* Available at www. dentalsimulations.com.

Willis, David O. 2013. *Business Basics for Dentists*, New York: John Wiley & Sons, Inc.

Websites

www.dentaleconomics.com/. *Dental Economics* home page.

www.sba.gov/. Small business administration, steps for starting a business.

www.aabacosmallbusiness.com/. Formerly Yahoo Small Business web site.

Learning Exercises

1. Describe the formula for each of the following statements:
    A. Balance sheet
    B. Income statement
    C. Cash flow statement
2. Describe the purpose for each of the following statements:
    A. Balance sheet
    B. Income statement
    C. Cash flow statement
3. Define pro forma statements and describe how they are used.
4. Discuss the use of financial statements.

Chapter 3
Practice Financial Analysis

David O. Willis

Financial analysis uses the "numbers" of the practice to identify areas that need improvement. These numbers are essentially quantitative measures of quality management for a general dental practice. The measures come primarily from the office financial statements and the office computer system. While some of these data may be used in raw form, other data need to be converted into financial ratios in order to be meaningful. By way of illustration, to say that someone weighs 200 pounds is meaningless unless we relate that weight to the person's sex, height, body frame, and previous weight.

The practitioner may want to analyze the finances of the practice for several reasons. If someone is considering purchasing the practice, s/he will want to know areas the practice does well, and areas of potential savings. The practitioner may want to analyze the practice to improve profitability. Finally, the practitioner may want to understand the office finances so that a merger, acquisition, or other office growth strategy can be successfully planned.

Dental Office Financial Analysis

The basic source for financial analysis is the profit and loss statement. It starts with the revenue produced, takes away all costs, and results in spendable profit (or loss) for the practitioner. The basic P&L statement breaks down into specific elements as in the following sections.

Dental Practice Revenues

Total (gross) practice revenues result from the number and type of procedures that the office does, the fee that is charged for each of those procedures, the number and type of adjustments granted from full fee, and the collection ratio shown by the office. If revenue is low, any of the four factors may be at fault. The following formula describes these relationships:

Gross Production = Number of Procedures × Fee
Net Production = Gross Production − Adjustments
Collections = Net Production × Collection Ratio

Dental Practice Transition: A Practical Guide to Management, Second Edition.
Edited by David G. Dunning and Brian M. Lange.
© 2016 John Wiley & Sons, Inc. Published 2016 by John Wiley & Sons, Inc.
Companion Website: www.wiley.com/go/dunning/transition

Gross production is the total amount of dentistry produced by the office for the period, charges at the full fee value before any discounts or adjustments. Production levels vary with the number and types of *procedures* done, and the *fee charged* for each procedure. Production numbers are obviously very important for a dental practice, for without production, no money flows through the office.

Adjustments are the amounts of money that the office "wrote off" for discounts because of insurance plans (such as preferred provider plans or PPOs), marketing efforts, or professional courtesies. The practice should track different types of adjustments to detect the impact that source has on the office finances.

Net production is gross production less any adjustments for insurance or other reasons. This is the amount of money that you would expect to collect if everyone (patients and insurance companies) paid all that they contractually owe you for work done. Practices that have a large amount of insurance write-offs (adjustments) need to produce more (gross production) to reach the same net production level as a comparable noninsurance practice.

Collections are the amounts of money (cash, checks, and credit cards) that crossed the receptionist's desk for the period. Some of this may be from production for this month, while the rest of it may be for dentistry performed several months ago but is being paid now. Individuals, insurance companies, or government programs may make payments. Technically, revenues are income from all sources. In most dental practices, collections for dentistry done is the major (or only) source of revenue, so the two terms are essentially equivalent.

The *collection ratio* is the percentage of accounts (net production) that have historically been paid in full for the services provided. Uncollectibles are the monies that the office has given up trying to collect. At some point (120 days, 6 months, 1 year) the office decides that the person who owes this money isn't going to pay, and they "write off" the account. They deem it uncollectible. If collections and net production are equal, then you have a 100% collection ratio, collecting all that you expect to collect.

Dental Practice Costs

Many people consider that any cost (or overhead) is bad. In fact, there is a cost of doing business, and that is overhead. Any cost that improves profitability is a "good" cost; any cost that decreases profitability is a "bad" cost. The key is to decide which is which. To accomplish this, most management experts compare a practice to norms, or "average" practices of a similar type. These may come from surveys published in the dental press or from proprietary information gathered by management or accounting firms. For example, every dentist has a cost associated with rental (or purchase) of office space. If the "average" dentist pays 6% of his or her production for rent and you are paying 9%, then some of your rent may be decreasing the profit of the practice. As another example, suppose a dentist hires a new staff member, paying him or her $15 an hour. That staff member allows the office to produce an additional $50 per hour. That is money well spent (or invested), a "good" piece of overhead. However, if the office does not increase production enough to make up for the additional costs, the additional money spent on the staff member would be "bad" overhead. This is simple in concept. The problem is trying to decide which costs are wasted and which contribute to the practice's profitability. That is what financial analysis is really about.

Dental practice costs fall into three basic categories: fixed, step-fixed, or variable.

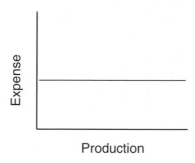

Figure 3.1. Fixed costs.

Fixed costs do not change with production. Whether the office produces $3,000 or $30,000 per month, fixed costs are constant. Examples include rent, dental association dues, and malpractice insurance premiums. These remain constant, regardless of how much production is done. (While these are not exactly the same from month to month, they are generally consistent.) Fixed costs are depicted graphically in Figure 3.1.

Fixed costs consist of the following:

Office space/equipment consists of all costs associated with operating the physical space and equipment of the practice, including rent payments and utility, tax, or repair charges associated with the occupancy of the building. Depreciation expense for office and equipment is included, since this represents wear and tear on those assets. The cost of a practice buy-in or equipment replacement program also represents an office space cost.

Other fixed costs include bank charges, office insurances, advertising, and legal and professional expenses.

Step-fixed costs (staff costs) vary with production, but only in discrete steps. The existing staff will work harder as production increases. Finally, the load becomes too great, and another staff member must be hired to help the office run efficiently. Costs jump in a discrete step when we hire the new person. Staff members are hired as entire people (or increments of people). These costs are considered "fixed" over their range, so that when another person is hired, a new set of fixed costs is established. Unless a staff member is hired or leaves, staffing costs will be relatively constant or "fixed" in the range of our analysis. Step-fixed costs are depicted graphically in Figure 3.2.

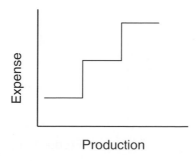

Figure 3.2. Step-fixed costs.

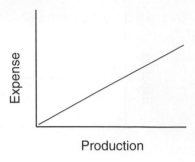

Figure 3.3.   Variable costs.

Staff costs include direct wages, benefits, payroll taxes, retirement plan contributions, hiring and training expense, and any other costs that are direct results of employing staff for the office. Labor costs can be divided into clerical (front office), hygiene, and chair-side assisting personnel.

Variable costs change directly with the production level. If the office produces $30,000 of dentistry 1 month, then the cost for dental supplies will be approximately 10 times more than a month with $3,000 in production. If the office has no production, then theoretically there will be no variable costs. Variable costs change with production, not collections. The office must still purchase supplies for procedures that they discounted or did not collect. The types of variable costs should be tracked separately. Variable costs are depicted graphically in Figure 3.3.

Dental lab costs are associated with contract laboratory work. The costs of laboratory supplies in the office (stone, waxes, etc.) are considered dental supplies. If the office employs a laboratory technician, all costs associated with the laboratory operation (salary, benefits, supplies, lab space rent, etc.) are included in this category.

Dental supplies are the materials used when doing dentistry. They include expendable supplies (cotton rolls, anesthetic, alloy, composite material) and small instrument replacement.

Office supplies are the costs associated with materials for the front desk operation. This includes paper products, computer program fees, postage, magazine subscriptions, pencils, and other items used in processing patient visits.

Total costs are the sums of fixed, step-fixed, and variable costs. Likewise, the diagram for total costs is the combination of these various types of expenses. Total costs are depicted graphically in Figure 3.4.

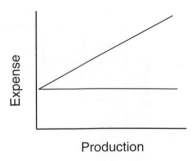

Figure 3.4.   Total costs.

Financial Analysis: Quantitative Measures of Quality Management for a General Dental Practice

Financial analysis uses the "numbers" of the practice to maximize profit from the practice. These numbers are gathered from financial statements or from the office computer system. The financial control process can be simple or complex. The possibilities for gathering data are endless. An office computer system can generate so many reports that the problem is deciding which reports and analyses are truly useful. Try to remember the acronym "KISS" (*keep it simple, stupid*). Do not inundate the analysis with information; keep it simple. Look for major problem areas first. Start with a basic ratio in each of the areas (production, patients, collections, managed care and costs), and look for problems in these areas. If there are no problems, there probably is no need to do any in-depth analysis. Conversely, your practice may be having problems in one certain area that needs particular, additional attention. Other areas may be functioning well and only require periodic monitoring. Table 3.1 summarizes the key areas where financial ratios can help determine practice success. Each key to practice success is provided in the list below, along with one or two common ratios used to assess accomplishment of the key. You can use these ratios either in assessing a practice to make it more efficient or to determine whether the practice is a healthy practice for a buying opportunity.

Most people only think of costs when they look at financial control. However, the revenue side is equally important. Since both output (revenues) and input (costs) help to set productivity, we obviously must control both to be productive. These indicators are summarized in Table 3.2. Management literature, research, and practice have emphasized *quality management* for many years. Importantly, these critical success factors are, in essence, quantitative measures of quality management for a general dental practice. It should also be noted that practice advisors and consultants may have slightly different opinions about some of the suggested targets listed in the right column of Table 3.2, and/or might suggest additional variables/targets. Market differences must also be kept in mind—for example, achieving lower overhead in a rural area may be more readily achieved than in a large city. Similarly, the extent of production from managed care may depend in part on the saturation of dental insurance in a given market. In the end, the key point is to continuously monitor practice performance in light of established goals and targets.

Office Production

Office production per month tracks the total amount of dentistry done by the entire office for the month. Assuming a solo practitioner, production should remain steady or rise each month. (Obviously, if the owner takes a week off, then production will be down for that month. Likewise, if you raise fees by 5%, then production should increase a

Table 3.1 Keys to practice success.

1. Increase office production
2. Generate patients for the practice
3. Maintain collections
4. Control managed care
5. Control costs

Table 3.2 Critical success factors.

Critical Factors in Practice Success and Their Measures		
Success Factor	Measure of Factor	Value of Measure
1. Maintaining Production		
Gross Production	Gross office production per month	Level or increasing
Net Production	Net office production per month	Level or increasing
2. Generating Patients		
Adequate New Patients	New patient ratio	1 NP/practitioner/day
Effective Recall System	Recall effectiveness	>90% recalls due
3. Maintaining Collections		
Accounts Receivable	A/R amount	1/2 to 1 month's production
Collections	Collection ratio	98% of net production
4. Controlling Managed Care		
Managed Care Plans (1)	Managed care 5f n5f netproduction percentage	<50% gross production
Managed Care Plans (2)	Managed care adjustments	<20% gross production
Single Plan Size	Managed plan size	<25% production in any one plan
Individual Plan Efficiency	Managed care efficiency	Highest efficiency
5. Controlling Costs		
General Cost Control	Overhead ratio	<65%
Specific Costs Control	Specific cost ratios	Staff ratio 25–30% Variable cost ratio 15–22% Office space ratio 8–10%

corresponding amount.) Many dentists set production goals for the office. This then becomes the production measure. In order to do production, the office must be adequately scheduled. "Adequately scheduled" does not just mean being busy. Instead, you need a good mix of highly productive procedures (such as crown and bridge) and preparatory procedures (such as restorations). Since fee schedules vary across the country, be sure to use a similar practice if you want to compare your practice with another. If your practice is in a Midwestern rural area, don't use a practice in a large metropolitan area as the comparable practice. Many savvy practitioners track both gross and net productions. This allows them to follow how much dentistry the office does, and how much they write off for insurance plans.

Generate Patients for the Practice

Since new patients present with most of the large cases in an office, the *new patient's ratio* keeps track of this statistic. Each practitioner should see at a minimum twenty new patients per month (or about one per working day) to keep the practice adequately busy. "New patients" implies comprehensive care patients, not emergency or episodic care patients. Young and growing practices need to show more new patients than established practices.

Recall effectiveness measures the percentage of patients due for recall in a month who were actually seen for recall visits. This ratio examines how effectively the practice encourages patients to return for periodic maintenance visits. In established urban practices, production resulting from the "recall" visit and subsequent findings accounts for 60–75% of the total production. Managing the recall program is obviously a very important component of overall practice management. Some patient attrition can be expected as people move from the area or find different reasons to switch dentists or forego dental treatment. Practices should strive to see 90–95% of the patients who are due for the month. If they fall short, the front office person or hygienist (whoever is responsible for recall management) should begin procedures to increase recall acceptance. (This is also, in part, a scheduling issue.)

Maintain Collections

The *accounts receivable amount* shows the proportion of production that you are not collecting. A raw amount for accounts receivable (A/R) (for example, $30,000) is meaningless. Was that from a practice that grosses $25,000 per month or one that grosses $80,000 per month? Accounts receivable will be larger for larger practices, all other things being equal. This indicator says that for any practice, about three quarters to one times the average month's net production is acceptable as an accounts receivable amount. (This assumes that you file claims electronically and keep up to date computer files of insurance plans.) Your credit and collection policies will have an obvious impact on this indicator. Easy credit policies will generate higher accounts receivable; stricter policies, lower. Practices that process a large amount of insurance (greater than 75–90% of patients) will also have a larger A/R as they wait for insurance companies to process and mail checks. Immediate fee-for-service practices are on the low end of this range.

The total *collection ratio* is the percentage of net production that the office collects. It should be at or above 98%. Ideally, everyone should pay you. In reality, you will be fooled by some patients who promise to pay but do not. Most dental offices collect between 95 and 99% of the billable amount. (Since you do not really expect to collect adjustments, these amounts are not included in this ratio.) A lower collection ratio may suggest problems with collection procedures or a temporary surge in production, resulting in an increase in accounts receivable and potential cash flow problems. A very high collection number may suggest a credit policy that is too strict, discouraging patients from accepting large treatment plans. This may be a particular problem in younger, growing practices. It may also be the result of a short-term surge in production from an unusual number of large cases or an unusually productive month.

Control Managed Care

The managed care percentage looks at the portion of your practice production represented by managed care. This describes, in large measure, for the difference between gross and net production. There are two options for this measure. First, if total managed care production exceeds 50% of total practice production, then managed care is simply too great a part of the practice. Not only are you losing a lot of money but you are also losing control of the schedule, as managed care patients replace full fee-for-service patients. Any one plan should not account for more than 25% of gross production. The practice may be seen to be in a "risky" position if this large program changes reimbursement schedules or cancels a provider contract. An alternative measure is to look at managed care adjustments. They should represent no more than 20% of the total office production. This takes into account the efficiency of all of the plans (in total) you are working with, but does not assess an individual plan. Both measures give similar results. The first is a bit easier; the second, more accurate. This indicator is very dependent upon local market conditions. Areas with a lot of managed care (discounted insurance) plans will have a higher percentage as dentists compete for patients. Areas with fewer managed care plans should see a lower managed care percentage.

Managed care efficiency determines the level of reimbursement for each individual plan. It asks the percentage of charges returned compared to a similar, full fee patient. This way, you know how much of a discount is implied with each plan. To calculate this measure, take the total collections from each plan (including any capitation payments) and divide by the full fee value. You need to track this regularly, as plan administrators change their reimbursements and rules, often without telling you. All other things being equal, plans with the higher efficiency lead to higher profit and income levels. While you might not track every plan, you should certainly track the ten largest plans in the practice. This indicator then is relative, comparing one plan with another.

Control Costs

The *overhead ratio* (OH ratio) rearranges the information contained in the income statement to give a very general cost ratio. Rather than showing how much profit the office makes, the overhead formula shows how much it costs for a given amount of work. It answers the question, what percentage of production went to pay the bills? This shows, in a rough way, the percentage of every dollar generated that pays the costs of the practice. The inverse (1 − OH%) represents the profitability of the practice. The profitability ratio then answers the question, what percentage of production was left as profit? If the overhead is 70%, then the profitability of the practice is 30%. Any money left after paying bills is considered profit. This assumes that we are looking at a solo proprietorship practice. It does not separate out doctor's salary as a separate cost item. Typical corporate/franchise practices may pay an associate 25–30% of net production. If we include that as a cost item, then the profit margins become much less (~10–20%+/−). (This is sometimes called business or entrepreneurial profit.) Solo practitioners often just lump these together and call them all profit. Multipractitioner offices and networks often include doctor compensation as a cost of doing business. They then view business profit as their appropriate measure.

In solo general dental practices, overhead (and the OH ratio) fall into ranges—more than 65% is high; less than 55% is good; and 55–65% is about average. This ratio balances for different parts of the country. High fee areas are also generally high-cost areas. If overhead falls into the "good" range, you may be satisfied, realizing that the trouble of additional analysis and control may not produce enough return to worry about. Conversely, you may want to maximize the potential profit from the practice and continue the analysis to detect areas to increase profitability further.

The overhead ratio depends upon the point at which the practice is in the practice cycle. In a start-up phase (with few patients and relatively high debts and expenses), the OH ratio will obviously be very high. New practitioners are often paying off buyout or start-up loans. The interest and depreciation expenses represented by this outlay are additional costs that established practitioners generally do not have. New practitioners in a buyout situation often must replace or update equipment, supplies, and materials at an additional cost. Finally, many new practitioners simply cannot do the volume of

Table 3.3 Specific costs.

Typical Dental Office Cost Breakdown	
Category	Percentage of Collections
Staff Costs	22–30
Wages, Benefits, Taxes, Insurance	
Variable Costs/Supplies	12–22
Lab, Dental Supplies, Office Supplies	
Facilities	8–10
Rent, Utilities, Depreciation	
Miscellaneous	9–14
Legal, Acctg, Adv, Taxes, Ins, Interest	
Owner's Expenses	8–10
Dues, Subscriptions, Auto, CE, Retirement	
Profit	35–45

dentistry that established practitioners do. This may be from the need to increase their patient pool or the new practitioner's clinical inexperience. Regardless, if production is less than a comparable established practitioner, then the OH ratio, and most other ratios, will appear to be out of line. New practitioners can expect an additional 5–8% overhead for debt service and other start-up costs while paying off loans. They may even run at a loss (more than 100% overhead) while building their patient pool.

Specific cost control looks at the same thing as the overhead percentage but begins to break it into specific units. There are typical ranges of costs for each area of cost allocation. These are shown in Table 3.3. These standards attach values to various components of the expenses of operating a dental practice. When using these numbers, you are comparing your practice to the "norm" or other similar practices. You can compare every cost if you want, but that is not a good use of time. Concentrate on the areas where a change can make the most impact. The three largest cost areas in most general dental practices are staff, variable, and facility costs. As with the recommended values in Table 3.2, marketplace demands must be kept in mind when developing realistic expectations for controlling overhead costs. For example, all other things being equal, labor and facility costs may be higher in large metropolitan areas compared to small towns or smaller cities.

Most overhead numbers are related as a percentage of net production. Costs are more closely related to production than collections. If we use gross production, then we have to introduce the new category of adjustments, skewing traditional numbers.

Practice Analysis

We can use these key indicators of practice health as the basis for a financial analysis of the practice. If a dental practice is not profitable enough, often dentists immediately look to decrease costs to improve profitability. As we have seen in the previous discussion, lack of profitability can be caused by a shortfall in any of the success areas. Simple cutting costs may lead to still lower profits as needed activities are not funded. If, for example, the real problem is lack of new patients, not excess expenses, then cutting marketing costs will lead to even fewer new patients, lower production, revenues, and profits. There is not a formula to decide where the problem and solution lie. Instead, understand the process and apply it to your particular case. An example is presented below.

Office Production

If gross office production is low, then all of the ratios will be above standards. This low production may be the result of seeing too few patients, or charging fees that are low for the area. Look at both gross and net productions to decide if there is a problem with insurance plans or general lack of patient visits. Compare fees for key dental procedures with average fees for the area to decide if the practices fees are in line with area fees.

Generate Patients for the Practice

New patients often come to the office with significant dental needs. They result in large cases that increase production significantly. Recall or periodic maintenance patients bring a steady stream of additional work for the practice. So, a lack of either of these types of patients can result in low office production numbers. If gross production and new patients are low, then there is a need to develop a marketing campaign to attract new patients to the practice. This may include advertising, insurance plan participation, or other external methods to attract new patients.

Maintain Collections

If collections are low but gross and net productions are acceptable, then there is a problem in the collection process. This may be from a credit or collection policy that is too loose (allowing low down payments or long payment periods) or from a front office staff that is too lenient with patients' payment plans. Low production and collections may indicate a credit or collection policy that is too strict.

Control Managed Care

If gross production is acceptable, but net production is low, then managed care (discounted insurance) plans are too large a part of the office production. This can be a tricky problem to solve, because decreasing insurance plans also decreases gross production. Look at the efficiency of each plan, decreasing or eliminating the least efficient plans. Develop a marketing plan that will bring additional private pay or acceptable insurance plan patients to replace those patients (and their corresponding production) lost by eliminating the lower paying plans. Participating in additional plans is a seductive way to immediately increase gross production, but follow profit closely to decide if the additional work leads to adequate profits.

Control Costs

The starting point for cost analysis is the overhead percentage. If overhead percentage is out of line compared with other practices, then there is a need to look further at the practice's numbers. Generally, the problem is that the OH ratio is too high, but it may actually be too low. This happens when the office is understaffed, when the analysis does not account for all costs (such as working spouses), when collections surge because of anomalies in the collection pattern, or when the office does not purchase adequate supplies, equipment, and material to keep up to date. Specialty practices have different acceptable ranges due to the different characters of those practices. This also assumes that the practice does not use tax avoidance strategies (for example, renting space from yourself or hiring family members at an unusually high compensation) that can skew results.

Example Analysis

As an example problem, assume that our dentist, Dr. Mary Doe, wants to gain a better understanding of her office finances. She has worked with her accountant to prepare an income statement for the previous year so that she can use the results for a more detailed analysis of the practice finances. (We are using round numbers for illustration.) From that statement, she allocated costs into the various categories and arrived at the following financial outcomes for the past year in her office. Notice that she did not have perfect (complete) information. There may be holes or gaps in the background information that you would want to complete an analysis. At that point, you need to decide if a more complete analysis is worth the work to get additional practice numbers. If you are doing a detailed, focused analysis, then the extra work is probably warranted.

Category	Amount
New Patient Visits	220
Accounts Receivable	$39,250
Gross Production	$650,000
Adjustments	$125,000
Net Production	$525,000
Collections	$518,000
Fixed Costs	$120,000
Step-Fixed Costs	$135,000
Variable Costs	$110,000
Total Costs	$345,000
Profit	$153,000
Overhead Percentage Gross Production	56.1%
Overhead Percentage Net Production	69.5%

Production Analysis

We do not have previous year's production numbers to see trends. We also do not have comparable practice data. If we find that Dr. Doe's fees and production are in line with comparable practices, then production appears to be fine.

Generating Patients

Dr. Doe's new patient visits average about 18 per month. This is below the desired target of 22 per month. The office did 1,496 recall visits last year, which is slightly less than 8 per working day. We do not know how many recall visits were due for the time.

Maintaining Collections

Dr. Doe's office does a good job collecting accounts. They collect 98.6% of net production. Note that they collect 79.6% of gross production, a seemingly terrible amount that is due to high adjustments, not collection procedures. The account receivable amount ($39,250) is slightly below one month's production, which is acceptable.

Controlling Managed Care

Dr. Doe wrote off 19% of gross production for managed care (insurance) plan discounts. She did not break out managed care production separately to analyze that number. Her adjustment percentage is high, approaching the problem level. If she could replace all of the discounted work with full fee paying patients, costs would remain the same, but collections (and therefore profit) would increase by $125,000.

Controlling Costs

Dr. Doe's overhead percentage (69.7% of net production) is above acceptable. Staff costs (27%) and variable costs (20.9%) are also at the high end of normal. Given that overhead is high, the problem appears to be low production numbers, brought about in part on the high amount of managed care/insurance write-offs in the office, and low number of new patient visits.

Break-Even Analysis

Proper allocation of costs gives a much more accurate understanding of practice costs than the simple traditional "percentage overhead" figure. A valuable tool for putting this information to use is through the "break-even analysis" technique. This financial analysis technique relates the office's costs to the production and profit of a practice. While, as its name implies, it can determine the point of zero profit and zero loss (the "break-even point"), it has a much wider use by providing insights into the cost behavior of the practice and the riskiness of many courses of action. The basic equation used in the break-even technique is

Collection – Variable Expenses – Fixed (incl Step-Fixed) Expenses = Net Income

The equation brings mathematical sense to an intuitive concept; namely, that all the money you collect, minus all your expenses (fixed and variable), leaves a profit or loss. If you know any three of the numbers, you can substitute in the equation to find the fourth number.

The break-even analysis can also be depicted graphically (Figure 3.5).

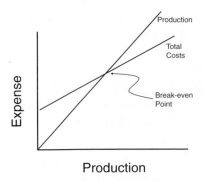

Figure 3.5.   Break-even point.

Essentially, this is the cost structure diagram superimposed on a production diagram. The point of intersection between the revenue (collection) line and the total cost line is the "break-even" point. Any production above this point results in profit; any production below this point results in loss. You can also see that production above the break-even point is "more profitable," since the fixed costs have been paid and you now incur only the lower variable costs. This also happens when a dentist takes an associate or in other ways offsets hours with another dentist. Fixed costs have already been paid; only step-fixed and variable costs remain. Any additional dentistry produced is on a better margin for the owner-dentist. The incremental cost of producing more is small in comparison to the initial cost ratio. This is also critical to understanding managed care or other reduced payment third-party plans. If there is slack chair time, then the only costs associated with the production are the variable costs, since fixed costs have already been paid. However, if these patients replace traditional, fee-for-service patients, then the cost must also include the loss from the foregone production on those traditional patients.

We can use our previous example to demonstrate the use of break-even analysis.

In our example, Dr. Doe produces $650,000 per year ($54,157 per month) and adjusts $125,000 for insurance. She collects 98.6% of net production. Variable costs are 20.9% of net production. Total fixed costs were $155,000 (fixed and step-fixed). Using the following formula and previously given cost data, her income for the year would be

Collections − Variable Expenses − Fixed Expenses = Net Income
$(0.98.6 \times \text{net production}) − (0.209 \times \text{net production}) − 255,000 = \text{Net Income}$
$\$518,000 − 110,000 − 255,000 = \text{Net Income}$
$\$153,000 = \text{Net Income}$

Dr. Doe netted $153,000 (before personal taxes) by producing $650,000 of dentistry, collecting 98.6% of accounts, and paying all fixed and variable expenses. Her actual production "break-even" point, where net income is zero, can also be found using

Collections − Variable Expenses − Fixed Expenses = Net Income
$(0.986 \times \text{net production}) − (0.209 \times \text{net production}) − 255,000 = 0$
$(0.777 \times \text{net production}) = 255,000$
Net Production = $328,185

That is to say, if Dr. Doe had a net production $328,185 of dentistry this year, she would pay all the bills but not take a dime home, having a net income of zero ($0). Since she adjusts 19.2% of gross production, she would need to produce $406,169 (gross) to break even.

Gross Production $\times (1 − 0.192) = \text{Net Production}$
Gross Production $= \$328,185/(1 − 0.192)$
Gross Production $= \$406,169$

Dr. Doe may decide that to buy a new house and join the local country club would require a net pretax income of $200,000. What production level corresponds to this net income level? Again the break-even analysis can be used:

Collections − Variable Expenses − Fixed Expenses = Net Income
$(0.986 \times \text{net production}) - (0.209 \times \text{net production}) - 255,000 = 200,000$
$(0.777 \times \text{net production}) = 455,000$
Net Production = $585,585
Gross Production × 0.808 = Net Production
Gross production = 585,585/0.808
Gross production = $724,733

Dr. Doe would need to produce $724,733 of dentistry per year ($60,394 per month) to "clear" the target income of $200,000. Can this be done given the existing staff, facilities, and fee structure? That decision is the essence of strategic practice planning and control. If not, then she should modify plans and reconfigure the estimates of fixed and step-fixed costs for the new configuration and repeat the analysis.

Once you understand and chart the cost and revenue structure of the practice (that is, once you develop a model), you can then look at various growth opportunities from a financial standpoint by asking the question, "what if?" What if I hire a hygienist and expand the office? What if I join the new insurance plan that is in town? What if I raise my fees by 10% and lose 5% of my patients? Applying the mathematical model of the practice can answer all of these questions from a financial standpoint. Many dentists have the ability, through computers and spreadsheet programs, to develop practice models that are very sophisticated. However, as already shown, we can develop a good working model of the break-even approach that uses a pencil and handheld calculator. Fortunately, even these now primitive tools can give good results with a minimal amount of time and effort. And sophisticated financial reports available through software certainly augment simpler tools.

Application to Associateships and Practice Purchase

Practice financial analysis has a foundational role to inform decisions about associateships and practice valuations/purchases. Consider the impact on an associateship in comparing solo-dentist practices A and B:

	Overhead	New Patients Per Month	Managed Care Production %	Managed Care Efficiency (as % of Fees)	Annual Revenue
Practice A	65%	40	40%	75%	$875,000
Practice B	80%	15	60%	65%	$675,000

Based on these variables and all other things being equal, Practice A appears much better positioned to hire an associate to work alongside the owner. The overhead of the office is lower, managed care is a smaller portion of the practice, and the managed care plans in this office are more efficient for the office. Practice B seems unlikely to be able to provide an adequate revenue stream to sustain an associate, due to the high levels of managed care, and their lower reimbursement rate. Anyone considering an associateship *must* evaluate that opportunity in light of key practice financial indicators such as those detailed in this chapter, including the laboratory expense and how it will be paid (by the owner and/or associate). The manner in which the laboratory expense alone is paid will directly impact an associate's income and the owner's overhead. Chapters 20 and 21 explore some of the financial dynamics related to associateships in traditional private practice and dental service organization settings.

Similarly, as especially explored in Chapter 5 (practice valuation), Chapter 6 (buying and buying-into a practice), and Chapter 9 (financing a practice), a practice's financial indicators have a *critical* impact on the viability of purchasing a practice. Lenders insist on the practice cash flow in view of not only the practice's overhead/profitability but also the borrower's personal/family budget. A practice's overhead percentage has a direct bearing on cash flow. In the example of Practices A and B above, Practice B will likely have a lower value not only because of having $200,000 less in annual revenue, but also because of a much higher overhead, fewer new patients per month, more managed care involvement, and lower managed care reimbursement.

References and Additional Resources

Books

Finkbeiner, Betty Ladley and Finkbeiner, Charles Allan. 2001. *Practice Management for the Dental Team*, 4th ed. Philadelphia: Mosby.

Pinson, Linda. 2001. *Keeping the Books: Basic Recordkeeping and Accounting for the Successful Small Business*, 5th ed. Chicago: Dearborn Trade Publishing.

Rattan, Raj. 1996. *Making Sense of Dental Practice Management: The Business Side of General Dental Practice*. Abingdon, UK: Radcliffe Medical Press.

Willis, David O. 2007. *The dental practice: a management simulation*. Available at www.dentalsimulations.com.

Willis, David O. 2013. *Business Basics for Dentists*. John Wiley and Sons, Inc.

Websites

www.dentaleconomics.com/. *Dental Economics* home page.

www.sba.gov/. Small business administration, steps for starting a business.

www.aabacosmallbusiness.com/. Formerly Yahoo Small Business website.

Learning Exercises

1. Describe the relationship between production and collections in the dental office.
2. Describe the types of costs and give examples of each.
3. Describe the five keys to practice success.
4. Give an example of an indicator (ratio) for each of the five areas.
5. Analyze the financial health of a dental practice based on the income statement.
6. Describe the uses of the break-even analysis technique.

Part 2
Ownership: Business Planning, Practice Valuation, Dental Equipment, Buying/Buying into a Practice, Starting a Practice, Financing a Practice, and Business Entities

Chapter 4
Business Planning: From the Perspective of the Dentist and the Banker

Nader A. Nadershahi, Lucinda J. Lyon, and Lisa Itaya

Failure to plan is planning to fail.

Anonymous

Upon acquiring your own dental practice, you will not only be a practicing dentist but also a small business owner. As such, you will be responsible for managing all aspects of your practice, which requires important time, study, and effort. One key to your success as a business manager is to continually think about the future and not rely on good things to just happen. What do you want to do? When do you want to do it? How will you accomplish it? How will you measure your success? Achieving success, then, is rooted in creating and implementing a well-researched and thought out plan, or as some would simply say *plan your work and work your plan*.

After studying this chapter, you will understand:

1. The importance of management and the management process,
2. The impact of thorough planning on a successful practice,
3. The essential features of a business plan,
4. Critical elements of the business plan from a banker's point of view.

The Management Process as a Foundation for Planning

Management is the effective and efficient planning, organizing, leading, and controlling of limited resources, in the face of a changing environment, to achieve organizational goals.

This definition reflects four important concepts: (1) the effective and efficient accomplishment of goals; (2) the limitation of resources; (3) the constantly changing

Dental Practice Transition: A Practical Guide to Management, Second Edition.
Edited by David G. Dunning and Brian M. Lange.
© 2016 John Wiley & Sons, Inc. Published 2016 by John Wiley & Sons, Inc.
Companion Website: www.wiley.com/go/dunning/transition

environment, both internal and external to the organization itself; and (4) the four basic management functions of planning, organizing, leading, and controlling.

Being *effective* means getting the job done—achieving your stated goal. Being *efficient* means using the fewest resources to accomplish that goal. For example, explaining a new procedure to each dental assistant one-on-one would be highly effective because you could ensure that each one fully understands it. However, it would not be very efficient because of the total amount of time you would spend. In contrast, you could be very efficient and explain the new procedure in a group setting, but that might not be as effective as one-on-one because some people may be reluctant to ask for clarification. Your job as a manager is to balance the two without having a negative impact on your operations. The second concept, *limited resources*, recognizes that there is a finite amount of all resources. There are, for example, only 24 hours in a day, a finite number of dental chairs in your office, and only one of you. A *constantly changing environment* is a reality of life, both outside and inside your practice. The question is not whether things will change, but at what rate they will change. Externally, new dental procedures and technologies are discovered virtually every day. The economy can impact decisions to purchase new technologies or to move to a new location. Internally, hiring new employees brings new skills and new personalities to your staff. Your decision to implement a new administrative (office) procedure can be seen as positive or negative by different employees. Figure 4.1 illustrates how the *four basic management functions* of planning, organizing, leading, and controlling interact as a process.

Clearly, the management process must begin with planning. Without a goal, it is impossible to determine how to organize your practice, how to lead your team, or how to control your efforts. After establishing your goals and creating a plan to achieve them, you must organize your practice and hire the right people to build the team to support you in achieving these goals. You and your management team must then lead your staff by creating a positive, shared culture with a unified vision and mission. Helping team members maximize their potential will support achievement of both individual and practice goals. Finally, you must monitor employees' progress to ensure the effective and efficient accomplishment of understood goals, taking corrective action

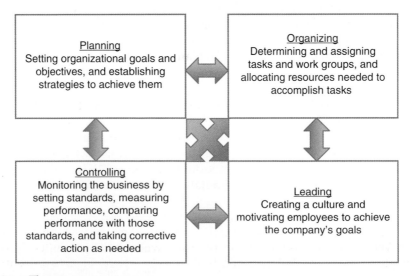

Figure 4.1.   The management process.

as necessary. In other words, the goals you established in the planning process become the standards against which you measure employee performance in the control, or evaluation, process. If all is going well, your job is to support team development and encourage continued good performance. However, if goals are not being met, you must take corrective action. You must evaluate both the goal in question and the employees' performance. Your evaluation might determine that the goal is still valid and employee behavior must be corrected. However, you may determine that the stated goal is no longer valid due to a changing environment. For example, after you wrote your goals, you purchased new technology, or you hired new employees with different individual needs, or your patient load increased or decreased. As a result, you need to raise or lower the bar—that is, change the goal. So, even though everything begins with planning, all four management functions are interrelated and are ongoing, and any one can have an impact on any other one.

Why Is Planning Important?

Overall, the primary purpose of planning is to offset future uncertainty by reducing the risk of an event catching you completely off guard. As important as your fully formed, completed business plan is, the process of researching and thinking about your business in a through, organized way is the larger benefit. A strong business plan

- attracts potential lenders,
- aids in attracting patients and strong employees,
- helps the enterprise succeed (but no guarantees),
- provides direction,
- helps the practice prioritize efforts and manage change,
- informs the performance of management functions, and
- helps to evaluate practice progress (the planning function becomes an integral part of the evaluation or control function by acting as the standard against which performance is measured).

Why Don't All Business Managers Create and Utilize a Plan?

Good planning is hard work.

Planning is long term, and we tend to be short-term oriented.

Planning is only one activity of many, and we are often too busy "putting out fires." Note the irony—perhaps better planning would prevent those fires from ever occurring.

A business plan may involve concepts of which we have minimal knowledge and understanding. It's often easier, though not necessarily wise, to play to our strengths— we know how to do the dentistry.

What Is a Business Plan?

A business plan is a written document that describes and analyzes a proposed or current business and includes a marketing plan, a management plan, and a financial plan. While there is no guarantee of success, a well-written plan offers business owners a greater probability of success simply because it requires them to think about virtually every aspect of their business in a systematic way. A business plan is a roadmap for your dental practice. On the other hand, having a business plan, even one that is highly detailed, does not guarantee success. Implementation matters—your plan must be a living, guiding document. As that anonymous someone once said, "Poor management can cause even a McDonald's to fail."

Why Write One?

The main purpose for writing a business plan should be to allow the entrepreneur the opportunity to gain an in-depth look at the potential for the business to succeed (or fail) and what it will take to achieve that success. In other words, your primary audience should be yourself. However, many entrepreneurs write their business plan solely to obtain financing. Well-written business plans can help you answer many questions, including the following:

- What specific products and services will you offer?
- Is the target market in your geographic marketplace large enough for the practice to be profitable, given the competition?
- What kind of marketing will be necessary to create and maintain an adequate patient base?
- What will your facility and technology needs, and resulting investment, be?
- How many support personnel will you need, when will you need them, and at what cost? What will be their job descriptions?
- Are the professional and support staff available in the current labor pool qualified at the service level you desire/require? If not, what resources will you utilize to train and develop team members?
- What revenue is required for you to break even in an average month? What is the practice's projected ability to generate that revenue.

In other words, given your proposed location and the services you plan to offer, a business plan can help you determine whether or not your practice has the potential to be successful. By putting together a thorough plan, you may discover that adjustment or changes may be warranted; for example, choosing a different location, offering different hours of operation, or partnering with another dentist or dentists (a second or third dentist in the same location only marginally increases the overhead costs).

How Long Should the Plan Be?

The short answer is, as long as it needs to be. The main body of most plans should be no more than 25–30 pages. Generally speaking, the higher the amount of financing you require, the more detailed the plan should be in order to justify the desired financing and to substantiate your ability to repay the lender/investor.

This is not a document you can expect to write over a free weekend. Nor should you expect the first draft to be the final draft. As with any important paper, you should do your research (using your business plan outline as a guideline) and then put together the first draft. Put it down for a day or two, and then read it as if you were the investor, making notes of possible changes. Then, rewrite it and put it down for a day or two before re-reading it. Go through this process until you are satisfied it is complete—that it tells the whole story. Then, go back and make sure it is grammatically correct, especially your cover letter. Remember, people often write like they speak, but the rules for speaking are different than for writing. You do not want to lose a potential investor because of errors in your plan. That shows a lack of attention to detail that will not bode well for you as a manager (and a seeker of funding). Additionally, you may wish to have a trusted colleague review your draft as well. Things that make perfect sense to the writer may be less obvious to the reader. Peer review can be a great way to uncover a need for clarification.

Another important point is to make sure that the end results—the numbers in your financial projections—are a result of your research, and not the other way around—that is, the "research" was developed to support the numbers that reflect a positive outcome. Making the numbers show a great cash flow and a large profit will often lead to difficulties later on. You might even convince the banker that your plan is accurate, but you, the practice owner, suffer the greatest risk and stand to lose the most, with inaccurate projections.

Business Plan Format

While every business plan is unique, and should be designed and written for a specific purpose, certain elements are universal. Figure 4.2 provides one such framework and is the basis for this discussion.

I. COVER PAGE
    A. Business name, address, telephone, and e-mail
    B. Names of principals
    C. Date
II. TABLE OF CONTENTS
III. EXECUTIVE SUMMARY (not to exceed 2 pages)
    A. Brief overview of the practice—owners, history, future projections
    B. Market opportunity
    C. Financial projections
    D. Loan request amount—including how you will utilize financing to support practice profitability and assure loan repayment
IV. PRACTICE DESCRIPTION
    A. Mission statement
    B. Goals/objectives/business philosophy
       1. What are your top short-term and medium-term goals or objectives?
       2. How does each goal support your mission?
    C. Describe briefly the business of dentistry—trends, challenges, how you will position the practice to respond to these.
    D. Describe your own professional experience, your management team, and professional advisors.
    E. Legal structure of the practice: sole proprietor, partnership, corporation.
V. MARKET RESEARCH: DEMOGRAPHICS/ECONOMIC PROFILE
    A. Product description
       1. What services will you offer? How will these differentiate you from your competition?
       2. What factors will provide you competitive advantage or disadvantage— for example: specific services, insurance networks, technology, languages spoken.

Figure 4.2. Business plan format.

      B. Industry analysis
- 1. What is the current status of the dental industry?
- 2. What opportunities and threats do you face; for example, are there any new products, markets, trends, and so forth that might affect the business either positively or negatively, particularly in the proposed geographic area where you plan to practice?
- 3. How could the following affect your practice: change in economy, local industry, government regulations, and technology.

      C. Market definition (target market)
- 1. Discuss primary market(s) and, if applicable, secondary market(s).
- 2. Develop market demographic, for example, age, education level, income, major industry/employers.
- 3. How many potential patients are there?
- 4. Given your competition and the average percentage of the population that seeks your type of services, what makes this market viable (potential sales)?

      D. Competitive analysis
- 1. Who are your top competitors (due to specialty and/or proximity)?
- 2. What is the dentist-to-population ratio?
- 3. What are their strengths and weaknesses?
- 4. How do *your* strengths and weaknesses compare to those of your competitors?

VI.   MARKETING CONSIDERATIONS/PLAN

      A. Place
- 1. Where is your proposed location—how will it affect your customers/patients?
- 2. Amount of space, type of building, zoning, and so on.
- 3. What are its advantages and disadvantages?
- 4. Will you lease, purchase, remodel, or build? What are the up-front and monthly costs?
- 5. Ongoing maintenance, utilities, and insurance costs?
- 6. Equipment serviceability/upgrade/replacement needs?
- 7. New technology necessary/desired?

      B. Price/fees
- 1. Compensation model(s): insurance types, fee for service.
- 2. What is your pricing policy/strategy; will fees be equal to, over, or below market average?
- 3. What are your product costs?
- 4. What will be your prices?
- 5. What are your competitors' prices?
- 6. What will be your credit/financial policies?

      C. Promotion
- 1. What are your advertising plans; for example, media, frequency, grand opening?
- 2. Develop your advertising budget for the first year.
- 3. Prepare a 3-month schedule of your promotional activities. Also discuss what will be done internally.

VII.   MANAGEMENT PLAN

      A. What business office and professional personnel will you need, for example, office manager, billing/insurance specialist?
- 1. For what function(s) will each team member be responsible/accountable for?
- 2. What background/qualifications/licensure will you seek in your team?

Figure 4.2. *Continued*

    B. Organization structure
1. Prepare an organizational chart indicating who will perform what functions.
2. Understand that the same person may perform more than one function.
3. Identify your professional advisory team, for example, accountant, the business's CEO (this may be the owner dentists), attorney if known, by name.

    C. Personnel management
1. Discuss factors such as recruiting, wage and salary structure, benefits, job descriptions, and evaluation against job description.
2. What is the current local market rate for your team members?
3. Indicate how many employees will be needed (include a typical work schedule).
4. Explain training/development methods, requirements, and associated costs.
5. What are your plans for employee performance evaluation?

    D. Systems and polices
1. Internal: for example, employee standards (that is, conduct and dress), financial controls, financial arrangement/collection policies, filing insurance claims, scheduling, managing accounts payable, and so on.
2. External: for example, credit and collections, check cashing.
3. On what resources will you draw to create an Employment Policy Manual?

    E. Legal
1. What will be the legal structure of your business?
2. What are the start-up and ongoing legal costs?
3. What other legal requirements might apply; for example, contracts, licenses, permits, lease/rent agreements, and workplace regulations?
4. If not a sole ownership practice, discuss provisions for such things as profit/loss distribution, adding or buying out partners, and business termination.

VIII.   FINANCIAL PLAN
    A. Turn-key costs
    B. Personal financial statement
    C. Pro forma cash flow (first year, by month)
    D. Pro forma income statements (3 years)
    E. Pro forma balance sheets (3 years)
    F. Break-even analysis for an average month
    G. Proposed financing
1. Summarize the total amount needed, including working capital until the practice breaks even and begins to generates owner income.
2. Indicate the proposed source(s) and use(s) of funds.
3. Indicate the security/collateral offered.

IX.   APPENDICES
    A. Résumés of key personnel
    B. Letters of recommendation or endorsement
    C. Market research
    D. Historical financial data
    E. Other items

Figure 4.2. *Continued*

Again, your business plan should be written to meet your needs. There is no "perfect" business plan format. The outline discussed here and the sample business plan appearing later in this chapter demonstrate this fact. To reiterate, the strength of the business plan is the process of researching, analyzing, and planning your proposed business in a systematic way—looking at past, present, and future. A strong plan will provide a living, guiding document to be referred to frequently as you build your practice.

Elements of the Plan

Cover Page

The cover page identifies the name, address, and phone number of the business and the owner(s), as well as the date the plan was submitted. If you are requesting funds from more than one source, also include a copy number.

Table of Contents

The table of contents provides a concise overview of the plan's contents and should list, as a minimum, each primary and secondary heading with its starting page number. For example, a major heading would be "Mission," and a secondary heading would be "Mission Statement."

Executive Summary

This introduction to your proposal must capture the attention of the reader with a convincing message to read the entire plan. It is a brief synopsis (not more than 2 pages) addressing the essence of your proposed business. Hence, even though it is the first thing read, it is the last thing written. While a lender might talk about having read, say, five hundred business plans, what the lender really read were five hundred executive summaries. Only a small percentage of those executive summaries successfully led to the full plan being read, so these introductory comments are critical and foundational.

Imagine that just you and a potential investor are in an elevator, and you have that person's undivided attention for maybe 1 minute. What would you say to convince this person that your proposal would be a great investment opportunity? The executive summary is simply a written version of an "elevator pitch" and should briefly describe the following:

- *The company and its founders:* Describe your service, what is special about it, and what the qualifications of the owner(s) are.
- *The market opportunity:* Describe the size and growth rate of your market and how it is currently being served.
- *The key financial highlights:* Summarize your sales and profit projections for at least the first year. Clearly state the total capital needed from all sources (including personal resources), what use will be made of each source's capital, and an anticipated repayment schedule. While you may not know the exact terms of the loan (such as the interest rate and length of the loan), you should make a reasonable estimate. For example, suggesting that a loan of $500,000 can be obtained at a 2% interest rate to be repaid over 4 years would not be reasonable. Finally, include when your business practice will financially break even.

Mission

Mission Statement

A company's mission statement answers the question, why do I exist? It is a short statement (twenty-five words or less) that tells employees, clients, and investors what you do and what you believe in. In other words, it gives direction to your practice, it sets strategic priority. Like your elevator pitch, your mission statement must summarize the very essence of your business clearly and succinctly. Consider a format that includes verb/target/outcome. Twitter's mission statement offers an example of this: *To give everyone the power to create and share ideas and information instantly, without barriers.* If you can't express your mission in less than twenty-five words, you probably don't yet have a handle on who you are and what you're all about.

Goals and Objectives

While the mission statement provides the broad overview of your business, goals and objectives are actually what help you achieve your mission. *Goals* are broad, long-range statements of what the practice would like to achieve. An example might be "to be the premier general dentist in Anywhere, USA." An *objective* is a very specific statement that is relatively short-term oriented and follows the basic formula "to do something, by a certain time, by some amount." For example, "to increase my patient base by 300 within 6 months" or "to reduce uncollectible accounts receivable by 2% by the end of the fiscal year." These goals and objectives give you and your practice a sense of direction and should, obviously, relate to your basic mission statement.

Marketing Plan

Having sound market research data and a well-designed marketing plan is crucial to your success, in terms of both acquiring needed funding and having a viable practice. Indeed, it is your market research and marketing plan that forms the basis of your financial forecasts. So, knowing your target market, defining your product, having an appropriate pricing strategy, selecting the right location, and developing a suitable promotion strategy are some of the most critical—and challenging—aspects of building your plan.

The Four "Ps" of Marketing—Product, Place, Price, and Promotion

These four factors are commonly known as the "4 Ps" of marketing (product, place, price, and promotion), and, together with your target market, create an image for your practice. All five factors must blend together; otherwise, your marketing message will not be consistent. If you change any one of them, you change the image people have of your practice, intentionally or unintentionally. For example, if an active periodontal recare system will be an important service and production cornerstone in your practice, then building an office in a community with high resident turnover, such as a military or college community, would not likely serve your best interests. Your location would be incompatible with the product you wish to provide.

Another important marketing concept is how you see, or relate to, the marketplace. Do you have a production orientation or a marketing orientation? A *production orientation* suggests that you already have a product, so you must now find the target market(s). A *marketing orientation* suggests that you determine your target market(s) first, and then you determine what product(s) the people in your target market need or want. In other words, the production concept says that you already have a product that, of course, you believe is the greatest thing since sliced bread, but you must now find a market that thinks the same way you do—not always the easiest thing to do. The marketing concept says that you have selected a market you wish to serve, and now you must find a product they need or want. Conventional wisdom says that having a product and trying to figure out how to convince potential customers they should buy it (the production orientation) is much more difficult than determining what someone wants or needs and then making it available to them (the marketing orientation). Knowing your orientation suggests which is most important to you: your product or your patient.

As you begin the process of starting your professional career, you have likely already determined what area of dentistry you will practice. Does that mean you automatically are relegated to a production orientation? Absolutely not! As your client base develops, based on what services you do or do not choose to provide, you will gain a more in-depth understanding of your patients' needs and desires, as well as an understanding of your own developing professional interests and potential continuing education demands. As these needs converge, you will be able to fulfill more and more of your patients' needs.

Product Description

A product is defined as goods, services or, most often, a combination of the two. A good is tangible; a service is not. For example, a routine semiannual exam would be a service; the toothbrush you give to a patient would be a good; the preparation for and the seating of a crown would be a combination of the two (preparing the tooth and seating the crown are services, but the crown itself is a good). Other "product offerings" might include convenient hours, options for financing dental care, or the latest technology. Knowing exactly what your total product offerings are (and being able to describe them in terms the average layperson can understand) will govern many decisions. For example, what skills will you seek in hiring new staff members (or in retaining current ones)? What promotional activities will your target market most likely respond to? How will you price your products? (Virtually every aspect of your product offerings has an associated cost, and you must ensure your pricing covers all of those costs.)

It is also important to clearly understand and describe how your product differs from that of your competition. That is, what is your *distinctive competency* or advantage—what sets you apart from your competitors—and how will that give you a competitive advantage? As a general dentist practicing in an urban business district, you might establish office hours so that your patients will miss very little work, for example, very early morning or evening hours.

Industry Analysis

Demonstrating an understanding of your industry tells the investor that you have an eye on the future. Briefly describe the current status of the dental industry. What opportunities and threats do you face (such as new products, markets, and trends) that might affect the business either positively or negatively, particularly in the geographic area where you plan to practice? How do you plan to take advantage of those opportunities and overcome the threats?

Market Definition

The term "market" has both a geographic and a people component, which, combined, constitute your target market. The geographic component refers to the physical area you plan to serve, for example, the entire city or county, or the area of the city bounded by certain streets. The people component is the demographic description of your potential patients (such as age, income, specific types of dental treatment required). The major question you must ask (and answer) is, how many potential patients (the people component) live/work in my geographic area (geographic component)? That is, about what percentage of the population requires or seeks the services you plan to offer? On average, how often might an individual patient seek those services? Given your competition (see the next section), what percentage of the total potential patient load can you expect to seek those services from you as opposed to one of your competitors? Given your proposed pricing schedule, what, then, are your potential sales? Is that enough to cover your total business costs and still leave enough for your personal needs?

Competition

Understanding your competitors is especially important if you are starting from scratch. And even if you are buying out or buying into an existing practice, you should consider how many practitioners there are in your area and what demographic changes, if any, there may be since the practice first started. Are there still enough patients to support the current practices plus yours? What is the current dentist-to-population ratio? Might current patients of the practice you are purchasing value a practitioner's years of experience versus "the new kid on the block"? Who, then, are your top competitors due to specialty and/or proximity? What are their strengths and weaknesses? How do *your* strengths and weaknesses compare to your competitors'? In promoting your practice, you want to emphasize your strengths and distinctive competencies that are different from your competitors' strengths. For example, because you just graduated from dental school, you might emphasize your knowledge of the latest techniques. Your competitors have much more experience than you do, so your emphasis should be on other competencies.

Place

While place generally refers to your location, it actually encompasses more than that. A better word might be *distribution*, but "4 Ps" sounds better than "3 Ps and a D." Certainly, your physical location, to include the physical structure, is a vital component of your business. However, the consideration is how you deliver your total product, both services and goods, to your customer. So, unless you have your own lab and fabricate your own crowns, for example, you must also include other businesses in your business plan. You may be able to choose from among several suppliers for various items. Which one(s) will you use and why? How will cost, financing arrangements, convenience, and quality play into your decision? While your banker may not necessarily want to know these details, you do. Choosing a supplier whose quality is less than you desire or whose turnaround time is slow can have a definite impact on your bottom line through the loss of patients. Remember, your patient does not really care that someone else made the poor-fitting crown or could not deliver it in the time promised.

Regarding the physical location, where exactly is it? What are its advantages and disadvantages, including, for example, age of the structure, available parking, room for expansion, proximity to clients? Are you going to rent or buy an existing structure, or will you build? What are the upfront and monthly costs?

Price

Your pricing structure, when multiplied by the number of the various procedures you and your team can perform, will ultimately determine your total sales. The following are the basic questions you must answer about fees:

- What is your pricing policy/strategy—are your fees equal to, over, or below market average?
- What are your product costs?
- What are your fees?
- What are your competitors' fees?

Chapter 12 is devoted to dental fees and patient financial policies, while Chapter 13 explores dental benefits/third-party insurance.

Promotion

When nonmarketing people see or hear the term "promotion," they usually think of advertising. However, promotion is more than that. It also includes personal selling, specialty advertising, and publicity. We do not normally think about dentists and physicians engaging in *personal selling*, but that is what you do when you present options for elective procedures such as teeth whitening. How you and your staff interact with patients is also part of personal selling, in that you are constantly "promoting" superior service, which translates into satisfied customers who will remain loyal patients. The giveaway items with your name and logo on them such as pens and toothbrushes are called *specialty advertising*. *Publicity*, sometimes thought of as "free advertising," is when your business (or you) is the subject of, or mentioned in a story in the mass media such as a newspaper article. Social media fits into this category and it is important to be aware of and manage it. These references may be positive or negative. For example, a reporter may choose to write a story about the opening of your new practice or include the fact that your office had 100% participation in a blood drive. On the other hand, the fact that you, or a member of your staff, were involved in a single-car accident and alcohol was cited as a contributing factor would be seen negatively. Including a reference to you was the media or commenter's choice, not yours. And since you do not pay for this publicity, you have no control over it.

Conversely, *advertising* is a site or space that you purchase, which means you control, to some degree, what is said and where it is placed; for example, your web page or print advertising.

In this section of your business plan, you should include (1) your initial advertising plans (e.g., media, frequency, grand opening), (2) a 3-month schedule of all your promotional activities, and (3) your advertising budget for the first year. You will discuss any internal promotion in this section. Chapters 17 and 18 respectively explore in detail external and internal marketing concepts and strategies.

Management Plan

Unlike the marketing plan, which has an external focus—your customers—the management plan has an internal focus—the structure of the business itself.

Key Management Personnel

What supervisory positions are necessary to ensure the efficient and effective operation of your practice, and, if known, who will fill those positions? Examples include an office manager or a billing/insurance specialist, positions that are not normally filled by an owner of the practice. Specifically, what will be the responsibilities of each of these positions? If there are multiple business owners, what function(s) will each owner control? What background/qualifications will you seek for each manager position? Chapter 23 includes some sample job descriptions.

Some forms of ownership require a board of directors—namely, corporations. Identify the members of your board by name if possible or, as a minimum, by qualification (for example, accountant and the business's CEO). If such a board is not required, you may wish to consider having a "board of advisors" whose function is basically the same as a board of directors.

Organization Structure

Preparing an organizational chart indicating who will perform what functions helps everyone to see how all of the various components of your practice interact. That is, it presents a clear picture of who does what and who reports to whom. Because some workers may have multiple responsibilities, especially in a small practice, one name will be in more than one "box."

Personnel Management

Arguably your most important asset, and one of your largest expenses, is your staff. If you are starting a new practice, you may need only two people, a dental assistant and a receptionist, for example. Those two names, along with yours, will fill all the boxes in your organizational chart. On the other hand, your practice may require several staff members. Indicate how many employees you need and in what positions. Also indicate if and when you plan to add additional staff. Include such factors as recruiting, wage and salary structure, benefits, and job descriptions. Chapters 22 and 23 provide insights about human resource compliance and staff management strategies.

Policies

Thinking about, and establishing, both internal and external policies at the outset can help you avoid making hurried decisions later on. Taking the time up front to consider *all* the pros and cons about situations that will likely occur on a regular basis will result in less stress for you and more consistent decisions later on. Examples of internal policies might include personnel issues (for example, coming to work late, use of alcohol, smoking, advances in pay) and financial controls (such as who collects payments, who makes deposits). External policies might include credit and collection policy (such as selling accounts over 90 days old to a collection agency). Recognizing what resources you may draw upon to create an Employment Policy Manual and employee performance evaluation protocols will be important. Chapters 16, 22, and 23 focus on preventing embezzlement, implementing sound human resource policies, and managing staff.

Insurance

What types of insurance will you require to protect your business assets, including yourself as the chief source of labor, and at what costs? While insurance is expensive, you may want to make sure you have enough of the right kinds. Chapter 25 provides a detailed discussion of personal and practice/business insurance needs.

Legal

What will be the legal structure of your business? What are the start-up and the ongoing costs? If it is not a sole ownership practice, discuss provisions for such things as profit/loss distribution, adding or buying out partners, and business termination. See Chapter 10 for an in-depth discussion of the various forms of business ownership.

In addition to the legal structure of your practice, what other legal issues are important and at what costs? For example, what are the terms of a lease/rent agreement? See Chapter 7 for more details about leases.

Financial Plan

The financial plan details your revenues and expenses. It shows how they translate into a profit (or loss) and how (and when) the money flows into and out of the business. It also shows the practice's assets and who "owns" them—you (owner's equity) or someone else (a liability). The financial plan is where the "rubber meets the road." In business terms, what's the "bottom line"? Virtually everything in your marketing and management plans must be quantified. What are your costs, when will you incur them, and when will you pay for them? For example, how many patients do you expect to see per month, and at what price (target market/fees)? What are your advertising costs (promotion plan)? What are your legal, insurance, and personnel costs (management plan)?

The three financial statements that you should understand (not necessarily be able to create them, but understand them) are the *cash flow statement* (which includes *turn-key costs* for a start-up practice), the *income statement* (sometimes called a profit and loss statement, an operating statement, or a statement of earnings), and the *balance sheet*. See Chapter 2 for an in-depth discussion of these financial statements.

Cash Flow and Turn-Key Projections

The cash flow statement is considered by many to be the most important financial statement for any business owner. It shows when money actually flows into the business and when money actually flows out of the business, not when the sale is made or the expense incurred, as is often the case with the income statement, which will be discussed subsequently. Say, for example, you provide a service on May 5 for which you charge $100, but you do not receive payment for it until June 10. Your profit and loss statement could show a $100 "sale" in May, but your cash flow statement will show the receipt of that $100 in June, when it actually flows into the business, not May. Similarly, if you order $100 of supplies in May, but pay for them in June, your profit and loss statement could show an expense of $100 in May, but your cash flow statement will show a $100 payment in June, when the money literally flows out of the business.

In other words, the cash flow statement is like your checkbook. It is a month-to-month accounting of your actual deposits and your actual withdrawals. A cash flow statement should not be confused with a "statement of cash flows" or a "sources and uses of funds" statement, which are often produced by accountants. While the latter two statements can be useful for an overview of the sources of the cash and how that cash was spent, they do not show how your cash "cycles" through your business on a month-to-month basis. Basically, if your practice cannot maintain a positive cash flow, all other financial monitoring information will be useless because you will not remain in business.

Your business plan should include monthly pro forma cash flow statements for the first 12–24 months. These pro forma statements forecast expected financial outcomes (see Figure 4.3f as an example).

Turn-key costs are all of the costs you incur before "turning your key in the door" to open it for business; for example, construction or renovation costs, legal fees, purchase of equipment and supplies, utility deposits, and the like. Some of those costs can be paid for after you open your doors, but some may require payment at the time of purchase. Ultimately, these costs will be reflected in the expense section of the income statement.

Income Statement

The income statement shows sales, expenses, and the resulting profit (or loss) for a specified period of time such as monthly, quarterly, or annually. Income statements can be on an accrual basis (when the sale or expense is incurred) or on a cash basis (when the money is received or expense is paid). As a minimum, your business plan should include monthly pro forma income statements for the first year and an annual summary for year 2.

Balance Sheet

The balance sheet shows the total assets of the business and who "owns" them—either you (owner's equity) or someone else (liability). Because all assets are owned by someone, total assets must equal total liability plus owner's equity. The balance sheet is a reflection of a single point in time; for example, the end of your fiscal year. Your business plan should include *pro forma* (projected) balance sheets for opening day and the end of years 1 and 2.

Break-Even Analysis

An important question to answer is, what level of sales, or production, must I have to cover total costs for an average month? Knowing your *break-even point* is particularly critical when there is a gap between the date of the sale and the receipt of payment. You should also be aware of when during an average month you expect to reach that point—that is, when do you anticipate actually receiving payments to cover your costs? For example, say your break-even point is projected to be the 20th of the month. It is now the 15th, and your receipts are only half that amount. Knowing the situation, you are in a better position to plan what you will do before you come face-to-face with the "end of the month crunch." Chapter 2 also discusses break-even analysis.

Also essential from your pro forma is an estimate of which month the practice will produce above and beyond overhead costs.

Proposed Capitalization

Finally, itemize your total proposed capitalization, or financing, from all sources, equity and debt. *Equity financing* is money that comes from the owner(s) and does not have to be repaid. It is called "risk capital" because the money could be lost if the business fails. *Debt financing*, on the other hand, is money that you borrow and must repay with interest. Indicate how the money from each funding source will be used, what security/collateral, if any, will be used, and your proposed terms of repayment. Financing your practice is covered in detail in Chapter 9.

Appendices

Include as appendices (or attachments) anything that adds useful detail to your proposal. Examples include, but are not limited to, résumés of key personnel, letters of recommendation or endorsement, market research, contracts, and historical financial data.

Your Business Plan from the Banker's Perspective

Bankable Traits

When considering granting a business loan, the loan industry frequently refers to the *Five Cs of Credit* as a framework for assessing credit worthiness and the financial viability of you and your business proposal. Are you and your business a good risk?

Character: This includes your reputation (and that of your partners) in the dental industry and the greater business community. Such things as your honesty, integrity, reliability, and borrowing history help the bank assess whether you can be trusted to act in good faith.

Capital: This is the amount of money, or equity, that the owner has invested in the business, relative to total business assets. The greater the owner's equity, the more vested they will be in the success of the business, the less likely they will be to default on the loan, and the better the credit risk will appear to the bank. The potential borrower's personal financial standing, assets, and credit quality will be analyzed.

Conditions: These reflect the environment in which your practice will be operating, including the overall economy, health of the dental industry, and the local marketplace. Strong industry growth and a positive economy support the practice's ability to thrive and repay the loan. The inclusion of thorough market research and a strong competitive analysis in your business plan will be important here.

Capacity (cash flow): This is the borrower's ability to generate sufficient cash flow to repay the loan interest and principle. A well-written business plan must demonstrate strong potential to meet business goals and service the requested debt.

Collateral: To secure a loan, the borrower pledges something he or she owns, which will be forfeited if the loan is defaulted. This may be commercial real estate, equipment, accounts receivables, the business itself, in addition to personal assets. If the business is unable to generate sufficient cash flow to repay the loan at some point in the future, the bank will liquidate the collateral and use the proceeds to pay off the loan.

Your Business Plan Through the Eyes of the Banker

Given the value of a well-conceived and crafted business plan to the success of your business, what are the most important things a banker will look for in your plan when considering whether granting you a loan would benefit their bank and it's depositors?

- A strong management team is desirable: Credibility and experience are helpful. Demonstrate that you know your business. Evidence of this might include not only description and backgrounds of you and your management team, but also sound information about your business model, products, services, and strategies.
- Explanation of why you believe you'll be successful and recognition of potential obstacles. Make a case for yourself and your proposed business.
- Strong market research: Is there interest and demand for your product? Document your claims. Clearly and realistically, explain your competitive advantage.
- Sound projections: Your balance sheet, profit and loss, and cash flow projections for the first 1–2 years are critical. Cash flow is the most important. Your figures should be realistic compared to industry norms. Do not underestimate costs or over-estimate profits.
- Amount of your loan request is well aligned with your business plan. Do not request more or less money than your business plan demonstrates you will need. Show how much you need and demonstrate how you plan to use funding.

Some loan officers may look only briefly over your plan, focusing primarily on the financial information you provide. Others will read it carefully, discuss it with you and, with good fortune, begin to build a mutually beneficial relationship.

Resources for Business Plans

There is a vast array of resources available to assist and guide you in putting together your business plan as well as to provide information and education about the various aspects of managing your own business, such as understanding financial statements. These resources range from one-on-one individual assistance from consultants to books and online self-help guides to attending classes and workshops. A small sampling of various resources follows below.

Business Consultants

Business consultants are people who offer advice to others about how to better run a business. Some consultants specialize in a particular industry, and some are generalists. Check the internet or local yellow pages in your phone book for "business consultants." Some state dental associations may also offer resources or referrals. You might talk to your business attorney or accountant. It is not unusual for them to assist in putting together business plans. Some may even have "how-to" booklets for business plans. There is also the Academy of Dental Management Consultants. This academy has experience-based requirements for member-consultants (www.admc.net).

Federal Government (SBA)

The Small Business Administration (SBA) is the federal government's agency specifically designed to assist small business people in finding financial assistance. More to the purpose of this chapter, however, is the management assistance they provide small business people through the Service Corps of Retired Executives (SCORE) and through a network of Small Business Development Centers (SBDCs).

SCORE

SCORE is an organized group of retired business executives with a wide variety of backgrounds who provide free consulting to any small business owner. Not all industries are represented in each local chapter, so be sure to ask for someone whose background is compatible with your needs. To find the SCORE chapter nearest you, check their website at www.score.org.

SBDC

The SBDC program is a cooperative effort of the private sector, the educational community, and federal, state, and local governments. Assisting with the development of feasibility studies (business plans for start-up businesses) is only one of the many services the program provides to anyone interested in starting a small business or improving or expanding an existing one. For more information on their services or to locate the office nearest to you, go to www.sba.gov and click on Local Assistance.

State and Local Agencies

Many states and local agencies offer a variety of assistance. Check out your city's chamber of commerce or economic development office for local information. Similarly, your state's economic development office will often have a myriad of resources and links to assist you.

Academic Institutions

Your local college or university may be a good source of assistance. First, some instructors or professors supplement their income by providing private consulting. Similarly, assisting in developing a feasibility study may be an excellent student project for a small business class or an internship. While the work is actually done by a student, it is supervised by the course instructor.

Books

There are literally hundreds of books on the market specifically designed to help put together your business plan. Some contain fill-in-the-blanks worksheets, some come with interactive CDs, and some simply give you the information. Check your local library or bookstore, or, for a more complete listing, check online with Amazon (www.amazon.com) or Barnes & Noble (www.barnesandnoble.com), keyword: business plans.

Key Points

- Developing knowledge about management and the management process is critical to the success and enjoyment of managing a business.

- The main purpose of a business plan should be the opportunity to gain an in-depth look at the potential for the business to succeed and what it will take to achieve success.
- The essential features of a business plan are fairly standard. A number of resources are available to help analyze your market and create accurate financial projections.
- Considering the elements of the business plan from a banker's point of view will help you shape yourself and your business for a win–win relationship.

One final key point: This chapter serves as a vital and complementary supplement especially to Chapter 7 (buying/buying into a practice), Chapter 8 (starting a practice from scratch), and Chapter 9 (financing a practice).

References and Additional Resources

AllBusiness Editors. 2015. *What do bankers look for in a business plan.* Available at http://www.allbusiness.com/what-do-bankers-look-for-in-a-business-plan-3508-1.html (accessed March 7, 2015).

American Dental Association. 2015. *Guidelines for developing business plans.* Available at www.ada.org (accessed July 15, 2015).

Armstrong, Gary, and Kotler, Philip. 2004. *Marketing: An Introduction*, 6th ed. Upper Saddle River, NJ: Pearson Education, Inc.

ATB Financial. 2012. *Your business plan, from a banker's perspective.* Available at http://www.atb.com/learn/articles/Lists/Posts/Post.aspx?ID=81 (accessed October 7, 2015).

Berry, Tim. 2005. *What bankers look for in a plan.* Available at http://www.entrepreneur.com/article/80170 (accessed March 7, 2015).

California Dental Association. Practice Support Center. Business Plan Template. Available at www.cda.org (accessed April 7, 2015).

Daft, Richard L. 2008. *Management*, 8th ed. Mason, OH: Thomson Higher Education.

Deloitte. 2013. *ABCs of a bankable business plan.* Available at http://www.kznfundingfair.co.za/wp-content/uploads/2014/08/Day_1_Topic_1_The_ABCs_of_a_bankable_business_plan.pdf (accessed July 15, 2015).

Hellweg, Eric. 2004. The eight-word mission statement. *Harvard Business Review.* Available at https://hbr.org/2010/10/the-eight-word-mission-stateme/?cm_sp=Article-_-Links-_-Comment (accessed May 7, 2015).

McKeever, Mike. 2007. *How to Write a Business Plan.* Berkley, CA: Nolo.

Scarborough, Norman M., and Zimmerer, Thomas W. 2006. *Effective Small Business Management*, 8th ed. Upper Saddle River, NJ: Pearson Education, Inc.

Strischek, Dev. 2009. The 5 Cs of credit. *RMA J* 91(8): 34–37.

Wells Fargo. 2015. Practice and Finance. Business Plan Template. Available at https://practicefinance.wellsfargo.com/dentists/practice-resources/ (accessed January 7, 2015).

Learning Exercises

1. Contact a dentist in your intended area of practice who recently began his or her practice (within the past 5 years) and who has the same type of business arrangement you plan to have; that is, they either started or bought a single-practitioner office, or started or bought into a multiple practitioner office. Did he or she prepare a business plan before starting the practice? Why or why not? How detailed was the plan? How long did it take to complete it? Who, if

anyone, assisted in the plan's preparation? Was creating the plan beneficial? Why or why not? If there was no plan, does he or she still agree with that decision? What advice does she or he have about writing a business plan?

2. Interview a local banker (or some other entity from which you might request a loan) and ask questions such as:

   A. How important is a well-prepared business plan?

   B. How important is being knowledgeable enough about the plan's content to discuss it with the banker, particularly the financial projections? How important is it to have a smooth presentation?

   C. What is a typical loan repayment schedule (about how many years to repay and approximately what interest rate) for the type and amount of loan you are seeking? (This is information you will need to know to prepare your financial projections.)

A Sample Business Plan (Figure 4.3)

This business plan was prepared by Dr. Lisa Itaya under the supervision of Dr. Nader Nadershahi as part of a course in practice management. The plan details the proposed establishment of a general practice in Foster City, San Mateo County, California. The plan demonstrates a slightly different organizational format than the one presented earlier in this chapter, illustrating that a business plan may be organized in various ways depending on the needs of the person developing the plan.

Confidential Business Plan
Lisa Itaya

Table of Contents

Executive Summary

Services

   Type and Characteristics of Services

Location Demographics and Economic Profile

   Region and City Location

   Population Demographics

   Regional and Local Economic Profile

   Industry Profile

Competitive Analysis

Marketing Plan

Lease and Setup Information

Personnel Management Plan

Figure 4.3. Sample business plan.

Executive Summary

Upon completion of graduation and State of California licensing requirements, Lisa Itaya intends to organize, establish, and operate a private practice in general dentistry as a limited liability or professional corporation. The practice will be located in Foster City, California, and serve a diverse base of patients throughout the metropolitan San Mateo County area.

This confidential business plan summarizes the nature of the practice to be established. Operations will commence after an initial funding of $75,000 is secured through a combination of private placements, bank loans, and/or access to Dr. Itaya's home equity line of credit. First year operations are summarized in Figure 4.3a.

Summary of First Year Operations Forecast	
Revenue	$194,600.00
Expenses	$232,624.00
Net Profit/(Loss)	($38,024.00)

Figure 4.3a. Summary of first year operations forecast.

The first year's net loss (before taxes) is largely attributed to the initial investment in equipment and supplies. Additionally, $20,400 is drawn from the annual operation for Dr. Itaya's initial salary. Although this plan only addresses the first year of operations, it is important to note that the operation is cash flow positive beginning the eighth month and thereafter.

Services

Type and Characteristics of Services

Dr. Itaya will establish a general practice dental office offering comprehensive care to patients of all ages. Based upon her experiences as a student at the University of the Pacific Arthur A. Dugoni School of Dentistry, she expects to offer services that will be of special appeal to patients with dental phobia, persons with disabilities, and the elderly.

Specialty services will include nitrous oxide sedation, cosmetic restorations, bleaching, emergency care, extractions, root canals, and dental implants.

In-office marketing programs (for example, a computer-generated silent commercial viewable in the reception/waiting area) will inform and educate patients about services that may be of potential interest to them.

Figure 4.3. *Continued*

Location, Demographics, and Economic Profile

Region and City Location

Incorporated in 1971, Foster City is a master-planned mostly white-collar community situated on the San Francisco peninsula midway between the metropolitan cities of San Francisco and San Jose. Foster City comprises a population of approximately 30,000 persons and is conveniently situated to serve potential patients from throughout San Mateo County (population 719,400).

San Mateo County's cities are low in crime, and Foster City has one of the lowest crime rates in the entire San Francisco Bay Area. The county schools rank among the highest in the state in academic achievement. The county has served as home to some of the richest residents in California and is home to many of the newest transplants to California. The county is one of the most desirable addresses in the state, owing much of its prestige to its history, its amenities, its topography, and its location. Foster City residences are mostly of newer construction, with the oldest structures only 40 years old.

There are over 2,000 businesses located in Foster City, the largest being in the bio-pharmaceutical and biotechnology sectors. The largest employer is Gilead Sciences with 7,000 employees worldwide and 3,400 in Foster City. VISA, Incorporated is headquartered in Foster City and employs approximately 7,500 people.

Population Demographics

About 91% of the county's approximately 700,000 residents reside in twenty cities; they are Atherton, Belmont, Brisbane, Burlingame, Coma, Daly City, East Palo Alto, Foster City, Half Moon Bay, Hillsborough, Menlo Park, Millbrae, Pacifica, Portola Valley, Redwood City, San Bruno, San Carlos, San Mateo, South San Francisco, and Woodside. Each of these communities is within 15 miles of Foster City. From 2010 to 2014, there was a 56% increase in the population of San Mateo County. This is significantly higher than the 1.2% increase during the prior decade from 2000 to 2010 and reflects robust growth in this region. San Mateo County is the epicenter of Silicon Valley, and benefits from the myriad types of business and services needed to service that population of highly educated and skilled workers.

According to the U.S. Census Bureau, Foster City residents enjoy an average household income of $114,300, while county-wide the average is a robust $88,200. As shown in Figure 4.3b, 59% of earned income is derived from so-called "white collar" professions (management, professional,

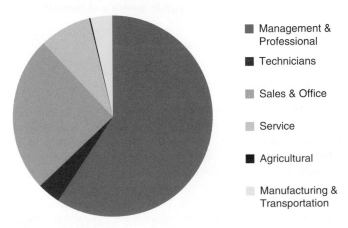

Figure 4.3b. How San Mateo County earns its money.

Figure 4.3. *Continued*

and sales). These groups are expected to be more likely than others to be motivated to attain and maintain good oral health.

Moreover, the county's high level of adult education gives further evidence of a pool of potential patients historically predisposed to seeking regular oral care (see Figure 4.3c).

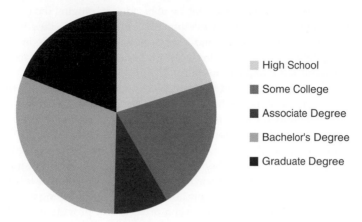

High School

Some College

Associate Degree

Bachelor's Degree

Graduate Degree

Figure 4.3c.   Education level of population age 18 and older.

Finally, the distribution of the county population indicates that general dental practices are necessary to accommodate the large number of working adults in the county. Population projections show retirees, both young and mature, as the largest growth segments (see Figure 4.3d). With more of the aging population retaining their teeth, general dentistry services will continue to be in demand.

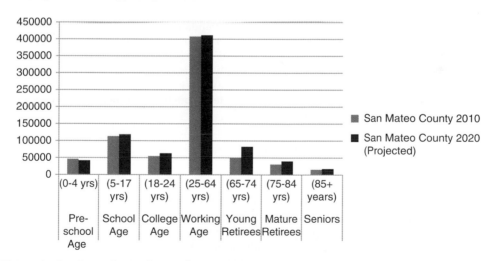

San Mateo County 2010

San Mateo County 2020 (Projected)

Figure 4.3d.   General population characteristics.

Regional and Local Economic Profile

The San Francisco Bay Area in general, and San Mateo County in particular, have been consistently robust economic regions. Although high-technology companies represent an extremely large and

Figure 4.3.   *Continued*

visible slice of the economic pie, the region is by no means dependent on any one industry. In addition to high technology, the area has strong influences from airlines, biotechnology, agriculture, media, petroleum, and telecommunications companies.

The California Department of Finance forecasts that by the year 2020, (1) the area's retiree population will increase from over 30% to over 140,000 people; (2) the county's total population will grow 7%; and (3) more than 1.4 million jobs will be added, bringing the regional total to 4.3 million. The Association of Bay Area Governments forecasts that cities with large senior populations will be required to provide more services with older people in mind, including health care. Clearly, there will be a growing need for geriatric dentistry, as the so-called baby boomers become a large aging population group.

Foster City's largest employer, Gilead Sciences, plans to increase its campus from 1.2 million square feet to 2.5 million square feet in the next 5 years. The plan includes new spaces for offices, laboratories, and warehouses (to include a new pilot plant). Along with the expansion is the corresponding intent to grow its workforce.

The City of Foster City currently has eleven major projects initiated by private land developers either in construction or under consideration to repurpose land to mix-use housing and retail. The redevelopment plans call for the construction of 1.8 million square feet of new commercial space for retail, dining, and offices and over 1700 new housing units. New housing will include units for low-income residents. The multitude of expansion projects will provide new opportunities for dental services in the area.

Industry Profile

According to the American Dental Association and the U.S. Department of Health and Human Services, the following points characterize the dental industry:

- Dentistry ranked 1 among the 100 Best Jobs and ranked 2 among the Best Paying Jobs by U.S. News in 2015.
- Dentists ranked fifth for their honest and ethical standards.
- Dental offices are the third highest ranking category of start-up businesses and most likely to survive.The average 2009 net income of general dental practitioners was about $175,400. Dentists rank in the 92nd percentile of U.S. family income.
- The success of preventive dentistry in reducing the incidence of oral disease has contributed to a growing older population that will retain their teeth longer and be even more aware of the importance of regular dental care.

Competitive Analysis

Although it has been suggested that the San Francisco Bay Area is saturated with dental practitioners, Dr. Itaya is optimistic that an active and profitable general practice can be established in Foster City. There are 523 general and pediatric practitioners in San Mateo County allowing for a 1:1375 dentist-to-patient ratio. In Foster City, there are 25 general dentists and 3 pediatric dentists. While the resident population supports a 1:1091 dentist-to-patient ratio, the large employers draw in thousands of additional professionals to the city each day (see Figure 4.3e). The daytime swell of business, research, and high-tech employees presents ample opportunities for new business by those who have more dental insurance and discretionary income than an average resident population of California or even San Mateo County.

Figure 4.3. *Continued*

	San Mateo County	Foster City
General Dentists	492	25
Pediatric Dentists	31	3
Total Dentists	523	28
Population	719,440	30,570
Penetration	1:1357	1:1091

Figure 4.3e. Dentist-to-patient ratio.

Marketing Plan

Within the context of a professional dental practice, marketing refers to activities that ethically promote the services to potential new patients and encourage additional and recall services with existing patients. For planning purposes, the plan identifies two broad classes of marketing programs.

Internal marketing programs refer to practices and procedures implemented within the office to promote additional services and satisfaction with existing patients:

- Recurrent training to encourage office personnel to solicit referrals from patients as well as the employee's own family, friends, and associates
- Availability of in-office printed material (brochure) describing the range of services, after-hours emergency care, and Saturday hours
- Referral bonuses to patients who refer new clients
- A posted mission statement that articulates the values of the practice (a promise of quality, excellence, and efficiency; a commitment to a healthy environment by exceeding OSHA regulations with respect to infection control and waste management; a pledge to excellent oral health through clear communications, education, and community involvement)
- Morning staff "huddles," including informal ongoing technical and administrative education (see Chapter 24 for information about morning "huddles")

External marketing programs include activities selected to increase community awareness of the dental practice and to acquire new patients:

- Become a member and referral of the San Mateo Dental Society and the Foster City Chamber of Commerce Better Business Bureau
- Create an office website and a Facebook page featuring educational topics and highlighting office staff
- Participate in 800-DENTIST
- Offer a patient referral bonus
- Sponsor the Foster City American Youth Soccer Organization which brings hundreds of youth and adults to Foster City each Fall
- Contact businesses with twenty or more employees and set up a lunchtime oral health wellness presentation with giveaways
- Join the Rotary Club of Foster City, as they participate and sponsor many of the local activities that draw large crowds in the city

Lease and Setup Information

The practice will operate at 1289 East Hillsdale Boulevard. This mature two-story medical/dental building is convenient to the city hall, a major shopping location, and the vibrant Metro Center, a

Figure 4.3. *Continued*

multiple high-rise building development housing many large and small companies. The office is a short drive from any location in the city, including residences and the headquarters of VISA, Incorporated and Gilead Sciences. The building has more than ample free parking and is directly accessible to patients in the county from nearby Highways 101 and 92.

Dr. Itaya is extremely fortunate in that the contemplated office suite has 1351 square feet of fully furnished useable space, including two operatories that are fully outfitted, a consult room, business office, and a restroom. As detailed in the financial exhibits, the facility is available on a 3-year lease basis at $3,310 per month, including water, sewer, electricity, and garbage utility services.

The office includes personal computer systems for the front desk receptionist, the business office, and in each operatory. Digital radiography equipment, electric handpieces, and sterilization equipment are available and all in good working condition. As revenue increases, 3D imaging machines for crown and bridge and implants will be added to improve efficiency and patient comfort.

Accounting Systems

Commercial software packages will be evaluated to select an accrual basis accounting system that could be integrated with the dental-specific functions of appointments, insurance claims processing, and patient records.

Income statements and profit and loss statements will be compared against the annual budget at the close of each month of operation. The reports will be analyzed by Dr. Itaya and the business consultant to manage the ongoing operation. Monthly income and cash flow projections for the first year of operations are included as Figure 4.3f in this plan.

Patient Systems

An electronic health record system will be selected to permit the complete electronic recording and retrieval of patient records. As noted above, the electronic health record system should be able to be integrated with accounting software that manages accounts payable, receivable, patient billing, and profit and loss.

The receptionist will have the responsibility to ensure that a patient's next appointment is secured before the patient completes his or her current office visit. The receptionist will also be responsible for reconfirming upcoming appointments.

Patient recalls will be semiautomatic through the above-described procedure and/or a reminder postcard with follow-up. The automated patient record and tracking system can easily alert the receptionist to patients who have unscheduled recalls coming due.

Personnel Management Plan

According to the Bureau of Labor Statistics, in the San Francisco Bay Area, dental office receptionists and dental assistants earn $20.00/hour and dental hygienists earn approximately $50.00/hour or $104,000/year. This plan seeks to balance what is needed to support the doctor and serve the patients against conservatism in committing to ongoing fixed costs in advance of a sustainable revenue run-rate. The practice will hire two essential regular employees at the onset of operations. There is high confidence that the following positions can be readily filled from the local employment pool without the use of expensive recruiting services.

- One front office receptionist at $20.00 per hour. This person will greet arriving patients, answer the telephone, make and reconfirm appointments, collect and log payments, and manage the daily operating schedules.

Figure 4.3. *Continued*

- One dental assistant at $20.00 per hour. This individual will greet and seat the patient, take x-rays, take and pour impressions, ensure sterilization of instruments, set up the operatory for planned procedures, and generally assist the doctor with four-handed dentistry. This employee must have state certification to make x-ray images.

The practice will add two additional employees when the indicated sustainable levels of production are achieved.

- One registered dental hygienist at $50.00 per hour. When office production reaches $50,000 per month, this licensed professional will join the team initially for 2 days a week to review patient medical history changes, take updated radiographs, perform prophylaxis and root planings, and carry out cursory hard tissue examinations. Prior to this hiring, Dr. Itaya will personally perform these procedures.
- One financial administrator. It is not yet determined when this individual will be required. It is planned that Dr. Itaya's husband, who has over 30 years of experience in new business development, will advise the practice on marketing ("promotion") activities and will personally maintain the accounting books. These services will be provided without charge until the practice can sustain a part-time bookkeeper.

In general, hired positions will be subject to the following terms, which are typical of the industry and region:

- Positions are full time and employment is "at will."
- An office policy manual will detail job descriptions, benefits, leave and sick policy, social media policy, and professionalism. Each employee will be given the office policy manual and will sign to indicate that they have read and understood its contents.
- Wages will be as noted above and paid semimonthly.
- Each employee shall earn 1 week of paid vacation after 1 year of service. Two weeks of paid vacation will accrue for 2–5 years of service, and 3 weeks thereafter.
- Employees will receive paid holidays for New Year's Day, Presidents' Day, Memorial Day, Independence Day, Thanksgiving Day (2), and Christmas Day. This policy is expected to be expanded as the practice grows.The practice will initially grant up to 5 sick days per year to each regular employee.
- The practice will seek to obtain group rates for medical and health insurance. Initially, these premiums will be fully paid by the participating employee.

Management and Organizational Plan

Dr. Itaya will make all executive decisions regarding the direction and operations of the office. Until revenues support the addition of an office manager and bookkeeper, Dr. Itaya will use the pro bono business consulting services of her husband. He will ensure that accounts payable and receivable are tracked correctly and in a timely fashion.

In order to attract patients who work in Foster City as well as the residents of Foster City, the office will be open from Tuesday through Saturday from 9 a.m. to 5 p.m. If it appears that the general patient base prefers different hours of operations, changes will be made. Marketing efforts will emphasize availability for people with dental emergencies to generate new business.

Pro Forma Income Statement/Cash Flow

Figure 4.3. *Continued*

Figure 4.3. *Continued*

23-Apr-16	Month 1 projected	Month 2 projected	Month 3 projected	Month 4 projected	Month 5 projected	Month 6 projected	Month 7 projected	Month 8 projected	Month 9 projected	Month 10 projected	Month 11 projected	Month 12 projected	Year 1 projected
REVENUES													
Dental Service Revenue	5,000.00	6,000.00	7,500.00	9,000.00	10,800.00	13,600.00	16,400.00	19,400.00	21,800.00	24,300.00	28,800.00	32,000.00	1,94,600.00
Bank Service Fees	0.00	0.00	0.00	0.00	0.00	0.00	0.00	0.00	0.00	0.00	0.00	0.00	0.00
Total Revenues	5,000.00	6,000.00	7,500.00	9,000.00	10,800.00	13,600.00	16,400.00	19,400.00	21,800.00	24,300.00	28,800.00	32,000.00	1,94,600.00
EXPENSES													
Variable Expenses													
Dental Supplies 8%	400.00	480.00	600.00	720.00	864.00	1,088.00	1,312.00	1,552.00	1,744.00	1,944.00	2,304.00	2,560.00	15,568.00
Laboratory Fees 9%	450.00	540.00	675.00	810.00	972.00	1,224.00	1,476.00	1,746.00	1,962.00	2,187.00	2,592.00	2,880.00	17,514.00
Total Variable Expenses	850.00	1,020.00	1,275.00	1,530.00	1,836.00	2,312.00	2,788.00	3,298.00	3,706.00	4,131.00	4,896.00	5,440.00	33,082.00
% of rev	17%	17%	17%	17%	17%	17%	17%	17%	17%	17%	17%	17%	17%
Fixed Expenses													
Accounting	0.00	0.00	0.00	0.00	0.00	0.00	0.00	0.00	0.00	0.00	0.00	0.00	0.00
Advertising	1,000.00	1,000.00	1,000.00	1,000.00	1,000.00	1,000.00	1,000.00	1,000.00	1,000.00	1,000.00	1,000.00	1,000.00	12,000.00
Continuing Education	0.00	0.00	0.00	0.00	0.00	0.00	0.00	0.00	0.00	0.00	0.00	0.00	0.00
Dues and subscriptions	165.00	165.00	165.00	165.00	165.00	165.00	165.00	165.00	165.00	165.00	165.00	165.00	1,980.00
Employee Benefits	0.00	0.00	0.00	0.00	0.00	0.00	0.00	0.00	0.00	0.00	0.00	0.00	0.00
Insurance- Disability	0.00	0.00	0.00	0.00	0.00	0.00	0.00	0.00	0.00	0.00	0.00	0.00	0.00
Insurance- Health	0.00	0.00	0.00	0.00	0.00	0.00	0.00	0.00	0.00	0.00	0.00	0.00	0.00
Insurance- Malpractice	100.00	100.00	100.00	100.00	100.00	100.00	100.00	100.00	100.00	100.00	100.00	100.00	1,200.00
Insurance- Workers Comp	0.00	0.00	0.00	0.00	0.00	0.00	0.00	0.00	0.00	0.00	0.00	0.00	0.00
Legal	400.00	400.00	400.00	400.00	400.00	400.00	400.00	400.00	400.00	400.00	400.00	400.00	4,800.00
Maintenance & Repairs	0.00	0.00	0.00	0.00	0.00	0.00	0.00	0.00	0.00	0.00	0.00	0.00	0.00
Office/Clinic Supplies 2%	15,000.00	120.00	150.00	180.00	216.00	272.00	328.00	388.00	436.00	486.00	576.00	640.00	18,792.00
Payroll Taxes 13.65%	1,178.54	1,178.54	1,178.54	1,178.54	1,178.54	1,178.54	1,178.54	1,178.54	1,178.54	1,178.54	1,178.54	1,178.54	14,142.49
Postage and delivery	0.00	0.00	0.00	0.00	0.00	0.00	0.00	0.00	0.00	0.00	0.00	0.00	0.00
Rent	3,310.00	3,310.00	3,310.00	3,310.00	3,310.00	3,310.00	3,310.00	3,310.00	3,310.00	3,310.00	3,310.00	3,310.00	39,720.00
Salaries-Staff Receptionist	3,467.00	3,467.00	3,467.00	3,467.00	3,467.00	3,467.00	3,467.00	3,467.00	3,467.00	3,467.00	3,467.00	3,467.00	41,604.00
Salaries-Dental Assistant	3,467.00	3,467.00	3,467.00	3,467.00	3,467.00	3,467.00	3,467.00	3,467.00	3,467.00	3,467.00	3,467.00	3,467.00	41,604.00
Salaries-Doctor	1,700.00	1,700.00	1,700.00	1,700.00	1,700.00	1,700.00	1,700.00	1,700.00	1,700.00	1,700.00	1,700.00	1,700.00	20,400.00
Taxes & Licenses	175.00	175.00	175.00	175.00	175.00	175.00	175.00	175.00	175.00	175.00	175.00	175.00	2,100.00
Telephone/Internet	100.00	100.00	100.00	100.00	100.00	100.00	100.00	100.00	100.00	100.00	100.00	100.00	1,200.00
Travel, Meals, Ent.	0.00	0.00	0.00	0.00	0.00	0.00	0.00	0.00	0.00	0.00	0.00	0.00	0.00
Utilities	0.00	0.00	0.00	0.00	0.00	0.00	0.00	0.00	0.00	0.00	0.00	0.00	0.00
Misc	0.00	0.00	0.00	0.00	0.00	0.00	0.00	0.00	0.00	0.00	0.00	0.00	0.00
Total Fixed Expenses	30,062.54	15,182.54	15,212.54	15,242.54	15,278.54	15,334.54	15,390.54	15,450.54	15,498.54	15,548.54	15,638.54	15,702.54	1,99,542.49
% of rev	601%	253%	203%	169%	141%	113%	94%	80%	71%	64%	54%	49%	103%
Total operating expenses	30,912.54	16,202.54	16,487.54	16,772.54	17,114.54	17,646.54	18,178.54	18,748.54	19,204.54	19,679.54	20,534.54	21,142.54	2,32,624.49
% of rev	618%	270%	220%	186%	158%	130%	111%	97%	88%	81%	71%	66%	120%
NET INCOME (LOSS)	-25,912.54	-10,202.54	-8,987.54	-7,772.54	-6,314.54	-4,046.54	-1,778.54	651.46	2,595.46	4,620.46	8,265.46	10,857.46	-38,024.49
% of revenue	-518%	-170%	-120%	-86%	-58%	-30%	-11%	3%	12%	19%	29%	34%	-20%
Bank Loan (Int Rate) 7.00													
Interest	438.00	438.00	438.00	438.00	438.00	438.00	438.00	438.00	438.00	438.00	438.00	438.00	5,256.00
Total Interest Payments	438.00	438.00	438.00	438.00	438.00	438.00	438.00	438.00	438.00	438.00	438.00	438.00	5,256.00
% of rev	9%	7%	6%	5%	4%	3%	3%	2%	2%	2%	2%	1%	3%
CASH FLOW CHECK	-$26,350.54	-$10,640.54	-$9,425.54	-$8,210.54	-$6,752.54	-$4,484.54	-$2,216.54	$213.46	$2,157.46	$4,182.46	$7,827.46	$10,419.46	-$43,280.49

Figure 4.3f. Pro forma.

80

23-Apr-16		Month 13 projected	Month 14 projected	Month 15 projected	Month 16 projected	Month 17 projected	Month 18 projected	Month 19 projected	Month 20 projected	Month 21 projected	Month 22 projected	Month 23 projected	Month 24 projected	Year 2 projected
REVENUES														
Dental Service Revenue		0.00	0.00	0.00	0.00	0.00	0.00	0.00	0.00	0.00	0.00	0.00	0.00	0.00
Bank Service Fees		0.00	0.00	0.00	0.00	0.00	0.00	0.00	0.00	0.00	0.00	0.00	0.00	0.00
Total Revenues		0.00	0.00	0.00	0.00	0.00	0.00	0.00	0.00	0.00	0.00	0.00	0.00	0.00
EXPENSES														
Variable Expenses														
Dental Supplies	8%	0.00	0.00	0.00	0.00	0.00	0.00	0.00	0.00	0.00	0.00	0.00	0.00	0.00
Laboratory Fees	9%	0.00	0.00	0.00	0.00	0.00	0.00	0.00	0.00	0.00	0.00	0.00	0.00	0.00
Total Variable Expenses		0.00	0.00	0.00	0.00	0.00	0.00	0.00	0.00	0.00	0.00	0.00	0.00	0.00
% of rev		0%	0%	0%	0%	0%	0%	0%	0%	0%	0%	0%	0%	0%
Fixed Expenses														
Accounting		0.00	0.00	0.00	0.00	0.00	0.00	0.00	0.00	0.00	0.00	0.00	0.00	0.00
Advertising		1,050.00	1,050.00	1,050.00	1,050.00	1,050.00	1,050.00	1,050.00	1,050.00	1,050.00	1,050.00	1,050.00	1,050.00	12,600.00
Continuing Education		0.00	0.00	0.00	0.00	0.00	0.00	0.00	0.00	0.00	0.00	0.00	0.00	0.00
Dues and subscriptions		173.25	173.25	173.25	173.25	173.25	173.25	173.25	173.25	173.25	173.25	173.25	173.25	2,079.00
Employee Benefits		0.00	0.00	0.00	0.00	0.00	0.00	0.00	0.00	0.00	0.00	0.00	0.00	0.00
Insurance- Disability		0.00	0.00	0.00	0.00	0.00	0.00	0.00	0.00	0.00	0.00	0.00	0.00	0.00
Insurance- Health		0.00	0.00	0.00	0.00	0.00	0.00	0.00	0.00	0.00	0.00	0.00	0.00	0.00
Insurance- Malpractice		105.00	105.00	105.00	105.00	105.00	105.00	105.00	105.00	105.00	105.00	105.00	105.00	1,260.00
Insurance- Workers Comp		0.00	0.00	0.00	0.00	0.00	0.00	0.00	0.00	0.00	0.00	0.00	0.00	0.00
Legal		420.00	420.00	420.00	420.00	420.00	420.00	420.00	420.00	420.00	420.00	420.00	420.00	5,040.00
Maintenance & Repairs		0.00	0.00	0.00	0.00	0.00	0.00	0.00	0.00	0.00	0.00	0.00	0.00	0.00
Office/Clinic Supplies	2%	1,644.30	1,644.30	1,644.30	1,644.30	1,644.30	1,644.30	1,544.30	1,644.30	1,644.30	1,644.30	1,644.30	1,644.30	19,731.60
Payroll Taxes	13.65%	427.23	427.23	427.23	427.23	427.23	427.23	427.23	427.23	427.23	427.23	427.23	427.23	5,126.74
Postage and delivery		0.00	0.00	0.00	0.00	0.00	0.00	0.00	0.00	0.00	0.00	0.00	0.00	0.00
Rent		0.00	0.00	0.00	0.00	0.00	0.00	0.00	0.00	0.00	0.00	0.00	0.00	0.00
Salaries-Staff Receptionist		3,640.35	3,640.35	3,640.35	3,640.35	3,640.35	3,640.35	3,640.35	3,640.35	3,640.35	3,640.35	3,640.35	3,640.35	43,684.20
Salaries-Dental Assistant		3,640.35	3,640.35	3,640.35	3,640.35	3,640.35	3,640.35	3,640.35	3,640.35	3,640.35	3,640.35	3,640.35	3,640.35	43,684.20
Salaries-Doctor		1,700.00	1,700.00	1,700.00	1,700.00	1,700.00	1,700.00	1,700.00	1,700.00	1,700.00	1,700.00	1,700.00	1,700.00	20,400.00
Taxes & Licenses		183.75	183.75	183.75	183.75	183.75	183.75	183.75	183.75	183.75	183.75	183.75	183.75	2,205.00
Telephone/Internet		105.00	105.00	105.00	105.00	105.00	105.00	105.00	105.00	105.00	105.00	105.00	105.00	1,260.00
Travel, Meals, Ent.		0.00	0.00	0.00	0.00	0.00	0.00	0.00	0.00	0.00	0.00	0.00	0.00	0.00
Utilities		0.00	0.00	0.00	0.00	0.00	0.00	0.00	0.00	0.00	0.00	0.00	0.00	0.00
Misc		0.00	0.00	0.00	0.00	0.00	0.00	0.00	0.00	0.00	0.00	0.00	0.00	0.00
Total Fixed Expenses		13,089.23	13,089.23	13,089.23	13,089.23	13,089.23	13,089.23	13,089.23	13,089.23	13,089.23	13,089.23	13,089.23	13,089.23	1,57,070.74
% of rev		0%	0%	0%	0%	0%	0%	0%	0%	0%	0%	0%	0%	0%
Total operating expenses		13,089.23	13,089.23	13,089.23	13,089.23	13,089.23	13,089.23	13,089.23	13,089.23	13,089.23	13,089.23	13,089.23	13,089.23	1,57,070.74
% of rev		0%	0%	0%	0%	0%	0%	0%	0%	0%	0%	0%	0%	0%
NET INCOME (LOSS)		-13,089.23	-13,089.23	-13,089.23	-13,089.23	-13,089.23	-13,089.23	-13,089.23	-13,089.23	-13,089.23	-13,089.23	-13,089.23	-13,089.23	-1,57,070.74
% of revenue		0%	0%	0%	0%	0%	0%	0%	0%	0%	0%	0%	0%	0%
Bank Loan (Int Rate)	7.00													
Interest		0.00	0.00	0.00	0.00	0.00	0.00	0.00	0.00	0.00	0.00	0.00	0.00	0.00
Total Interest Payments		0.00	0.00	0.00	0.00	0.00	0.00	0.00	0.00	0.00	0.00	0.00	0.00	0.00
% of rev		0%	0%	0%	0%	0%	0%	0%	0%	0%	0%	0%	0%	0%
CASH FLOW CHECK		-$13,089.23	-$13,089.23	-$13,089.23	-$13,089.23	-$13,089.23	-$13,089.23	-$13,089.23	-$13,089.23	-$13,089.23	-$13,089.23	-$13,089.23	-$13,089.23	-$1,57,070.74

Figure 4.3f. (*Continued*)

Figure 4.3. *Continued*

81

Appendices

A. Curriculum Vitae (withheld from sample plan)
B. Personal Balance Sheet
C. Personal Living Budget
D. Sources of Information

Appendix B: Personal Balance Sheet (Figure 4.3g)

ASSETS	
Cash	$500.00
Bank Accounts (Checking/Savings/Money Market)	$1,500.00
Securities (Stocks/Bonds/Other)	$0.00
Accounts/Notes Receivable	$0.00
Life Insurance (Cash surrender value)	$0.00
Auto (s)	$5,000.00
Real Estate	$0.00
Pension/Retirement Plan (vested)	$0.00
Personal Property (Art/Jewelry,Furniture/Etc.)	$27,000.00
TOTAL ASSETS	**$34,000.00**
LIABILITIES	
Accounts Payable (Credit/Revolving Accts/Etc.)	$0.00
Contracts Payable (Installment Payments)	$0.00
Notes Payable (Auto…)	$0.00
Real Estate Loan Principal Balances	$0.00
Student Loan Principal Balances	$241,000.00
Other Liabilities	$0.00
TOTAL LIABILITIES	**$241,000.00**
NET WORTH (Total Assets - Total Liabilities)	**-$207,000.00**

Figure 4.3g.   Personal balance sheet.

Figure 4.3.   *Continued*

Appendix C: Personal Living Budget (Figure 4.3h)

PERSONAL MONTHLY BUDGET	
Regular Monthly Payments	
Rent or Mortgage	$2,500.00
Automobile Loan	$0.00
Appliances	$0.00
Personal Loans	$0.00
Educational Loans	$1,700.00
Auto Insurance	$0.00
Other Insurance	$0.00
Miscellaneous	$0.00
Total Regular Monthly Payments	**$4,200.00**
% of Total Expenses	76.85%
Household Operating Expenses	
Telephone	$100.00
Utilities	$100.00
Other Household Expenses	$0.00
Total Household Operating Expenses	**$200.00**
% of Total Expenses	3.66%
Meal Expenses	
Dining at home (Groceries)	$0.00
Dining out	$300.00
Total Meal Expenses	**$300.00**
% of Total Expenses	5.49%
Personal Expenses	
Clothing, cleaning, laundry..	$100.00
Pharmaceuticals	$0.00
Medical/Dental	$50.00
Charitable Gifts and Donations	$0.00
Travel	$0.00
Subscriptions	$0.00
Auto expense fuel/maintenance/parking	$100.00
Other spending allowances	$0.00
Total Personal Expenses	**$250.00**
% of Total Expenses	4.57%
Tax Expenses	
Federal and state income taxes	$500.00
Property taxes	$15.00
Other taxes	$0.00
Total Tax Expenses	**$515.00**
% of Total Expenses	9.42%
TOTAL MONTHLY EXPENSES	**$5,465.00**
Non-Business Income (Significant Other / Spouse / Investment)	$3,765.00
NET MONTHLY PERSONAL CASH NEED	**$1,700.00**

Figure 4.3h.   Personal budget.

Figure 4.3.   *Continued*

Appendix D: Sources of Information

U.S. Census Bureau, 2010 Census

City of Foster City, Crime Stats, www.fostercity.org/projectsandinitiatives/crimestats.cfm

Manta, Companies in Foster City, http://www.manta.com/mb_51_ALL_1NP/foster_city_ca

San Jose Mercury News, 2011: Gilead Sciences expansion in Foster City grows, www.mercurynews.com/business/ci_18871114

U.S. Census Bureau and County QuickFacts, 2013, http://quickfacts.census/gov/qfd/states/06/0625338.html

Metropolitan Planning Group, Foster City General Plan Update 2011: Snapshot Workbook, http://www.fostercity.org/departmentsanddivisions/communitydevelopment/PlanningCodeEnforcement/Planning-Commission.cfm

County of San Mateo, 2012–2013 Profile, http://www.co.sanmateo.ca.us/bos.dir/budget/recommend2012/county/a-19.pdf

California Department of Finance, Report P-1: Summary Population Projections by Race/Ethnicity and by Major Age Groups, http://www.dof.ca.gov/research/demographic/reports/projections/P-1/

City of Foster City, Amendment to the Gilead Sciences Corporate Campus Master Plan, http://www.fostercity.org/departmentsanddivisions/communitydevelopment/Features/Gilead-Sciences-General-Development-Plan-Project.cfm

Best Health Care Jobs-Dentist, U.S. News & World Report, http://money.usnews.com/careers/best-jobs/dentist

Newport, F. Congress retains low honesty rating; Nurses have highest honest rating; Car salespeople, lowest. 2012 Gallup Poll http://www.gallup.com/poll/159035/congress-retains-low-honesty-rating.aspx

ADA, 2010 Survey of Dental Practice, http://www.ada.org/~/media/ADA/Science%20and%20Research/HPI/Files/10_sdpi_highlights.ashx

May 2014 Metropolitan and Nonmetropolitan Area Occupational Employment and Wage Estimates for San Francisco-San Mateo-Redwood City, CA Metropolitan Division, http://www.bls.gov/oes/current/oes_41884.htm

Figure 4.3. *Continued*

Chapter 5
Understanding Practice Valuation

C. Steven Wolff, DDS

Introduction

The subject of business valuation—and for our more specific purpose, dental practice valuation—consumes many textbooks and is the focus of both undergraduate and postgraduate programs. We cannot within the confines of a single chapter expect to cover this entire subject; instead, we hope to provide the reader with enough information about the terminology and techniques to allow some working knowledge on the topic. We have no doubt that at some time during the course of your career you will need to have some idea about how a dental practice is evaluated. "We" is used throughout this chapter because the process of practice valuation as described typically involves a team effort.

The Internal Revenue Service's definition of fair market value is this: what a willing buyer will pay and what a willing seller will accept when neither is under any compulsion to act and both have been advised of all information needed to make a decision. It would be convenient if the IRS's definition would allow parties to always arrive at some mutually agreeable price. However, the market does not always work that way, and consequently, an appraiser should be retained to determine the starting point for negotiation between the parties.

Before we get too far down the road concerning the process and techniques, let's clarify a common misunderstanding. The terms "valuation" and "appraisal" are frequently used interchangeably when in fact they have significantly different meanings. A valuation is used primarily to determine an appropriate asking price for a practice placed on the open market. In real estate, this might be referred to as a BOV or broker's opinion of value. After collecting and reviewing practice, market and financial data, the valuator may recommend a range of value (sometimes based on the perceived urgency of the sale), allowing the ultimate decision regarding the asking price to rest with the seller. However, in the case of a true appraisal, the valuator will present a substantial, often bound, document to the client specifying a dollar value, and as a result of his or her experience and credentials, would be prepared to defend that number. That defense might be given to a potential buyer with counsel, a financial institution, or in litigation. As you might expect, an appraisal document involves considerable time and expense, but in the post-Great Recession world of practice,

Dental Practice Transition: A Practical Guide to Management, Second Edition.
Edited by David G. Dunning and Brian M. Lange.
© 2016 John Wiley & Sons, Inc. Published 2016 by John Wiley & Sons, Inc.
Companion Website: www.wiley.com/go/dunning/transition

transition has become the *necessary starting point* for both financing and sales. Obviously, several other chapters in this book complement the content of this chapter, and the reader is strongly encouraged especially to read Chapter 6 (dental equipment), Chapter 7 (buying/buying-into a practice), and Chapter 9 (financing a practice).

Overview of the Process

There are four distinct steps leading up to determining a specific or range of valuation depending on the nature of the assignment. Each step is vitally important to the credibility and accuracy of the project and demands considerable detail on the part of both the valuator and the client.

Step One

First, the purpose and scope of the assignment must be determined. Is the work being done to place the practice for sale on the open market, or is it being done because of litigation between two partners? What is the effective date, and to whom will this information be revealed? Does the client understand the fee for these services, and what are the time constraints for the completion of the project?

Step Two

The second step involves the collection of all necessary financial and demographic data regarding the practice. The client is asked to complete a questionnaire about the practice and to provide statistical and cultural information about the area in which the subject practice is located. In addition, we will need a current profit and loss statement, as well as complete business federal tax returns for the last 3–5 years. We normally schedule a complete physical inventory and guide the client through a hands-on count of instruments, handpieces, and supplies.

Step Three

In the third step, we spend a considerable number of hours processing the data in order to use it in subsequent valuation computations. We determine the in-place, functional, and productive value for all equipment based on our experience and familiarity with the market. Be advised that this number will not be the same as the retail, wholesale, "book," or liquidation price and in most cases will amount to less than 35% of the total value of a typical dental practice.

A significant task necessary in the processing phase is referred to as the "normalization" of the tax returns. While doctors and their tax preparers may have taken great pains to find as many legitimate deductions from gross income as possible, our job is to separate necessary operating expenses from the perks of business ownership in order to determine the true cash flow, entrepreneurial profit and excess earnings. Excess earnings are defined as cash available after normalized overhead is paid and after the owner/provider receives fair compensation for producing dentistry. In larger business valuation conversations, this is often referred to as EBITDA or earnings before interest, taxes, depreciation, and amortization. In a perfect world, that amount would be equal to 10–15% of gross revenues. This is a critical process that will be used in subsequent valuation methods.

Let's divide these expenses subject to normalization into three categories: doctor's personal expenses, judgment calls, and disappearing items.

1. *Doctor's personal expenses:* These are sometimes referred to as lifestyle expenses or perks. To give an example, a trip to Hawaii for an 8-hour continuing education course is allowable as a legitimate business expense and is deducted from the gross income of the practice. Those 8 hours of training could also be had from various online study courses at a fraction of the cost. While continuing education is a necessary expense for the ownership of a dental practice, a standard has to be determined by the valuator, and adjustments are made accordingly. Other personal expenses may include the following:
   a. Auto expense
   b. Charitable contributions
   c. Insurance
   d. Retirement contribution
   e. Travel and entertainment
2. *Judgment calls:* There are recognized industry standards for certain overhead categories available from a variety of sources. If the practice varies too far from these guidelines, we investigate and adjust accordingly. Be advised that the adjustments can be both up and down:
   a. Supplies
   b. Telephone
   c. Payroll
   d. Laboratory
3. *Disappearing items:* All of the disappearing items are adjusted to zero. In the case of interest expenses, it is assumed that all assets of the practice are being transferred free and clear and that the buyer's only interest expense will be for the practice mortgage and any subsequent capital improvements.
   a. Depreciation of purchased tangible assets (for example, equipment)
   b. Interest
   c. Amortization of purchased intangible assets (such as "goodwill")

There are probably as many variations in tax returns as there are accountants preparing them. Careful analysis of the return is necessary in order to give an accurate picture of the funds available to pay overhead, taxes, living expenses, and debt service. It also helps to have at least a rudimentary knowledge of the different business models commonly used in Dentistry. These would include the sole proprietorship, a limited liability company (LLC), a Subchapter S Corporation, and in rare occasions when dealing with mature practices, a C Corporation. Please refer to Chapter 10 for additional information about business forms/entities.

Now the process of applying the various methods of valuation begins. These methods, which we will discuss in greater detail shortly, range from purely mathematical computations to very subjective techniques based on the experience of the appraiser. Some, all, or perhaps even a weighted combination of several methods may be used to arrive at a conclusion. Dentists love formulas, so while a strict by-the-numbers technique would probably be most appreciated by our clients, the fact remains that most appraisers are going to use some combination of art, science, and mathematics to develop their conclusions.

Step Four

The fourth step in the process involves the writing of a report either as specified by the requirements of an actual appraisal or to advise a prospective seller/client about the feasibility of placing the practice on the market. The letter will briefly review the comparisons made by the valuator of the target practice to other similar practices. Based on his or her experience in the market, a market price will be recommended to the client. The urgency of a sale may have considerable effect on the final decision regarding the listing price. In the case of a true appraisal, the final report will be presented in several bound copies and will go into considerable detail about the qualifications of the appraiser, the methods of valuation used, the "weight" of those methods, and finally, a number that represents the valuator's professional opinion as to the specific value of the practice.

Appraisal Methods

As mentioned earlier, the methods of appraisal range from pure mathematics to the valuator's instincts. We also discuss a frequently used term in business valuation and how it may or may not apply in dentistry. The most common methods used to determine the value of a dental practice include summation of assets, comparable sales, capitalization of earnings, and its first cousin, the excess earnings to retire debt calculation. Let's discuss them individually after setting a few ground rules. For this text we will confine our discussion to the valuation of single-owner practices selling assets (not stock) and expecting to get cash at closing. Variations on that theme will be discussed later in the chapter.

Summation of Assets

Being familiar with the market and having previously determined the value of the tangible assets, the appraiser performs a build-up of values based on the comparison of the subject practice to a standardized practice model. This scoring includes items such as location, staff experience, equipment, hygiene efficiency, patient count and demographics, cash flow, and profitability as they relate to a statistical norm. For example, is the active patient count more or less than you would expect to see for a typical general practice? Is the practice located in a suburban neighborhood or is it in a more isolated rural area? There may be as many as 20–25 data points that will figure into this equation. The results of this method are a product of a proprietary program maintained by the appraiser.

Comparable Sales

All qualified appraisers should have access to a database that will track what similar practices with similar revenues have sold for in similar markets. While accepting the fact that all dentists are unique, and consequently their practices are unique, five or more data points in two or three different databases can be very convincing in determining a practice's place in the market. We frequently use the real estate analogy: if you knew what fifty homes with 1,500 square feet of living space, three bedrooms, and two bathrooms on one half of an acre in a suburban neighborhood of a city sold for, you could probably come very close to knowing the market value for the fifty-first next such home.

Capitalization of Earnings

This method utilizes a computation based on a calculated rate of return on the practice's profits. This rate of return is referred to as the cap rate and involves a variety of factors outside the scope of this chapter including present dollar values, risk of the market, fixed securities return, and so forth. For now, let's think of the cap rate as the rate of return on the excess earnings of the practice. Once those earnings are determined from the normalization of the tax return, an appraiser can use that derived cap rate to work backward into the value of the practice.

Let's simplify this by using the example of a certificate of deposit of unknown value. Pretend that you just received a notice from your bank that you have been credited with the annual proceeds from a long-forgotten CD in the amount of $6,000 at 5% annual percentage rate. By using the following formula, you could determine that the value of the CD is $120,000.

$$\text{Value} = \frac{\text{excess earnings (\$6,000)}}{\text{cap rate (5\% = 0.05)}} = \$120,000$$

Don't let the example mislead you, however, as historically the cap rate for dental practice earnings is several multiples of 5%, generally in the 20–35% range.

Excess Earnings to Retire Debt

This calculation uses an amortization schedule (loan payment schedule) in reverse to calculate how much debt our previously determined excess earnings could support using industry standards for acquisition financing. As an example, let's suppose that our calculations resulted in excess earnings of $70,000. Given an interest rate of 8% and a loan amortization/length of 7 years, the buyer could service a loan amount of almost $375,000. Since most buyers will also need to have some operating capital to fund the practice's expenses until the revenue stream begins, the sales price will have to be 10–15% less than the total loan amount. This test is sometimes referred to as the "sanity test" to check the validity of the numbers derived from the other methods and to quickly determine the plausibility of the transaction.

Other Methods

Sometimes appraisers will make a value determination based on what costs could be avoided by purchasing the seller's practice. The national average cost of a three operatory build-out and start-up is currently in excess of $350,000. Thus, serious consideration is sometimes given to what costs the buyer could avoid by purchasing and moving to another office that, while lacking adequate cash flow for typical valuation methods, may have some inherent value just because it already exists and is ready to go. There may be some strategic value in purchasing a nearby practice, either for control of a local market or as a means of increasing practice revenues without having to increase marketing costs or agreeing to participate in preferred provider organizations (PPOs) with potentially significant adjustments/write-offs.

A simplified version of the summation of the assets method depends on access to a national database that tabulates the value placed on the intangible or soft assets, which include a patient base, "blue-sky" or "goodwill," a covenant not to compete, a trained and available work staff, and a recognizable ongoing business concern. This database, known as the Goodwill Registry published by The Healthcare Group, expresses the allocation of intangible value as a percentage of the most recent year's gross revenues. The resulting amount can then be added to the known hard (tangible) asset values for equipment, furniture, instruments, and supplies to give a valuator another indicator of the value, less any liabilities of the practice.

Rule of Thumb

Another frequently discussed idiom in this industry is the rule of thumb. No less of a resource than the ADA's *Valuing a Practice* refers to multipliers that are based on 5 years of data. These multipliers are used in conjunction with gross revenues and net income. These data, while interesting, can be very misleading to both buyers and sellers. Let me use the following examples to illustrate the need for caution when considering averages and multipliers. If you stand a 5 foot 2 inch dental student next to a 6 foot 4 inch student, a 5 foot 6 inch student, and a 6 foot student, a rule of thumb might claim that all dental students are 5 foot 9 inches tall. Understandably, while that may be close, it is not accurate.

A more on-point example should further illustrate the need to look beyond this method in determining a practice's value. Let's assume the Smith and Jones practices each have gross revenues of $600,000. Would the practice values be the same given these details?

1. The Smith practice has a 100% fee-for-service patient base, and the Jones practice has 50% Medicaid patients.
2. The Smith practice has a solid below-market-rate 7-year lease, and the Jones practice was going to be relocated due to an eminent domain proceeding with the city.
3. The Jones practice has a 20-year history in the community with steadily increasing revenues, while the Smith practice has had peaks and valleys due to numerous associate doctors with varying skills.
4. The Smith practice has a long-term, well-trained staff, whereas the Jones practice has been plagued by constant turnover.

It should be obvious from these extreme (and yet very real) examples of valuation points that these practices could not have the same value. In the Midwest market, we have seen practices sell for as little as 25% and for almost 85% of gross revenues. We're told that practices in some areas of the country sell for over 100% of revenue. Our advice would be to *use rule of thumb as a check mechanism* to examine the reasonableness of an appraisal, asking price, or offer. If the numbers are outside of the expected range, some explanation may be required.

Factors Affecting Practice Value

We would not pretend to be able to create a complete list of all of the factors that can influence the value of a dental practice. We would only need to wait for the next transition to find a new one. However, *there are some key variables that have been consistently shown to affect both the price and marketability of a practice.* Certainly, the most important are *cash flow and profitability*. Businesses are purchased for the purpose of making money. If a practice does not produce adequate revenue to pay overhead, a fair wage to the producer, some return on investment capital, and to service the debt, it will have less than hoped-for value. The longer the history of adequate revenues, the less risk to the potential buyer, and therefore, a higher value can be placed on the practice. Likewise, the more transferable the revenue stream to the new owner, the higher the value.

Probably the next most important factor in practice value would be *location*. Location factors considered in a practice analysis would include metro versus rural, placement and visibility within a trade area, and patient demographics of the area.

The *number of active patients of the practice, a favorable lease, new patient development, the availability of a trained staff along with the overall curb appeal of the office, and equipment* are all important issues that can have a dramatic influence on a practice's value. Even issues such as fees, procedure mix, and the percentage of PPO contracts have to be considered. We will blend all of these and many other issues together in a valuation exercise later in this chapter.

We have been asked if there is some discount factor that needs to be taken into consideration with regard to patient retention. It has been our experience that a well-orchestrated transition will result in little if any patient loss above and beyond the normal attrition rate of a practice. While hard data are difficult to obtain, anecdotally we think the typical loss of patients in a practice purchase is at around 10%. This number is probably high for rural offices and potentially a little low for metro practices. There is always some patient attrition even without a practice purchase. Patients move, die, or just aren't compatible with the personality of the practice. So, with a healthy influx of new patients, most buyers notice little if any net loss. Assuming the practice has a long history of new patient flow, the net loss will not likely even be noticeable. Since the market has already accounted for any consideration that might be given to this issue, there is no further discount factor in the practice value due to patient attrition.

Historical Performance versus Future Earnings

Practices are appraised on the basis of performance over a period of time. While cash flow projections can be an effective marketing tool in attracting a buyer, they would figure *only marginally* in the process of evaluating a practice. However, projections of cash flow and profitability may figure much more prominently in financing a practice. It is certainly of some comfort to a potential buyer and his or her lender that there is a long-standing history of positive and adequate cash flow. That history implies a reduced risk of losing that cash flow and, therefore, a stronger value. Just as most other investments carry a disclaimer stating that past performance is no guarantee of future earnings, the same can be said for investment in a dental practice. The buyer has to show up, do the work, and run the business in order to enjoy the benefits that were available to the previous owner. The economic world of business and finance is unpredictable—for example, sales based on rosy projections in 2007 have often brought pain and disappointment when the Great Recession in many cases forced revenues down below practice averages. While revenues generally go up over a long period of time, they do not necessarily go up every year and expectations regarding cash flow should be conservative.

Notwithstanding, astute buyers may recognize and leverage the potential for growth over time, increasing profitability in a given practice. Sharp population growth, reduced competition, or the ability to expand the procedure mix may indeed make for a good buying opportunity. These factors are very difficult to quantify and consequently are generally beyond the scope of both an appraisal and an opinion of value.

Other Issues in Practice Appraisals and Sales

As mentioned earlier in this chapter, most of our discussions have centered on the premise that the target practice involved a solo owner/operator buying or selling assets, not stock, and with the expectation of a cash exchange at closing. In addition, we are further biased by the fact that all of our work has been confined to the Midwest. Obviously, there is room for a discussion of market variations throughout the country.

We would point out that comparable sales data can vary significantly from one part of the country to another. Population density, competition among recent dental graduates, and cost of living variables can make for vastly different prices for similarly sized practices. Likewise, in our work we notice differences between metropolitan and rural practices in spite of the fact that the office environment and equipment may be identical and that profitability may be higher in the rural office. As a general rule, metropolitan practices will appraise for a higher value. *Always* ensure that the appraiser who has been retained has recent experience in the specific market of the target practice.

The discussion of stock versus asset sales is nearly moot because the overwhelming majority of transactions are conducted as asset sales. If it is at all possible, we suggest this approach because it results in a much cleaner, more financeable, tax-friendly transaction. Stock sales generally involve larger group practices and the acquisition of a new partner. While recognizing that this type of a transition may not be as common, please do not overlook the need for qualified counsel to assist in the process. Group practices appear to be on the rise, and thus purchases involving stock may increase over time. Refer in particular to Chapter 7 (buying and buying-into a practice), Chapter 9 (financing a practice), and Chapter 10 (business entities/forms).

While such was not the case only a decade or so ago, most practice appraisals and valuations are based on a "cash at closing" value. With the current attitude of capital lenders, sellers are seldom expected in the current market to "carry back" (or finance) any or all of the purchase price in the form of a note (loan). If sellers were so required, especially by lenders/banks, the uncertainty of payment would involve more risk, and since risk equals reward, the value of the practice may have to be increased. Payment in full at closing removes that risk of future payment and may reduce the appraised value.

The last item for discussion in this chapter involves the valuation of nonmajority interest in a dental practice, and the subsequent discount applied to that value. Any ownership percentage less than 100% results in some lack of control and marketability. Several factors come into play. Financing of a percentage ownership interest is more difficult, as the lender may not be able to have an adequate collateral position to support the loan. Nonmajority owners cannot exercise the same control over their destiny as can the majority or solo owner. By the same token, majority owners might find their interest to be less desirable to the market due to the presence of the minority third-party owner. Every circumstance would have to be very closely examined, but it may not be unreasonable for the discounted value to be 25–40% less for the proportion of the practice purchased by a nonmajority purchaser.

Valuation Exercise

Just for fun, let's see if we can place a listing price on a hypothetical four operatory general practice located in the Midwest. Rest assured that there will be no absolutely right or absolutely wrong answers, as there will be too many unknown variables. As a matter of fact, we're going to violate one of the fundamental rules of practice valuation by not being able to make a physical inspection of the facility. The way an office looks, feels, and smells can have a tremendous impact on its price and marketability. All that being said, let's look at the practice numbers and description and see if we can arrive at a projected asking price.

The subject practice was built in 1983 in a professional building that was at that time on the outskirts of the city. The city's growth has left this location about halfway between "downtown" and the outer borders of the metro area. The office has four nice-sized operatories in 1,700 square feet, along with a lab, sterilization center, and employee lounge. In addition, the doctor has a nice-sized private office that is plumbed and could be converted to a fifth operatory. The equipment was upgraded in 2005 and is very well maintained. The office uses digital radiography but retains the use of paper charts. A recent redecorating effort with contemporary colors and materials leaves the office looking very up-to-date and comfortable.

The four-member staff is a mixture of long- and short-term employees, with the receptionist having the longest tenure, at 12 years, and a recently hired chair-side assistant having been with the practice less than 6 months. The receptionist is probably at the top of her pay range. The patient base of almost 1,800 "active" patients has grown older with the seller and over half are over the age of 60. The practice has only a small preteen component. (*Note:* Active patients are commonly defined as those patients who have been in the office for a billable visit within the last 18 months and are not known to have moved away or died.) The hygienist sees between 30 and 35 patients during a 3.5-day work week. The doctor has a desire to retire. He and the staff work 4.5 days per week.

The gross receipts for 2015 totaled $712,000, which was about the same as 2014. Up until 2008, the practice has always had steady annual revenue growth of 2–3%. Normalized expenses for 2015 were $433,000, which resulted in a gross profit of $279,000. A salary of 28% ($200,000) would allow excess earnings of approximately $79,000. (*Note:* We would use a salary allowance of 30% if the doctor was working without a hygienist.) The seller recently signed a new 3-year lease with two options of 5 years each. The rate seemed to be comparable to other properties in the neighborhood. Due to the presence of a couple of large employers in the area, the office does participate in several different PPO plans. The office does not accept Medicaid or any other discount services plan.

All in all this is a very attractive practice that would most likely do very well on the market. It is not without issues, however, as just about every potential listing has a few warts. We have mentioned numerous items that need consideration regardless of whether we are analyzing this practice or others. In this case, is the location still vital or is the neighborhood declining? The equipment is now at least a decade behind the curve—will immediate upgrades be needed for the buyer to perform comfortably? Can you or can you not afford to pay a receptionist at the top of her salary range? Will the practice struggle if she is no longer there to greet patients? Although the overhead seems well controlled, will the buyer be able to do a comparable procedure mix that will maintain the current level of profitability? Will the age range between the new doctor and the majority of the patients be an issue? Will the landlord be agreeable to a lease assignment, or will he see this as an opportunity to make a dramatic increase in the terms? What if all of the custom cabinetry was configured for a left-handed dentist and most potential buyers are right- handed? All of these issues plus many other questions will have an effect on the final results, whether building up a summation of assets value or strictly performing a financial analysis.

Since the reader will not have access to computer models or statistical databases, we will provide the following numbers for this exercise.

Summation of assets: $462,650

Comparable sales price to gross revenues: $474,000 (the average of five similarly sized and located Midwest practices)

Comparable sales price to net income: $418,500

Excess earnings capitalized: $395,000 (20% cap rate)

Excess earnings would retire debt of approximately $593,000 (10 years @ 6%)

Given these numbers, what would be your asking price for this practice?

Remembering that there is no absolutely right or wrong answer, we would probably recommend that this practice be offered to the Midwest market somewhere between $460,000 and $490,000. We would guesstimate the probable selling price to be around $475,000. We would expect this practice to be on the market less than 1 year. Assuming all else besides market comparables being equal, the sales price would probably be less in our rural areas and much higher on either coast. The high value for excess earnings to retire debt is a function of the practice's well-controlled overhead and subsequent profitability. Had the excess earnings resulting from a 65% overhead been used instead of a 61% overhead, the resulting debt service number would only be about $370,000. This is another example of why overhead control is so important. Among others, keep especially Chapter 2 (financial statements) and Chapter 3 (practice financial performance) in mind in evaluating a practice opportunity.

The intent of this exercise is not to make you an expert appraiser but rather to further reveal the number of potential issues that must be taken into account in order to establish a working value for a practice. Please do not forget that we are working with a Midwest bias and that markets are different in other parts of the country. The methods used to calculate value are important, but every method may not be useful in every case. Curb appeal is still a strong component of a buyer's motivation and is difficult to quantify. The valuator must blend his or her experience with both objective and subjective information in order to ensure a fair price and successful transition.

Conclusion

Dental practice transitions and appraisals can be very delicate assignments. Sometimes seen by lenders as "mom and pop"-sized businesses, the owner/seller is placing his or her life's work on the line and, consequently, may have an emotionally inflated opinion about its value. Too high of an asking price results in frustration as the practice lingers on the market while the seller's motivation to keep the practice vital and productive wanes. Buyers may see the seller as being potentially unreasonable in other matters of the transition if they feel the asking price is too high. Too low of a value results in a reduced estate for the seller. The young buyer may have never purchased anything more costly than a second-hand car and cannot understand how a room full of used dental equipment can be worth much at all. The appraiser must maintain as objective of an opinion as possible about the value of the practice based on sound financial calculations, thorough research, and knowledge about the local market.

References and Additional Resources

Basic Business Appraisal. 1984. Boynton Beach, FL: Raymond Miles Southeast Business Investment Corporation.

Baumann, Paul and Berning, Randall. 2013. *The ADA Practical Guide to Valuing a Practice: A Manual for Dentists*, Chicago: American Dental Association.

Domer, Larry and Berning, Randall. 2006. *Valuing a Practice: A Guide for Dentists*, Chicago: American Dental Association.

Gabehart, Scott and Brinkley, Richard. 2002. *The Business Valuation Book*, New York: AMACOM.

Hill, Roger. 2006. *Transitions: Navigating Sales, Associateships and Partnerships in Your Dental Practice*, Chicago: American Dental Association.

http://www.healthcaregroup.com/general-dentistry.html

Pratt, Shannon, Reilly, Robert, and Schweihs, Robert. 1998. *Valuing Small Businesses and Professional Practices*, 3rd ed. New York: McGraw-Hill.

Learning Exercises

1. Determination of excess earnings
   A. Let's assume that the practice grossed $624,500 in collections in the last calendar year. The adjusted overhead was 57.4%. The practice has a hygiene staff that accounted for 30.5% of total revenues.

   What was the amount of excess earnings?

   B. The practice had gross revenues of $425,000 and the adjusted overhead was 61%. The doctor worked without a hygienist.

   What was the amount of excess earnings?
2. Normalization of expenses
   A. Which of the following would most likely NOT be adjusted to $0.00 in the process of normalizing a profit and loss statement or tax return?
      a. Depreciation of intangible assets
      b. Charitable donations
      c. Business interest
      d. Continuing education
   B. Which of the following may be adjusted by the evaluator to conform to industry standards?
      a. Dental supplies
      b. Advertising
      c. Property taxes
      d. All of the above
3. Excess earnings to retire debt (the sanity check)
   A. If a practice had gross revenues of $550,000 and an adjusted overhead of 58% without a hygienist, how much debt could the excess earnings support if we assume a 10-year loan at 6.0% interest?
   B. If the same practice increased revenues by $100,000 and reduced overhead to 56%, how much debt could be supported assuming the same loan terms?

Answers

1. A. Excess earnings
      Income: $624,500
      Overhead @ 57.4%: $358,463
      Net income: $266,037
      Dr. salary @ 28%: $174,860
      Excess earnings: $91,117
   B. Excess earnings
      Income: $425,000
      Overhead @ 61%: $259,250
      Net income: $165,750
      Dr. salary @ 30%: $127,500
      Excess earnings: $38,250
2. A. Normalization of expenses
      d. Continuing education
   B. Normalization of expenses
      d. All of the above
3. A. Sanity check
      Income: $550,000
      Overhead @ 58%: $319,000
      Net income: $231,000
      Dr. salary @ 30%: $165,000
      Excess earnings: $66,000
      Debt @ 6.0% for 10 years: $495.400
   B. Sanity check
      Income: $650,000
      Overhead @ 56%: $346,000
      Net income: $304,000
      Dr. salary @ 30%: $195,000
      Excess earnings: $109,000
      Debt @ 6.0% for 10 years: $818.100

Chapter 6
Dental Equipment

Mike Wacker

Tips on Buying New Equipment

This section addresses tips on purchasing what is considered large equipment items for a dental practice. Large equipment items consist of patient chairs, doctor's and assistant's seating, dental units, patient lights, dental cabinetry, sterilizers, intra-oral x-rays, 2D and 3D panoramic x-rays, x-ray film processors, intra-oral x-rays, phosphorus plate systems, digital sensors, air compressors, and vacuum systems.

When it's time to purchase new dental equipment, there are some important factors to consider, such as what best matches your needs and/or budget. There are some often overlooked or less obvious factors such as ergonomics, ease of use, operating expenses, and equipment maintenance to consider as well.

In some cases a piece of equipment you currently use may have a specific function or feature you feel you must have when purchasing a replacement. Be sure to discuss this need with a dental equipment specialist in order to avoid any disappointment with your purchase.

Seating

One area of dental equipment that has received much-needed manufacturer attention is seating ergonomics for the doctor, assistant, and the patient. There is a history of neck and back discomfort associated with practicing dentistry over an entire career; and manufacturers have worked diligently to revamp seating to help mitigate neck and back troubles. Figure 6.1 depicts correct posture for a dentist and dental assistant.

It is advisable to select doctor seating that has an adjustable seat and back. Avoid seating that has 90° corners and a nontilting seat bottom. Instead, purchase seating with a waterfall front edges on the seat bottom as well as a seat tilt feature. When the seat is properly adjusted you will not interrupt circulation in your legs. An adjustable seat back, when properly adjusted, will keep your back and neck from being hunched over. When purchasing doctor seating, keep in mind that one size does not fit all, so be sure to try out seating at a dental equipment supplier showroom or trade show.

The same is true for assistant seating regarding neck and back pain over an entire career of dental assisting. Assistant seating consists of a seat and upper body support. If

Dental Practice Transition: A Practical Guide to Management, Second Edition.
Edited by David G. Dunning and Brian M. Lange.
© 2016 John Wiley & Sons, Inc. Published 2016 by John Wiley & Sons, Inc.
Companion Website: www.wiley.com/go/dunning/transition

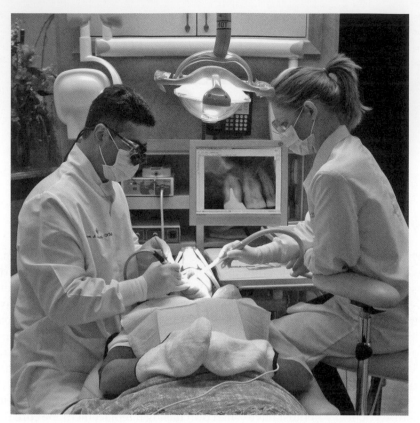

Figure 6.1.   Doctor in treatment: the treatment area must allow both the doctor and the assistant to see the operating field. Instrumentation must be easily transferred from the assistant to the doctor's finger rest.
Source: Photograph courtesy of Unthank Design Group, www.unthank.com.

your practice regularly performs lengthy procedures, the purchase of assistant seating with an optional backrest is recommended to help eliminate back and neck fatigue. As with the doctor's seating, waterfall front edges and seat tilt features are highly recommended for assistant seating.

Patient chair ergonomics has also undergone numerous studies and refinements for the benefit of the doctor as well as the patient. The recommended method of testing a patient chair is to place the chair into your working position (with someone in the chair if possible). Then, see if you can get close enough to the patient without straining your neck and back and also without pinching or trapping your legs under the reclined seat back. Also, check the accessibility of the patient chair controls while you are in the working position.

Patient comfort is also clearly important when considering the purchase of a patient chair. If the patient chair is too short or too narrow, has poor arm, lumbar, or shoulder support, or if the upholstery is too firm, the patient will become restless and unnecessarily tense. This causes the patient to frequently reposition themselves and, in turn, compromises your productivity. It is recommended you try out patient chairs at a dental equipment supplier showroom or tradeshow before making the purchase.

Dental Units

The dental unit is available as over-the-patient, orbit (also called left/right) unit, side delivery (wall or cabinet mount), and 12 o'clock (cart, wall, or cabinet mount). If you are undecided as to which to purchase, consider the following to help inform your decision. If your practice has both left-handed and right-handed doctors and hygienists, you might want to consider an orbit (left/right) dental unit, a cart with the left/right feature, a 12 o'clock wall-mounted unit, or a 12 o'clock cabinet with the left/right dental unit option. These units easily convert to left-handed or right-handed dentistry by simply rotating or sliding the unit from side to side.

Over-the-patient units, by contrast, are attached to either the left-hand or the right-hand side of the patient chair by way of a fixed steel bracket known as a chair adapter. In order to convert the unit to the opposite side of the patient chair, the unit must be removed from the chair. The steel chair adapter attached to the patient chair must be removed and reconfigured, or in some cases a new chair adapter must be purchased. The chair adapter and dental unit are then reinstalled onto the opposite side of the patient chair. Keep in mind that there are labor and possible parts costs associated with such a conversion.

If you practice four-handed dentistry, you can choose from the cart, 12 o'clock wall-mounted unit, or 12 o'clock cabinet with dental unit. It is recommended that you visit a dental equipment supply showroom or a dental tradeshow to study examples of these items. Refer to Figures 6.2 and 6.3.

Patient Lights

Another area with multiple choices is the patient light. Lights are available as ceiling-mounted, track (ceiling-mounted), wall-mounted, cabinet-mounted, orbit (also called left/right), chair-mounted, and unit-mounted.

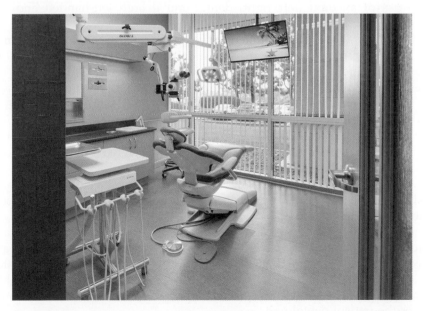

Figure 6.2. A single dual-function flexible rear delivery unit serves both the doctor and assistant.
Source: Photograph courtesy of Unthank Design Group, www.unthank.com.

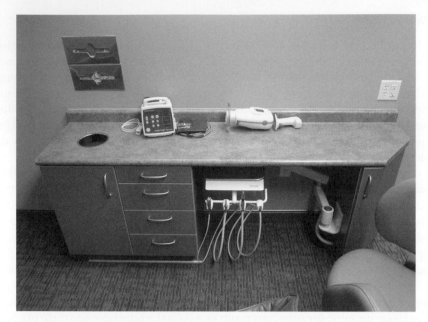

Figure 6.3.   Doctor's side delivery: when delivering the doctor's devices from the side wall or side cabinet, it locks the treatment room into being "handed." An opposite handed person cannot provide services with this arrangement.
Source: Photograph courtesy of Unthank Design Group, www.unthank.com.

The ceiling-mounted patient light is permanently attached to the ceiling on either the left-hand or the right-hand side of the patient chair and requires extra ceiling support or framing above the finished ceiling. The ceiling-mounted light is not recommended with the use of an orbit (left/right) dental unit if both left-handed and right-handed operators will be using this operatory.

The track light is also mounted to the ceiling and has a patient light mounted to a trolley that can be rolled toward the toe or head of the patient chair. This style of light can be used for left-handed or right-handed dentistry. Track lights also require extra ceiling support or framing above the finished ceiling.

The wall-mounted patient light attaches to a side wall, and the side depends on whether you practice left-handed or right-handed dentistry. The wall for this type of patient light has specific wall construction requirements that must be built. This style of light is not recommended if you are using the orbit (left/right) dental unit or if left-handed and right-handed operators will be using this operatory.

Cabinet-mounted patient lights are mounted onto a center island cabinet (center island cabinets are used in open concept style dental offices) and can be used with orbit (left/right) dental units.

Orbit (left/right) patient lights are attached to the patient chair and can be rotated from side to side around the toe end of the patient chair. This style of patient light is recommended when a practice has left-handed and right-handed operators.

Chair-mounted patient lights are attached to either the left or the right side of the patient chair. The same left/right conversion procedure applies here as outlined in the over-the-patient dental unit.

The unit-mounted patient light attaches to the over-the-patient dental unit that is attached to either the left or the right side of the patient chair. The same left/right conversion procedure applies here as outlined in the over-the-patient dental unit. It is recommended that you visit a dental equipment supply showroom or a tradeshow to see examples of these items.

Sterilizers

There are three types of dental sterilizers: dry heat, chemical, and steam.

Dry heat means the sterilizer uses heat only (no chemicals or water).

Chemical sterilizers use heat and chemicals for the sterilization process. The use of a charcoal filter helps to reduce the chemical odor emitted during operation.

Steam sterilizers use heat and distilled water for the sterilization process and are the most popular of the three types of sterilizer options. There are two types of steam sterilizers: recirculating and non-recirculating, offered as either manual or automatic models. The recirculating steam sterilizer reuses the distilled water each time a cycle is run. This type of sterilizer requires a frequent maintenance schedule. The non-recirculating steam sterilizer uses the distilled water for only one cycle. At the end of the cycle, the water is purged from the sterilizer into a container or into a drain. This type of sterilizer has higher distilled water usage but requires less maintenance.

Another version of the steam sterilizer is the "dry-to-dry" model. It is offered in the recirculating and non-recirculating versions as well. With this model, the instruments and/or handpieces are dried after the ultrasonic/disinfecting process and then placed into the sterilizer. The items inside the sterilizer go through an entire sterilization process, then a drying cycle, and then the sterilizer door opens when the sterilization cycle is complete. This type of steam sterilizer is more costly compared to other sterilizers and the sterilization process is longer due to the drying cycle. However, the contents are dry when the door opens at the end of the cycle.

After you have determined which type of sterilizer you want, you need to determine an appropriate size and whether you need more than one sterilizer. For example, if you use instrument cassettes, you will need a larger sterilizer. If you use sterilization pouches for instruments and/or handpieces, they should be laid in a single layer on the tray. If you use a cassette-style sterilizer, the pouches should be laid in a single layer on the bottom of the cassette. If pouches are multilayered, the middle layers will not completely sterilize, and if you have a dry-to-dry sterilizer, the middle layers will not dry. Also, multiple layers can shift and slide off to the side and touch the sterilizer chamber wall. This will result in burnt pouches and possible cycle failure. It is recommended that you have a larger sterilizer for larger loads and a smaller sterilizer for quick turnaround items (handpieces, specialty instruments, etc.). This also gives you the benefit of a backup sterilizer in the event one of the sterilizers breaks down. See Figure 6.4 for an example of a sterilization area.

Intra-Oral X-Ray Units

Intra-oral x-rays are offered as wall-mounted, mobile (mounted on a mobile stand), and handheld.

Intra-oral x-ray units produced today are capable of either film or digital x-ray imaging. When using film the exposure time is increased, resulting in a longer radiation exposure. In contrast, digital x-ray requires a lower exposure time, resulting in a much lower radiation exposure.

When setting up a new office or clinic, costs and cost savings are always an issue. Intra-oral x-rays can be set up in an x-ray room, one x-ray per operatory, in a pass-thru

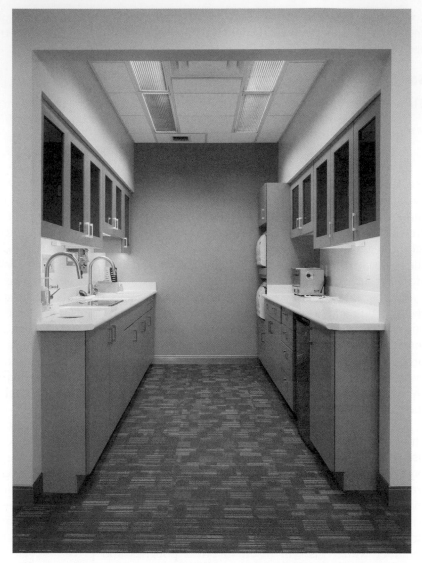

Figure 6.4. Sterilization: the sterilization area should provide a continuous flow of the instrumentation from the "contaminated" side to the "clean" side. Smoke glass upper cabinetry allows the team to see what each cabinet contains while patients simply see it as attractive cabinetry.
Source: Photograph courtesy of Unthank Design Group, www.unthank.com.

cabinet, or mounted on a center island. Consequently, the most expensive setup will be one x-ray unit in each operatory, and the use of an x-ray room will be the least expensive to set up. There are, however, other things to consider. Depending on the size of the practice, an x-ray room could cause a slowdown in productivity due to waiting for the room to become available. The pass-thru or center island option utilizes one x-ray unit mounted between two operatories, which will reduce costs. While this option will help reduce equipment costs, keep in mind that if that x-ray unit breaks down, two operatories will be unavailable for taking x-rays.

The handheld x-ray offers many benefits. It's a lower KVP and MA x-ray. When building a new office or adding operatories to an existing space, there is no need for specific wall construction or high- and low-voltage electrical wiring. The handheld is portable; so if in addition to your main office you have a satellite location, you can carry the handheld between the two locations. This reduces the number of wall-mounted x-rays to purchase as well as the number of x-rays registered with the state. The downside is this: if you have only one handheld x-ray and it gets dropped and knocked out of commission, you're unable to take x-rays until repairs are completed.

Panoramic X-Ray Units

Panoramic x-ray units produced today are capable of either film or digital x-ray imaging. Digital panoramics are available in 2D or 3D models. Exposure time between film-based and digital models is about the same. The reason for this is the distance the radiation must travel (from the tube head to the film/sensor) and the radiation must travel through the spine. If you purchase a film-based panoramic x-ray with intentions of upgrading the unit to digital in the near future, be sure to inquire whether a conversion will be possible for that unit. Also, it may be more cost-effective to purchase a digital panoramic unit initially instead of purchasing a film-based unit and then doing a digital conversion at a later date.

The panoramic x-ray is the one mechanical piece of equipment in the dental office that has the ability to pay for itself and continue to generate a significant income for the practice. Keep both your current and future needs in mind, purchasing the unit that best fits those needs. To keep costs down, do not purchase a unit that can be upgraded for features you will not use. For example, if you plan to take only panoramic x-rays, then try to purchase a unit that will do only panoramic x-rays. This unit will have a lower purchase price because it will not have the extra internal components necessary for the addition of a cephalometric. If you anticipate needing to take cephalometric x-rays in the near future, then purchase a unit that has the ability to add the cephalometric option. This type of unit will have the necessary internal components for a cephalometric upgrade but will also have a higher purchase price.

X-Ray Film Processors

X-ray film developing can be accomplished manually with the use of dip tanks, or automatically with the use of an automatic film processor. The dip tank method requires manually handling films through the entire developing, fixing, and rinsing process before exiting the darkroom. The automated film processor allows you to feed the films into the film processor, and once they are completely inside the machine, you can exit the darkroom. If a darkroom does not exist, the film processor can sit on a stand, cabinet, or countertop where space allows and will require purchasing an optional daylight loader. This is a small compartment that attaches to the film entry end of the processor for the handling of films without exposing the film to light.

Automated film processors are offered in an intra-oral only version and an intra-oral/extra-oral version. Intra-oral automatic film processors develop only intra-oral x-rays. These units are smaller, require less space inside the darkroom, and are less expensive to purchase than the intra-oral/extra-oral models. If you have a panoramic or panoramic/cephalometric x-ray, you will need the larger automatic film processor in order to develop both intra-oral and extra-oral films. Automatic film processors can be purchased as a plumbed or stand-alone model. The plumbed model is hooked up to a cold water supply line and a drain. The stand-alone model is totally self-contained, meaning the chemicals and water are pumped in and out of containers. These models use pumps to circulate the chemicals and water from containers into the automatic film processor, and then back into the containers. The stand-alone unit with a daylight loader offers the flexibility of placing an automatic film processor virtually anywhere within the dental practice. They are, however, more expensive than the plumbed automatic film processors.

The film-based x-ray process has a significant ongoing operating expense in the form of x-ray film, processing chemicals, and cleaning chemicals. Also, consider the amount of staff time required for the frequent maintenance of automatic film processors.

Lastly, the purchase of duplicating film and a film duplicator is necessary in order to send film(s) to another dental practice, insurance company, and so forth. Duplicating film is another item to be added to the list of ongoing operating expenses. The film duplicator will require a space in the darkroom.

X-ray film and x-ray film processors have had a steady decline in sales due to the technological advancements with phosphorus plate and digital sensors.

Digital X-Ray

There are two forms of digital x-ray available to the practitioner: phosphor plate technology and digital sensor technology. Determining which one is best for your practice involves understanding what each one has to offer.

Phosphor plate technology uses a phosphorus plate that is nearly the same size and shape of an x-ray film. Preparing to take an x-ray has the same setup steps as that of an x-ray film-based process. Once the image is captured on the phosphorus plate, it is placed into a light-proof container and carried to the scanner. The plate is removed from the container and placed into the reader. The reader is connected to a computer and monitor, and you are able to watch the image come up on the monitor as the phosphorus plate is being read. Processing a phosphor plate image is quicker than film-based processing but longer than digital sensor processing.

Digital x-ray software offers numerous features that allow you to manipulate images in a variety of ways as well as send images electronically. Phosphor plates are available in intra-oral and extra-oral sizes. Phosphor plate technology eliminates the need for duplicating film, a film duplicator, processing chemicals, cleaning chemicals, and the need for staff to perform routine maintenance. Care must be taken with the phosphor plate to avoid scratching or bending it. Phosphor plates are not repairable and do have a limited lifespan.

Digital x-ray uses a digital sensor with a wire coming out of the sensor that is connected to a computer to capture and show images. Once the x-ray is taken, it is available for viewing within seconds on the computer. The sensor is much thicker than film or phosphor plate and can be uncomfortable in smaller mouths or the posterior region. Digital x-ray software offers numerous features that allow you to manipulate images in a variety of ways as well as send images electronically. This technology replaces the use of x-ray film, a film processor, duplicating film, a film duplicator, and darkroom. Digital x-ray has a greater start-up cost (computers in each operatory, server, imaging software, etc.) but a considerably lower ongoing cost compared to its film-based counterpart. With ever-increasing improvements in image quality, reliability, increased manufacturer competition, and competitive pricing, digital sensors have become the preferred choice.

Dental Software

There are a number of practice management software systems available to the dental practitioner, and many of them offer you the ability to purchase only the modules you need. There are modules for scheduling, intra-oral imaging, panoramic imaging, and intra-oral cameras. It's a matter of finding a software system that fits your needs and budget and then working with a computer specialist for the installation. Many full-service dental companies offer software sales and installation of their software. Or, software not sold by a dental dealer can be installed by qualified independent computer specialists with a strong dental software background. Also, when shopping for software, coordinate with the software company about what hardware will be used. Some hardware and software combinations might require purchasing an additional bridge in order to allow the hardware and software to work together. Chapter 11 discusses technological integration in more detail.

Air Compressors

Air compressors are available as both lubricated and lube-free units, and both offer various sizes of units that are then matched to the number of users. Dental air compressors have built-in filtering systems in order to provide clean and dry air into the oral cavity. The lubricated models are quieter and usually less expensive than the lube-free models; however, they do require annual oil changes. On the other hand, the lube-free models do not require annual oil changes, and there is no risk of compressor oil ever getting into the air lines and dental unit(s). They do run a little louder than the lube-free models.

When purchasing an air compressor, consideration must be given to where the air compressor is placed within the facility and the decibel level generated from the unit. It might be necessary to purchase an optional sound cover that will help to reduce the decibel level.

Note: With the increasing reliability, quieter operation, and lack of potential oil contamination, some manufacturers have completely discontinued production of their lubricated air compressors.

Vacuum Systems

Dental vacuum systems are offered in two versions known as "wet-ring" or "dry." Both systems are sized based on the number of users. The wet-ring version is available as a single pump or dual pumps. Because of the compact size, especially the single pump, this system will fit into very small areas. A cold water supply line must be run to the pump(s), and the water is then injected into the operating pump(s). These pumps are offered in a water recycling version that reduces water consumption to approximately one-half (or less) of the nonrecycling versions.

The dry vacuum systems use an electric motor to drive a pump to create suction. While they use no water to create suction, they are larger and are more difficult to fit into confined spaces.

In terms of purchasing and ongoing costs, the wet-ring vacuum systems are less expensive to purchase than the dry vacuum systems. There is, however, a significantly increased water bill associated with the wet-ring vacuum system. In contrast, the dry vacuum systems have no impact on water bills, although their upfront purchase price is higher than the wet-ring vacuum pump option.

What to Look for in Used Equipment

This section provides you with important information if you're in the market for used dental equipment. As with anything used, it is important to know what questions to ask and what to watch out for. While some very good used dental equipment is offered for sale, you may also see some very old and even obsolete equipment for sale. In the case of buying or buying-into a practice (Chapter 7), it is critically important to have input from an independent equipment specialist when assigning value to the tangible and probably used equipment included in the practice sale.

Your Needs

As discussed in the new dental equipment section, you must first determine your dental equipment needs. If you are unsure of your needs, you can use the "Tips on Buying New Equipment" section above as a guide. The various types of dental equipment are explained and can help you determine your needs. It is very important to take time to carefully consider your equipment needs and not let yourself "settle" for something you may regret purchasing.

Age of Equipment

When considering the purchase of used dental equipment, it is to your benefit to research its age. If it is newer equipment, there may be the balance of a factory warranty still in effect. If it's older equipment, some parts or the entire unit may be obsolete, meaning that it may not be repairable (see below a more detailed discussion on obsolete equipment). Do not hesitate to ask the seller if he or she can produce documentation showing the purchase date. If the seller is unable to provide proof of the purchase date, the next step is to get the item model and serial number, manufacturer name, and, where applicable, model name. With this information, a dental equipment supplier should be able to give you at least a general idea of the manufacturing period. If you have at least a manufacturer name, model name (if applicable), and model number, the internet is another helpful resource. With this information, you should be able to learn the general manufacturing period. In some cases, having the serial number(s) during your internet research could also provide you with the year and month of manufacture.

Condition of Equipment

There are a number of things you can do to determine the condition of dental equipment. The most obvious is looking at the equipment's appearance. Look for missing or broken parts. If it's upholstered, is it discolored or torn? Dips in seat backs and seat cushions could indicate breakdown of the foam padding. If the surfaces are painted, look for discoloration, chipping, and flaking. If the surfaces are laminate, look for discoloration and chipping. Other red flags are sounds such as squeaking, grinding, snapping, rattling, leaks, or a loud electric motor hum. In some cases a squeak might be nothing more than a part needing to be cleaned and lubricated. A grinding or snapping sound might indicate a fatigued part or parts that could lead to costly repairs. Some equipment has been very well maintained but just needs some updating. An example of this is patient chairs, doctor seating, and assistant seating that has outdated or worn upholstery. Before you make a purchase, you should check with a dental equipment supplier on the availability and price of replacement upholstery packages.

Another area in which to exercise caution is with dental equipment that is, or has been, stored in a non-temperature-controlled storage in a freezing weather climate. If dental units and wet-ring vacuum pumps do not have the water purged with air before going into storage, the freezing temperatures will rupture water lines and crack metal parts. Needless to say, these are costly repairs, and in some cases the cost of parts and labor far exceeds the value of the unit.

If you purchase used dental equipment and intend to do some refurbishing, be aware of your total investment in the project. Remember, you are most likely refurbishing what is known to need attention. All other parts could still be original. After an initial purchase and refurbishing, you could end up putting as much as one-half (or more) of what new would have cost, and yet the used item is not completely refurbished and has no warranty.

Furthermore, consider the image your practice presents to your patients and prospective job applicants. Let's say you have one operatory you're going to equip with used dental equipment. You end up purchasing doctor seating, assistant seating, and a patient chair from three different sellers and may also end up with three different upholstery colors. There is also a good chance some or all of these upholstery colors may not match your operatory decor. Some new upholstery packages could make these items look as good as new for considerably less than purchasing all of these items new. Providing quality dental work to the patient is first and foremost. However, a neat, clean, updated facility and equipment are extremely important in creating a positive impression with patients, job applicants, and staff.

Red Flags

Obsolete dental equipment is knowingly and unknowingly offered for sale. In the "Age of Equipment" section of this chapter, tips were given for determining equipment age. A product is deemed obsolete when a manufacturer decides to stop producing it or if a manufacturer ceases to exist. Once the manufacturer's parts inventory is depleted, that source for parts is now gone. The next option would be checking for after-market parts companies that offer new replacement parts for a number of different equipment brands. However, not all parts are manufactured in the after market due to high manufacturing costs, low demand, or exclusivity to the original manufacturer. If you should happen to purchase obsolete dental equipment and new parts are not available, you can always shop the internet for replacement parts. Remember, the part you are looking for is probably going to be used and as old as the part you are replacing.

Other red flags are poorly performed repairs, air leaks, and fluid leaks. Look for electrical wires that have been taped. This could be covering bare or broken wires, and if this is part of a wiring harness, it could mean costly part(s) and labor repair. If you are looking to purchase a dental unit and the dental unit and junction box are still hooked up and in use, listen for air leaks and look for water leaks. When looking at a wet-ring vacuum pump, if at all possible try to hear it run because a loud squealing sound and/ or water leaking indicate needed repairs. If you are looking to purchase a used sterilizer, run one cycle from a cold start (first run of the day), and as soon as that cycle has finished, immediately run another cycle. On both cycles, note if the sterilizer reaches sterilization temperature or if it took a lengthy amount of time reaching sterilization temperature. Also check for leaks around the door or cassette and drips under the unit. If you observe any of these red flags, the sterilizing unit requires repairs.

Older hydraulic patient chairs are susceptible to hydraulic fluid leaks over time. Hydraulic hoses can split, and hydraulic cylinder seals can fail, which allows hydraulic oil to leak onto the chair base and/or floor. If parts are available, parts and labor costs range from moderate to expensive.

Air compressors also require a close inspection. They can have obsolete parts, rusty tanks, faulty electrical components, and slow recovery times. Lubricated compressors can have oil consumption issues that will allow oil to saturate filters and drying systems. This can also cause contamination of air lines and damage parts inside dental units, as well as emit oily-smelling air from the handpieces and the air side of the air/water syringe.

Valuation of Used Dental Equipment/Determining Fair Market Value

It is difficult to place a value on used dental equipment. The seller, who probably purchased the equipment new, remembers that it was very expensive when it was brand new. Even though the item might be 10 years old, the seller feels it's in great condition for its age, so it should be worth at least one-half (or more) of the new price. Another technique a seller may use is to ask a dental equipment dealer how much a like item costs today, then place his or her own value on the item. A buyer looking at the equipment may have a totally different opinion of the condition and value, and the result could be a no sale.

Because a used dental equipment price guide does not exist, a number of factors are considered in trying to determine a fair market value. The considerations are age, condition, parts availability, popularity, colors, and the cost if purchasing a new like item today. Oftentimes a buyer has already shopped the new equipment market prior to turning to the used market. The point here is this: as a seller you need to have some idea of what a fair price is but be willing to settle for what the market will bear. As a buyer, once you find what you're looking for, do your research before making an offer. Whether you are the buyer or seller, it is to your advantage to utilize available resources as a guide in determining a reasonable value for used equipment. One resource is your ADA chapter. The ADA distributes a newsletter that includes a "for sale" section that always has used dental equipment listed.

Another resource is internet auction sites. Individuals wanting to sell and companies that refurbish used dental equipment often post on auction sites. In either case you can't actually see the item(s) in person, so ask for photos from various angles and don't hesitate to ask questions. Keep in mind that in addition to the winning bid amount, you will most likely incur shipping and insurance expenses. Always cover yourself by asking for a written return and full refund guarantee in the event the item has missing parts or does not work upon receipt. This is especially important when purchasing any equipment that is easily damaged in shipment. For example, replacement circuit boards, if still available, are quite expensive. The filament in a used x-ray tube head is very fragile, and rough handling can ruin the tube head. If the tube head can be repaired or replaced, the repairs are extremely costly and in most cases will far exceed the value of the x-ray unit.

One other obvious resource for guidance on used dental equipment is dental equipment suppliers. They might be able to provide you with approximate time frames of manufacture dates, tips on what to look out for, information on reliability issues, and parts availability.

Maintaining Equipment

How to Maximize the Life of Your Equipment

Dental equipment requires a significant financial investment, so you will want to perform the necessary maintenance in order to maximize its life. As with anything mechanical, periodic maintenance is necessary, and it's simply a matter of getting a routine schedule set up and sticking to it. Because of the demands that will be placed on your time, you should assign equipment maintenance tasks to staff members as part of their job descriptions. Additionally, ask that your staff note and inform you if they hear air leaks or see water leaks, or if normal operating sounds change (that is, handpieces, air compressor, vacuum pump, etc.).

Oftentimes air compressors and vacuum pumps are placed in small closets or share a space with the furnace and water heater. Most of the time these rooms are not temperature controlled, so heat and humidity can be very high, especially in the summer. This causes the air compressor filtering system to become saturated with moisture, which will necessitate more frequent maintenance and higher maintenance costs. It is recommended to have a heating/air conditioning duct run to this space, with the duct open in the summer for the cold air. The duct should be closed for winter in order to keep additional heat out. Air leaks can be another source that will cause unnecessary stress and an early demise of your air compressor. Air leaks are most commonly found in the junction box where the dental unit connects to the plumbing and in the delivery unit. Air leaks are also possible where air-operated accessories are connected and within the accessory itself. Air leaks will cause your air compressor to run more frequently, causing unnecessary wear and tear.

If you own a lubricated air compressor, the oil level should be checked monthly. There is a sight glass on the side of each compressor head with a "FULL" indicator line next to the sight glass. To obtain the most accurate reading of the oil level, you should check it in the morning before the compressor is started. Checking the oil level when the compressor is cold will ensure all of the oil has drained down. Overfilling the air compressor with oil can cause damage. Each month when the oil is checked, you should also check for moisture in the tank. This is accomplished by slowly opening the valve at the bottom of the tank a few turns. Water (and sometimes air) may leak out. If water is coming out, let it drain completely and then close the valve tight. Failure to tighten the valve will result in an air leak.

The patient light is another item that when not cared for properly will result in costly repairs. The lens shield and the reflector should be cleaned with only water and a soft cloth. Glass cleaners or all-purpose cleaners will ruin the coating on the reflector, and paper towels will scratch the lens shield and reflector. You should never attempt to clean a patient light reflector that was just in use. The glass will be extremely hot and will crack if touched with a damp towel. Replacement reflector prices vary, but even the least expensive reflector could cost several hundred dollars.

Handpieces should never be placed in the ultrasonic cleaner or be doused with spray disinfectant, as this also causes expensive repairs. You should keep and post handpiece maintenance procedures for each manufacturer and type of handpiece you own. Maintenance procedures can vary by manufacturer, so care must be taken to follow their maintenance steps so as not to void any warranty and prolong the life of the handpiece. Any debris not removed prior to sterilization will be baked, possibly permanently, onto the handpiece and/or fiberoptics. There are some duties that need to be performed, but that are not part of the manufacturer's recommended maintenance schedules. The next section will cover setting up maintenance calendars for various manufacturers' equipment.

Some of the following duties are to be performed daily:

- If you have a chemical or steam sterilizer, at the start of the business day, you should check the fluid level in the reservoir. If the level is low, fill the reservoir to the "FULL" mark.
- If you use water bottle systems to supply water to delivery units and air/water syringes, fill the bottles with distilled water at the start of each business day. This will help to avoid running out of water during a procedure.
- If you have a plumbed-in nitrous system, turn the system on and check the gauges on the nitrous and oxygen tanks for pressurization and tank levels.
- Turn the air compressor on and check in the operatory, at the dental unit, for air to the handpieces and air/water syringe.
- Turn the vacuum system on and check in the operatory for suction to the assistant's utilities.
- At day's end, a vacuum line cleaner should be run through all saliva ejectors and high-volume evacuators (HVEs), which will disinfect the vacuum lines.
- Change or clean the solids collector in the operatory at day's end.

There is also a simple test you can perform semiannually that can tell you if there are air leaks that may be causing your air compressor to work harder than necessary. To perform this test requires a minimum of one hour and a time when dental units and air-operated accessories are not in use, so a lunch hour is ideal. After the last patient is seen just before lunch, run some handpieces and air syringes until the air compressor starts. Place the syringes and handpieces back on the dental unit and leave the dental units, any air-operated accessories, and the air compressor on. For the next hour listen to see if the air compressor starts up, and if so, note how many times it starts within that hour. If the air compressor starts at all during this hour, there are definitely air leaks that must be serviced in order to maximize the life of the compressor.

Manufacturer's Maintenance Schedules

With the purchase of any new equipment, you will receive a manual that covers use and care instructions. Oftentimes some pieces of equipment with specific maintenance requirements will have a separate maintenance document that can be posted near that unit as a reminder to perform maintenance. It can't be stressed enough to always follow the manufacturer's recommended maintenance procedures. Documented maintenance is critical in the event of a repair during the warranty period. By following the manufacturer's maintenance schedule, you will maximize the life of the equipment. Because each piece of equipment might be on a different maintenance schedule, you should set up a maintenance calendar to keep track of the various schedules.

Air compressors have an annual maintenance (under normal operating conditions). Annual maintenance for a lubricated air compressor is an oil change and filter(s) and drying system maintenance. Annual maintenance for a lube-free air compressor is filter(s) and drying system maintenance. Wet-ring vacuum pumps should have the solids collector cleaned (or replaced if using a disposable solids collector) each week at week's end.

The sterilizer door gasket should be checked daily for proper fit and for any cuts or tears. The gasket and chamber opening surface should be checked for debris. A worn, cut, or dirty door gasket and/or chamber opening surface will cause the sterilizer cycle to fail before the instruments and/or handpieces are sterilized. If you have a recirculating sterilizer (the distilled water is used over and over), you will need to perform a thorough maintenance procedure after several cycles. The use and care guide will provide you with the specific number of cycles you can run before this maintenance must be performed. Failure to comply will result in an extremely dirty-looking chamber and water reservoir and in premature failure of some of the internal components and costly repairs.

Upholstery Care and Maintenance

Doctor and assistant seating upholstery, as well as the patient chair upholstery materials, are offered today in vinyl or ultraleather. While both materials are very durable, vinyl has a stiffer feel to the touch while ultraleather has much softer feel. A patient chair with ultraleather upholstery is very appealing and relaxing to the patient. There are some things you will want to do to get as much life as possible from your upholstered items. Before seating the patient in the patient chair, try to notice if any sharp objects are in their back pockets. There are numerous horror stories about sharp objects in back pockets that puncture a hole in the patient chair upholstery. Ink pens are a double threat because they can puncture or cause ink stains. Also be watchful for leather apparel that has been freshly dyed, as this has been known to stain upholstery as well.

As for cleaning of the doctor and assistant seating upholstery and patient chair upholstery, avoid disinfectants with high alcohol content. Repeated use will discolor and crack upholstery and will significantly reduce the useful life of the material. Many dental offices now use a plastic barrier on the patient chair, which eliminates using harmful chemicals. The barrier is discarded after each patient, and a new barrier is placed on the patient chair before the next patient.

On a final note, most new doctor and assistant seating upholstery and patient chair upholstery have a 1-year warranty against manufacturing defects.

Final Helpful Hints

The "Tips on Buying New Equipment" section covered purchasing new equipment. If you plan on acquiring more than one bid for dental equipment, make sure bids are for *the exact same equipment*. One dental equipment supplier may have brand "X." Another dental equipment supplier may have brand "Y" and may tell you it's just like brand "X." If brand "X" is what you really want, try to find another dealer that carries that brand.

Lastly, a word of advice is needed for those of you building a new practice or remodeling space. Consistent and clear communication is absolutely essential within your team—you, your staff, your dental equipment supplier, your architect, and construction contractors. Confirm that everyone on the team is literally on the same page and has the same understanding from conceptualization/planning to each phase of actual construction. This will help avoid potentially very costly mistakes that may be made because of errant assumptions.

References and Additional Resources

Some Manufacturer's Websites

A-dec: http://us.a-dec.com/en/
Belmont: www.belmontequip.com.

Brasseler: http://brasselerusa.com/
DentalEZ: http://www.dentalez.com/products/dentalez
Gendex: http://www.gendex.com/home-pages-1.php
KaVo: www.kavousa.com
Marus:http://marus.com/.
Midmark: www.midmark.com.
Pelton and Crane: www.pelton.net.
Premusa: http://www.premusa.com/home/default.asp
American Dental Association, Review of dental manufacturers by name, location, and
   product:
http://www.ada.org/en/publications/ada-professional-product-review-ppr/
   manufacturers-and-distributors

Some Supplier Websites

Benco Dental: www benco.com
Goetze: www.goetzedental.com.
Patterson Dental: www.pattersondental.com.
Sullivan-Schein Dental: www.henryschein.com/us-en/DENTAL/default.aspx.

Other Sources

Internet auction sites.
State dental associations.

Learning Exercise

Assume that you are going to purchase your own dental practice. You have a
building with a favorable lease, but the existing dental equipment is in need of
replacement. Now you are in the process of making the decision to buy equipment.

1. Describe the decision-making process that you will employ.
2. Review and if necessary expand the following partial list of questions you
    need to answer:
    *   How much can you spend?
    *   What used, in-place equipment can be/should be purchased?
    *   What is the fair market value of the used equipment you plan to purchase,
        and how will you determine or negotiate its sales price?
    *   What new equipment will you need to buy?
    *   Will someone help you decide or recommend what to replace?
    *   Will the replacement equipment be new, used, or a combination of both?
    *   How will you price the equipment?
    *   What type of service agreement will you need?
    *   Will you remodel? If so, how long will it take to remodel the office?
    *   Will you replace the units one at a time or all at once?
    *   What other issues need to be addressed?
    *   What other questions need to be asked?
    *   What other information do you need to make decisions?

Chapter 7
Buying/Buying into a Practice
Nader A. Nadershahi and Lucinda J. Lyon

Business, more than any other occupation, is a continual dealing with the future; it is a continual calculation, an instinctive exercise in foresight.

Henry R. Luce

For most dentists, the choice of purchasing a practice is one of the top three largest decisions you will make in your life. This is true if you take the perspective of how it can affect your quality of life, finances, and professional satisfaction. This is exactly why it is important to spend the time necessary to make a well-informed decision based on a thorough evaluation of each opportunity.

In this chapter, we explore two of the most common paths of entry into dental practice. The first path we discuss is buying a dental practice, where the owner sells the entire dental healthcare service business to the buyer. The second path is buying into a practice where the owner is selling a share of the business to the buyer, who will become a partner or shareholder. Many other chapters in this volume complement key points in this chapter, particularly: financial statements (Chapter 2), practice financial analysis (Chapter 3), business planning (Chapter 4), practice valuation (Chapter 5), financing a practice (Chapter 9), and personal and business insurance (Chapter 26).

Our learning objectives are that after reviewing this chapter, you should understand the following:

1. The different variables that should be considered in choosing the location of practice
2. The difference between buying and buying into a practice
3. What to look for in each transaction
4. How to work with other professionals to protect your interests

In modern business it is not the crook who is to be feared most, it is the honest man who doesn't know what he is doing.

William Wordsworth

Dental Practice Transition: A Practical Guide to Management, Second Edition.
Edited by David G. Dunning and Brian M. Lange.
© 2016 John Wiley & Sons, Inc. Published 2016 by John Wiley & Sons, Inc.
Companion Website: www.wiley.com/go/dunning/transition

Choosing the Right Location

This section is intentionally placed first in the chapter because it is a critical part of the decision-making process in the purchase of a practice but is often overlooked. If you find an outstanding opportunity in an area that does not provide the elements that will allow for a happy personal and professional life, it is not the right opportunity for you. Whether you decide to buy a practice or buy into a practice, the first decision should be to find the general area where you want to live and work.

Quality of Life

With some of the changes that are occurring in licensure in the United States, such as larger regional examinations and reciprocity between states, a doctor is not locked into one location as much as in the past. What you must do is to start globally and begin to narrow down the area where you want to establish your professional roots. There are many questions to consider as you make this quality-of-life decision:

1. Do you want to be near certain friends or family members?
2. Do you and your family like living in a rural area, the suburbs, or a big city?
3. What recreational outdoor activities are you interested in, such as snow sports, water sports, or hunting?
4. Do you want to have access to certain cultural activities such as the opera, theater, or sporting venues?
5. Are you looking for an area to live where there are certain schools or other options available to you?
6. Does the community offer work in your spouse, or significant other's profession?

These and many other questions pertaining to the quality of life you will have are critical in narrowing down your options of where you will start your search for a practice to buy or buy into.

Professional Environment

After you have decided on some specific areas and communities that meet your personal needs, it is time to consider the professional environment. A specialist will want to locate a practice in an area where there are sufficient general practitioners and an appropriate population to maintain a healthy referral practice. As a general dentist, you would like to ensure that there are other professionals that you can work with to create a provider team as necessary for your patients. For example, if you believe some surgical procedures are outside your range of expertise or if you choose not to include them among your list of services, you should ensure that there are an adequate number of oral and maxillofacial surgeons or periodontists whom you can work with to serve the treatment needs of your patients.

You will also want to ensure that there is access to other professionals who may be valuable in the coordinated, interprofessional treatment of your patients, or as a source of referral and support for your practice. This team might include, for example, physicians, public health nurses, pharmacists, psychologists, and others.

Business Environment

The next area of evaluation is the business environment. This can be divided into the internal and external business environments. We touch on the internal environment in other areas of the book as we discuss issues associated with employees (Chapters 22–24), systems (such as scheduling appointments in Chapter 14), and other internal aspects of a dental practice. The focus of this section is the *external* business environment.

When choosing the right location to practice, you should look at all of the stakeholders in the business environment that have some effect on the practice of dentistry. In *Business and Its Environment*, Baron (1996) describes the external environment as the "market environment" that would include effects on your production, relationship and response to your patients, innovation, and incorporation of new procedures and techniques into your practice. Chapters 12 and 13 highlight some of the marketplace implications of dental fees and dental benefits. The "nonmarket environment" is the interaction with public institutions that are not driven by the private markets. Examples of nonmarket influences include environmental protection (EPA), health and safety (OSHA), other regulations (HIPAA, radiation safety, etc.), public responsibility, and ethics. These influences have slowly increased the demands placed on the management of a practice. Chapter 15 discusses some areas of government compliance.

It is important to ensure that you have an idea of what regulations and forces will affect your dental practice and to ensure that there are no regulations or forces from the external environment that would make it difficult to succeed in your small business. For example, some cities or towns will be more welcoming of professional businesses, and others create regulatory obstacles and costs that would discourage you from maintaining a practice in that location.

Alignment with Goals

Finally, as you narrow down your decision of where to practice, you want to ensure that the location will allow for a practice that is aligned with your personal and professional goals. This step would arguably be the first to consider, but all of the items discussed in this section hold equal weight in the decision-making process. Chapter 1 introduced you to some life goal questions.

Planning and goal setting are key components of success. You may have heard someone describe a study conducted at Yale University on the class of 1953, where researchers surveyed the seniors and found that only 3% of them had specific written goals. After 20 years the researchers found that the 3% with specific goals had accumulated more financial wealth than the other 97% of the class combined. Now whether this story is true or not (most likely not, since several articles have been written challenging the veracity of this story including Tabak (1996/1997) in *Fast Company*), setting goals is an important step toward personal and business success.

If you have not done so already, it would be wise to consider setting both short- and long-term goals for yourself. These goals can be broken down into 1-year and 3-year ones and then separated into personal and professional. There are many who subscribe to SMART goals, attributed to George T. Doran (1981). These are goals that are

- specific—clear, concise, simple,
- measurable—ensure tangible evidence that you've accomplished your goal,

- achievable/actionable—goals should include a stretch, but be attainable,
- relevant—consistent with your needs, and
- time-bound/trackable—include due dates to increase accountability.

Your personal goals may include health, family, retirement, travel, or recreation. Professional goals may include quantitative items such as number of new patients seen, revenue, or size of staff. They may also include qualitative goals such as practice image, range of services provided, how much time you will devote to providing care for the underserved in your community, or who your target market will be. Goal setting is discussed in Chapter 22 with respect to staff management and in Chapter 25 with respect to financial planning.

Choosing a location that will allow you to achieve as many of your personal and professional goals as possible will support more satisfying progress towards a successful practice career. If you intend on providing care for pediatric patients, you should avoid areas that have a population demographic that shows a continued growth in the older age ranges with little growth of children, new families, and new schools. On the other hand, if you intend to build a practice that is geared toward comprehensive prosthodontics, implants, or aesthetic dentistry, you will need to ensure that all of the demographics and the professional environment will support such a practice.

Deciding to Buy out or Buy into a Practice

In this chapter we are assuming that you have chosen not to start a practice from scratch. The scratch practice may include taking on more risk initially, with a potential for much larger rewards. It may also offer the opportunity to build a practice in exactly the way that you want, and to grow the business and equity more quickly. Practice start-ups will be covered in more detail in Chapter 8. Alternatively, many individuals will choose the path of entering a business that is already a going concern so that there is a built-in cash flow on day 1, as opposed to starting from scratch and building the cash flow. That is what we will focus on throughout the remainder of this chapter. There are several broader issues to consider in making your decision that we discuss initially and then compare and contrast some specifics about each type of transaction.

Opportunity Cost

Buying a practice, buying into a practice, and starting a practice from scratch are the three most common forms of practice entry. Practice valuations are discussed in Chapter 5 and financing a practice in Chapter 9. All of these discussions usually focus on the actual cost, or how much we are paying out of pocket or through the attainment of a private, commercial, or federally backed small business loan. Another concept of cost that is commonly overlooked in the dental practice marketplace is *opportunity cost*. In the text *Essentials of Corporate Finance*, Ross et al. (1996) describe opportunity cost as "the most valuable alternative that is given up if a particular investment is undertaken." In other words, when you are deciding to buy a practice, you should look at what other options, and potential gain, you are giving up for that dollar amount. What other options exist in the marketplace for a buy-in or practice start-up for that same $500,000 that you are planning on investing in a practice purchase? Another example would be if you already have an established practice and are looking at another that is for sale. What is the cost of everything you are giving up in your existing practice? Will you choose to sell your practice, the equipment, and the patient charts, or move some of your assets to the new location? An understanding and assessment of opportunity cost will allow you to evaluate all other alternatives as you strive to make the most informed choice when selecting a buyout or buy-in transaction.

Solo Practitioner or Partner

Another very important decision to make early in your decision process has to do with the type of practice that you want. Do you want to work in an office by yourself as the solo doctor, or do you want to be in a setting where there are other general practitioners and/or specialists? This decision should be made based on your personal style and professional interests.

A solo practitioner has the flexibility of making all of the decisions and serving as the leader in the practice. He or she will create the vision, mission, and goals for the practice, and then create an environment where those goals can be achieved. The solo practitioner also owns all of the responsibility when it comes to the management of staff, practice systems, finances, and all other aspects of the business operation.

Over time, more and more dentists appear to be pursuing partnership or group practice opportunities. In some ways, these options probably afford a practitioner the ability to focus more on performing the dentistry and less on the management of the business operations. A partnership or group practice may also create a built-in professional support system for the practitioner. The business management responsibilities and leadership roles may be shared or divided in a way that allows for each individual to take advantage of his or her personal strengths and focus on what he or she is interested in doing in the practice. Being in a partnership or a group does, however, require that you come to a consensus or compromise about important business decisions such as major purchases or employee issues. There needs to be clearly delineated roles for each doctor to avoid confusion among the partners or the staff about how decisions are made and work is completed.

Once you have made the choice to be a sole proprietorship (buying) or a partnership (buying-in), you need to consider, with the help of your accountant and attorney team, the type of business that already exists in the practice and what business entity you want to establish. The most common forms of business structure for a healthcare practice in the United States are as a sole proprietor, a partnership, a limited liability company, or a corporation. Details about these options are discussed further in Chapter 10.

Transition Considerations

Your decision on which transition route to choose may have to do with your current situation or options. At this time, or in future, you may have the opportunity to work in a practice as an associate, leading to partnership or a buyout. If this is the case, then you must have a clear understanding of what that transition period will look like. You and the current practice owner should discuss the details and create a *written agreement or memorandum*, with legal advice, that is attached to your employment contract. This memorandum will prevent any misunderstandings on the part of either party as time passes. Items to incorporate in this memorandum include, but are not limited to, the length of time before a purchase option is available, how and when practice value will be determined, details of how the purchase will be paid off, what the business entity will become after the transition (partnership, sole proprietor with or without an associate, corporation, etc.), and what the role of the selling doctor will be in the practice after the purchase has occurred.

Other Doctors Who Will Remain in the Practice

If the practice that you are considering buying or buying into has other doctors who work in the office, there are several questions that you will need to consider.

1. What is the configuration of the employment arrangement? Are these doctors employees or independent contractors? There are several considerations here that have different tax and legal implications, so you will want to ensure you have the proper advisors as you review this information. Table 7.1 describes some general differences between an employee and an independent contractor.

    Additionally, you will need to ensure that there is an employment agreement with each associate or employee and that it is transferable to you as appropriate. For example, if you are paying for a practice with the production of associates used as part of the determination of a final price, you will lose equity immediately if the covenant not to compete does not transfer to you and the associates take their patients and production to another office.
2. What is the relationship between the seller and these doctors? It's a good idea to assess this relationship and determine why this individual or individuals did not purchase the practice. Maybe they were not interested because of some problems that you have not noted yet, or maybe they are upset that the selling doctor did not give them the opportunity to buy in or buy the practice. You will have to manage that relationship after you take over.
3. What is the contact between the remaining doctors and the patients? The evaluation here would be to see whether these doctors have been seeing the patients in the practice on a regular basis and determine whether there is a greater chance that the patients would want to see them instead of you after the selling doctor is out of the practice.

    Chapters 20 and 21 respectively discuss associateship career paths in traditional private practice and dental service organization contexts.

Table 7.1   General comparison of employee versus independent contractor.

Employee	Independent Contractor (IC)
Paid by employer in regular amounts at slated intervals	Employer pays on formula or flat rate
Employee may receive benefits	No benefits
Employer pays taxes	Employer pays no taxes
Employer hires staff	IC hires staff
Employer responsible for equipment and supplies	IC responsible for equipment and supplies
Employer has the right to direct or control the way the work is done	IC has full control—sets own hours, controls how to accomplish tasks

Due Diligence

Due diligence is a noun and has to do with the process that a reasonable person will use to avoid harm financially and personally as he or she collects and evaluates all of the necessary information before making a business transaction. In the purchase of a dental practice or buying into a dental practice, you will need to consider a number of things in your due diligence process. The following sections discuss in more detail the cash flow considerations, operational systems, facilities and equipment, and personal considerations related to the selling doctor or other partners.

Cash Flow Considerations

In real estate, we know that the three most important considerations are location, location, and location. Well, in business, the three most important considerations are cash flow, cash flow, and cash flow. Now, we understand that this is a simplistic view of a healthcare practice and that there are many other considerations, not the least of which being the oral health of the patient and the public. However, if you do not manage the cash flow of your business, you will not be able to provide your great services to anyone in your community. Bear in mind the importance of cash flow in previous chapters, especially Chapter 2 (financial statements) and Chapter 4 (business planning).

In any transaction to buy or buy into a practice, you will want to closely review the financial status of the practice and create a *forecast or pro forma income statement*. These tools will allow you and your accountant to make some informed decisions on the likelihood that the practice opportunity you are evaluating will be able to support the practice overhead, service the debt you may incur on the practice, and provide you income to meet your personal living budget.

You will want to ask the selling doctor for several financial items to review as you are evaluating any purchase transaction: the last 3–5 years of financial statements (income statements and balance sheets), tax returns for the same period, bank statements to reconcile with the financial statements, an accounts receivable report including aging, and copies of any leases that are in force. Let's discuss each of these items and what you are generally looking for with each.

Financial Statements and Tax Returns

When you review the financial statements and tax returns from the last 3–5 years, you should first look at any trends that are displayed by the practice. For example, has the production decreased over the last few years, or have expenses suddenly increased? You will need to dig a little deeper and find out the reasons behind such changes and then decide if they are acceptable to you in making the final transaction. You and your accountant can also look at some bank statements if the seller is willing to review them with you to ensure that the financial statements, tax returns, and bank statements reconcile with one another.

Let's look at a few examples and discuss the kind of information you would request in addition to what is provided.

Practice A (see Table 7.2) is located in a large suburban city that has seen great growth and rising income levels. The selling doctor has been in this practice for 15 years and is

Table 7.2   Sample Practice A.

	2016	2015	2014	2013	2012
Revenue ($)	698,733	641,039	588,110	539,550	495,000
Expenses ($)	647,132	562,724	489,325	425,500	370,000

Table 7.3   Sample Practice A with net income/profit.

	2016	2015	2014	2013	2012
Revenue ($)	698,733	641,039	588,110	539,550	495,000
Expenses ($)	647,132	562,724	489,325	425,500	370,000
Net Income ($)	51,601	78,316	98,785	114,050	125,000

retiring from dentistry to focus on family and other interests. The patient base is made up almost entirely of employees from a transistor design and fabrication company. The existing doctor does minimal marketing and is only working with one preferred provider plan and other indemnity-type insurance plans.

The good points about this practice are the sustained growth of the area and the fact that the growth has translated to increased productivity with minimal resources put into marketing. However, there are two areas where you will want to go deeper for more information.

First, as you can see from Table 7.3, once you do the calculations of net income, the practice has become less profitable over the years despite the growth of revenues. As a matter of fact, the expenses have grown at a rate of 15%, where revenue has only grown at a rate of 9% annually. You will want to see if this is a trend that you could have any control over changing or if it is due to the rising cost of salaries and rent, which would be difficult for you to affect with closer management. The second area of concern is when you go into an area where the growth and patient base are related to only one major employer. You need to assess the risk of this semiconductor company going out of business, downsizing, or sending its fabrication business offshore. Any of these actions could have a significant impact on your ability to maintain a viable dental practice because the large majority of patients come from this business.

Practice B (see Table 7.4) is located in a rural area that has seen little growth and stable income levels from farming.

The selling doctor has been in this practice for 12 years and is selling to move her family to a different state. The patient base is made up of employees and residents in a 50-mile radius from the practice. The existing doctor does minimal marketing and is compensated by cash payment or indemnity insurance payments.

In this example the first thing you will notice is that the productivity has been somewhat erratic, with a significant drop in 2014 When you complete the calculations

Table 7.4   Sample Practice B.

	2016	2015	2014	2013	2012
Revenue ($)	540,250	495,642	359,250	539,550	495,000
Expenses ($)	466,475	405,630	420,219	425,500	370,000

Table 7.5 Sample Practice B with net income.

	2016	2015	2014	2013	2012
Revenue ($)	540,250	495,642	359,250	539,550	495,000
Expenses ($)	466,475	405,630	420,219	425,500	370,000
Net Income ($)	73,775	90,012	−60,969	114,050	125,000

for net income you will see in Table 7.5 that the practice actually suffered a loss during that year. So although this practice had in 2012 an identical financial pattern as Practice A, there was a large change in 2014. When you ask more questions you find that this doctor suffered a personal injury in 2014 that she was not comfortable revealing in the early phases of disclosure. She has shown good growth again since the injury, so this may be a good opportunity for you to pursue further.

In these two examples, you see some variations from the usual steady growth in profitability that occurs with many practices, but they illustrate the fact that you need to review the financial statements and use them as a source to continue a deeper evaluation of the practice you are considering.

Accounts Receivable

The accounts receivable (A/R) report will help you obtain a better understanding of the efficiency of the office and the systems that are in place for the financial management of patient accounts. The first item to evaluate in the A/R report is the quantitative aspect, which is the size of the A/R. For example, if the practice has an average production of $35,000 per month and the A/R report shows a total A/R of $100,000, there are some red flags about the collection processes and financial arrangements that are made in the office (see Chapter 12 for recommendations about collections and financial arrangements). An A/R of almost three times the monthly revenue is not a healthy number for an office to maintain, and this places a huge strain on the cash flow of the practice. You will want to look for a number that is closer to an A/R to revenue ratio of 1. The following examples illustrate what we are talking about:

$$A/R \quad = \$100,000$$
$$Revenue \quad = \$35,000$$
$$A/R/Rev = \$100,000/\$35,000 = 2.86$$

$$A/R \quad = \$35,000$$
$$Revenue \quad = \$35,000$$
$$A/R/Rev = \$35,000/\$35,000 = 1.00$$

Next you will want to make a qualitative assessment of the A/R. You should receive an A/R aging report, which gives you the A/R by the length of time since that receivable was accrued or when the treatment was posted to the patient's account. Patient financial arrangements should be in writing and reside within each patient's digital or paper chart or alternatively established location.

Let's look at the example of Practices C and D (see Tables 7.6 and 7.7). Both practices have monthly revenues that average $46,000 and A/R of $88,000, giving us a slightly

Table 7.6   Sample accounts receivable aging report for Practice C.

	<30 days	30–60 days	60–90 days	>90 days	Total
Accounts Receivable ($)	45,000	23,000	8,000	12,000	88,000

Table 7.7   Sample accounts receivable aging report for Practice D.

	<30 days	30–60 days	60–90 days	>90 days	Total
Accounts Receivable ($)	38,000	10,000	0	40,000	88,000

high A/R/Rev ratio of 1.91. On the surface, these two practices would look the same. However, as you look at the A/R aging report, you will see that Practice D is doing a really good job of collecting in the first 3 months, but there is a history of bad debt that is over 90 days old. Practice D has almost half of its A/R tied up in the over-90 category, which is much harder and less likely to be collected than the shorter term receivables. This may be due to a change in financial policies in the practice, or a new staff member who has come in and cleaned up the accounts. It is unlikely that you would want to purchase this A/R from the selling doctor, as you have only a small chance of getting a few pennies on the dollar with debt that goes out that far without more extensive collection processes, which you do not want to incur as a new owner in the practice.

If the practice participates in third-party payer agreements, for example, HMOs, PPOs, capitation programs, and so on, these will influence cash flow and account receivables. Chapters 12 and 13 will help you understand these reimbursement models more thoroughly.

Existing Equipment Leases

The final item we mentioned above that you would request from the selling doctor is information on any existing equipment leases. In this case, whether you are buying or buying into the practice, you should understand how the business is committed to these leases and if you are going to take over the responsibility of such leases. We do not recommend this as a first option, but you must discuss that as part of your negotiation of the purchase price. For example, you have agreed that the equipment has a value of $180,000, and the dental units and a CAD CAM machine are included in that price. These items have another 8 years of payments remaining, so your first choice would be to ensure those obligations are paid off as part of the transaction, or you can work with your accountant and come up with a value that would account for the depreciation and the net present value of the remaining payments. This can become complicated, so it is in the best interests of all parties to pay these leases off as the transaction comes to a close.

Financial Forecasting

After you have obtained and reviewed, to your satisfaction, all of the financial information and reports from the selling doctor, the final step in performing your due diligence as it relates to the cash flow is financial forecasting. This is another area where your accounting professional can help you with his or her experience.

One financial forecasting document that is created for a business is referred to as the *pro forma income statement*. This is basically the same as a standard income statement except for the fact that it is an educated guess of the forecast income, expenses, and profit or loss based on the historical information that you have at hand. This exercise of developing a pro forma income statement will help you evaluate the financial return potential of different purchase opportunities. It is also one of the financial documents that any lender will require if you are asking for a business loan. Figure 7.1 is an example of a pro forma income statement for a fictitious practice showing that this specific practice purchase would break even in terms of total expenses in the fifth month and eventually meet the personal living budget of the doctor (in Figure 7.2) in month 11.

Operational Systems

The first and arguably most important management system has to do with staffing. As you evaluate the practice, you should review the number of staff members in each position and decide if the office is over- or understaffed. For example, if the one-doctor practice you are looking to buy has three people working at the front desk, but the revenue and activity in the practice only support one position, this may be an area where you could decrease expenses in the future. The opposite may also be true with a general practice that has a need for more staffing to maintain growth. Another staffing consideration is if there is a family member of the selling doctor or a partner working in the office. This may create some conflicts or loyalty issues that should be considered and addressed in the beginning of the negotiation process. The turnover of staff is also important to note. Staff who have been in the office for a short period of time will not have the same connection with patients, and an entirely new team of doctors and staff may lead to a larger-than-normal attrition of patients after the transition. Staff who have been with a doctor for many years will take longer to develop a relationship of trust with the new owner as well. Finally, you should ensure that there is a good employee policy manual. This is important to outline some of the policies and procedures for the office and also to meet some of the nonmarket environmental regulations we discussed earlier. The bottom line with staff will be that they are the ones who help you succeed and you need to understand them, build a relationship with them early, and empower them to help you succeed. Chapter 23 includes a suggestion for individual staff interviews with the new practice owner.

The practice management software system in the office will also provide you with some other valuable office systems information to review. You can look at the fee schedule in the office and make a decision on the appropriate nature of those fees. You can also review reports such as demographics on where patients are coming from and the service mix of procedures that are most commonly performed by the office to ensure a fit with your professional goals. The system can also provide information on the number of new patients seen, cancellations, no shows, and the continuing care frequency and efficiency. All of this information will be important for you to understand how carefully patients are followed up and the growth of the practice through new patients. Chapter 11 reviews the incorporation of technology in a practice.

Facilities and Equipment

Now that you have reviewed most of the information that can be obtained before visiting the office, it is time to go to the facility if you have not already spent some time there. You can start by getting a feel for the neighborhood and look for things like

PROFORMA INCOME STATEMENT

	Month 1 projected	Month 2 projected	Month 3 projected	Month 4 projected	Month 5 projected	Month 6 projected	Month 7 projected	Month 8 projected	Month 9 projected	Month 10 projected	Month 11 projected	Month 12 projected	Year 1 projected
REVENUES													
Dental Service Collections	45,000.00	45,000.00	45,000.00	45,000.00	50,000.00	50,000.00	50,000.00	55,000.00	55,000.00	55,000.00	60,000.00	60,000.00	615,000.00
Total Revenues	**45,000.00**	**45,000.00**	**45,000.00**	**45,000.00**	**50,000.00**	**50,000.00**	**50,000.00**	**55,000.00**	**55,000.00**	**55,000.00**	**60,000.00**	**60,000.00**	**615,000.00**
EXPENSES													
Variable Expenses													
Dental Supplies 8%	3,600.00	3,600.00	3,600.00	3,600.00	4,000.00	4,000.00	4,000.00	4,400.00	4,400.00	4,400.00	4,800.00	4,800.00	49,200.00
Laboratory Fees 9%	4,050.00	4,050.00	4,050.00	4,050.00	4,500.00	4,500.00	4,500.00	4,950.00	4,950.00	4,950.00	5,400.00	5,400.00	55,350.00
Total Variable Expenses	**7,650.00**	**7,650.00**	**7,650.00**	**7,650.00**	**8,500.00**	**8,500.00**	**8,500.00**	**9,350.00**	**9,350.00**	**9,350.00**	**10,200.00**	**10,200.00**	**104,550.00**
% of rev	17%	17%	17%	17%	17%	17%	17%	17%	17%	17%	17%	17%	17%
Fixed Expenses													
Accounting	1,500.00	150.00	150.00	150.00	150.00	150.00	150.00	150.00	150.00	150.00	150.00	1,200.00	4,200.00
Advertising	500.00	500.00	500.00	500.00	500.00	500.00	300.00	300.00	300.00	300.00	300.00	300.00	4,800.00
Continuing Education	0.00	0.00	0.00	0.00	0.00	0.00	0.00	0.00	0.00	0.00	0.00	0.00	0.00
Dues and Subscriptions	150.00	150.00	150.00	150.00	150.00	150.00	150.00	150.00	150.00	150.00	150.00	150.00	1,800.00
Insurance–Disability	200.00	200.00	200.00	200.00	200.00	200.00	200.00	200.00	200.00	200.00	200.00	200.00	2,400.00
Insurance–Health	400.00	400.00	400.00	400.00	400.00	400.00	400.00	400.00	400.00	400.00	400.00	400.00	4,800.00
Insurance–Malpractice	400.00	400.00	400.00	400.00	400.00	400.00	400.00	400.00	400.00	400.00	400.00	400.00	4,800.00
Insurance–Workers Comp	450.00	450.00	450.00	450.00	450.00	450.00	450.00	450.00	450.00	450.00	450.00	450.00	5,400.00
Legal	2,000.00	0.00	0.00	0.00	0.00	0.00	0.00	0.00	0.00	0.00	0.00	0.00	2,000.00
Office Supplies	400.00	400.00	400.00	400.00	400.00	400.00	400.00	400.00	400.00	400.00	400.00	400.00	4,800.00
Payroll Taxes 8%	1,941.92	1,941.92	1,941.92	1,941.92	1,941.92	1,941.92	1,941.92	1,941.92	1,941.92	1,941.92	1,941.92	1,941.92	23,303.04
Postage and Delivery	250.00	250.00	250.00	250.00	250.00	250.00	250.00	250.00	250.00	250.00	250.00	250.00	3,000.00
Rent	2,500.00	2,500.00	2,500.00	2,500.00	2,500.00	2,500.00	2,500.00	2,500.00	2,500.00	2,500.00	2,500.00	2,500.00	30,000.00
Salaries–Office	4,864.00	4,864.00	4,864.00	4,864.00	4,864.00	4,864.00	4,864.00	4,864.00	4,864.00	4,864.00	4,864.00	4,864.00	58,368.00
Salaries–Assistant	3,040.00	3,040.00	3,040.00	3,040.00	3,040.00	3,040.00	3,040.00	3,040.00	3,040.00	3,040.00	3,040.00	3,040.00	36,480.00
Salaries–Hygiene	6,000.00	6,000.00	6,000.00	6,000.00	6,000.00	6,000.00	6,000.00	6,000.00	6,000.00	6,000.00	6,000.00	6,000.00	72,000.00
Salaries–Associate	0.00	0.00	0.00	0.00	0.00	0.00	0.00	0.00	0.00	0.00	0.00	0.00	0.00
Salaries–Doctor	10,370.00	10,370.00	10,370.00	10,370.00	10,370.00	10,370.00	10,370.00	10,370.00	10,370.00	10,370.00	10,370.00	10,370.00	124,440.00
Taxes & Licenses	500.00	500.00	500.00	500.00	500.00	500.00	500.00	500.00	500.00	500.00	500.00	500.00	6,000.00
Telephone	50.00	50.00	50.00	50.00	50.00	50.00	50.00	50.00	50.00	50.00	50.00	50.00	600.00
Travel, Meals, Ent.	150.00	150.00	150.00	150.00	150.00	150.00	150.00	150.00	150.00	150.00	150.00	150.00	1,800.00
Total Fixed Expenses	**35,665.92**	**32,315.92**	**32,315.92**	**32,315.92**	**32,315.92**	**32,315.92**	**32,115.92**	**32,115.92**	**32,115.92**	**32,115.92**	**32,115.92**	**33,165.92**	**390,991.04**
% of Revenue	79%	72%	72%	72%	65%	65%	64%	58%	58%	58%	54%	55%	64%
Total Operating Expenses	**43,315.92**	**39,965.92**	**39,965.92**	**39,965.92**	**40,815.92**	**40,815.92**	**40,615.92**	**41,465.92**	**41,465.92**	**41,465.92**	**42,315.92**	**43,365.92**	**495,541.04**
% of Revenue	96%	89%	89%	89%	82%	82%	81%	75%	75%	75%	71%	72%	81%
NET INCOME (LOSS)	**1,684.08**	**5,034.08**	**5,034.08**	**5,034.08**	**9,184.08**	**9,184.08**	**9,384.08**	**13,534.08**	**13,534.08**	**13,534.08**	**17,684.08**	**16,634.08**	**119,458.96**
% of Revenue	4%	11%	11%	11%	18%	18%	19%	25%	25%	25%	29%	28%	19%
Bank Loan (Rate%) 10													
Principal ($) 575000.00													
Total Bank Loan	**5,181.85**	**5,181.85**	**5,181.85**	**5,181.85**	**5,181.85**	**5,181.85**	**5,181.85**	**5,181.85**	**5,181.85**	**5,181.85**	**5,181.85**	**5,181.85**	**62,182.17**
% of Revenue	12%	12%	12%	12%	10%	10%	10%	9%	9%	9%	9%	9%	10%
CASH FLOW CHECK	-$3,497.77	-$147.77	-$147.77	-$147.77	$4,002.23	$4,002.23	$4,202.23	$8,352.23	$8,352.23	$8,352.23	$12,502.23	$11,452.23	$57,276.79

Figure 7.1. Pro forma income statement.

PERSONAL MONTHLY BUDGET	
Regular Monthly Payments	
Rent or Mortgage	$2,500.00
Automobile Loan	$600.00
Appliances	$0.00
Personal Loans	$0.00
Educational Loans	$2,000.00
Auto Insurance	$150.00
Other Insurance	$0.00
Miscellaneous	$0.00
Total Regular Monthly Payments	**$5,250.00**
% of Total Expenses	50.63%
Household Operating Expenses	
Telephone	$70.00
Utilities	$200.00
Other Household Expenses	$0.00
Total Household Operating Expenses	**$270.00**
% of Total Expenses	2.60%
Meal Expenses	
Dining at Home (Groceries)	$150.00
Dining Out	$100.00
Total Meal Expenses	**$250.00**
% of Total Expenses	2.41%
Personal Expenses	
Clothing, Cleaning, Laundry, ...	$75.00
Pharmaceuticals	$50.00
Medical/Dental	$175.00
Charitable Gifts and Donations	$0.00
Travel	$0.00
Subscriptions	$100.00
Auto Expense Fuel/Maintenance/Parking	$200.00
Other Spending Allowances	$0.00
Total Personal Expenses	**$600.00**
% of Total Expenses	5.79%
Tax Expenses	
Federal and State Income Taxes	$2,500.00
Property Taxes	$1,500.00
Other Taxes	$0.00
Total Tax Expenses	**$4,000.00**
% of Total Expenses	38.57%
TOTAL MONTHLY EXPENSES	**$10,370.00**
Non-Business Income (Significant Other / Spouse / Investment)	$0.00
NET MONTHLY PERSONAL CASH NEED	**$10,370.00**

Figure 7.2. Personal budget.

growth in housing, new schools, crime rate, and businesses in the area. Are there any issues with the lease or changes planned for the zoning of the area that may interrupt your business? A thorough demographic analysis will help you uncover the answers to these questions. What is the duration of the current lease and will you have the opportunity to assume it. You should also evaluate the actual structure from the outside and inside. Is there adequate parking for patients and staff? Is this the place you would love to get up and go to every morning? It is a good idea to take your digital camera and take a few photos or digital videos so that you can remember the details and go back to them as needed. Another consideration is room to grow, if that is part of your future plans.

Next, look at the equipment (see Chapter 6 for additional information). What is the condition of the equipment, and how has it been maintained? You want to ensure that you are not paying a high price for equipment that you will have to replace in a few short years. You also want to ensure that the equipment you will need is available for the treatment that you plan to provide for your patients. Do you need to have a computerized office with digital radiography? Do you need a CAD CAM machine or lasers? As you become serious about the transaction, you will also require an independent appraisal of the equipment value. Also, as discussed previously, ensure that there are no outstanding leases on the equipment that would remain after the transaction.

The charting system is also a critical evaluation. There are several things to look for here. Does the office use paper or digital charting? Make sure there is adequate notation and charting available that will not create a legal problem for you later. What are the referral patterns? What is the quality and thoroughness of the charting? Are there adequate radiographs of good quality for each patient? What kind of work has been completed on the patients? For example, are most patients fully restored, so you will have no work remaining on existing patients, or are most patients being monitored or "patched" and may see your treatment plans as aggressive? Another important part of this chart audit and evaluation is to actually make a count of *active patients*. This is an important step that also shows the health of the practice. There is no one right answer to this, and many varying opinions, but a one-doctor practice would be in a good position with 2,000 active charts, defined as patients seen in the last 2 years.

Evaluate how OSHA compliant the office is with the proper documentation manuals, material safety data sheets, and stickers warning of any hazards that may reside in the practice. Your visit to the office should give you a good sense of how well the office will fit with your personal style and goals.

Selling Doctor or Partners

Finally, you will want to look at the qualitative fit you will have with the selling doctor if buying the practice, or the selling doctor and remaining doctors if buying into the practice. A big mistake that can be made in this area is going into a practice where your personality style clashes with the culture of practice. For example, you are relatively introverted and quiet and tend to concentrate with little chitchat while you are providing treatment for a patient. You buy a practice from a doctor who was well known by the staff and patients as someone who was extroverted and would never stop talking. He would tell stories and jokes throughout the entire appointment and sometimes run over because of this characteristic. It is possible that after you go into the office, you will start losing patients because they had come to expect and look forward to the banter with the selling doctor, or they suddenly think you do not like or care about them and that is why you are being so quiet. This same dilemma may occur if you are buying into a practice where you may lose patients to other partners or never gain the support of the staff. As simple as this may seem, the personality matches within a practice in transition (and otherwise) are vitally important. Some practitioners routinely utilize personality assessments as part of hiring staff and team building.

You should also attempt to understand why the doctor is selling the practice and ensure it does not have to do with the decline of the business. If the doctor is moving, rather than retiring, where is his or her intended new location? Will their patients of record tend to follow them to their new location? You may also have the opportunity to assess his or her interest in negotiating a price. Most doctors will want to be fair and come up with a transaction that will maintain the health of their patients and create a real win-win transaction for the buyer and seller.

Common Transactions

Buying into a Practice

When you are buying into a practice, there will usually be two or more practitioners who remain in the office. You may be buying a share of an existing practice and creating a new partnership or buying out an existing partner who is leaving the group. You will have some form of a legal entity created after the transaction. The practice you are buying may exist as a sole proprietorship, limited partnership, general partnership, C or S corporation, or a limited liability company or partnership. After the purchase, you would go into the practice as a new shareholder, general partner, or limited partner depending on what structure you choose with your advisory team. See Chapter 10 for a discussion of various forms of ownership. In most cases, there will be a shared patient base and shared liability. Solo group and space-sharing agreements are not true partnerships, so they will most likely not be part of the final transaction.

Buying a Practice

When you are buying a practice, you will usually replace the existing doctor in the business. Unlike the buy-in option above, the final formulation of the business may include the sole proprietorship option as well.

Contracts

The *purchase agreement* for a healthcare practice is subject to several rules and regulations, *so any time you are reviewing and signing a contract, you should obtain the appropriate legal advice from the team of professionals you establish as part of your business support group.* You should also take care not to use the same attorney or accountant as the selling party, since your goals in some cases will be in direct conflict with one another. Some of the federal and state laws that will affect your transaction include but are not limited to those in the following list (Johnson 2002):

1. The state dental practice act and any other laws regulating the type and manner of ownership allowed for a healthcare practice in your state
2. Confidentiality laws such as the U.S. Department of Health and Human Services' Health Insurance Portability and Accountability Act of 1996 (HIPAA) that affect the privacy of patient information

3. State domestic property and divorce laws affecting the rights of a spouse to interests in the dental practice
4. Laws governing the covenant not to compete and liquidated damages
5. Statutes that relate to patient abandonment that could affect the transition process between treating doctors and how the patients are notified
6. Laws affecting the purchase of securities on the state or national level
7. Malpractice and professional liability laws and regulations
8. Laws affecting antidiscrimination at the state and federal level that could involve any portion of the transaction that relates to gender or ethnicity issues

Buying into a Practice

Buying into a practice will have some slight differences from buying a practice. The contracts for both will include the negotiated sale price, which will be a bit more complicated if you are already in the practice and growing it for the other owner(s). Some of the general contents of a practice buy-in or partnership agreement include the following:

1. The offering will outline what you are buying and what portion of the business and profits will be attributed to you. The calculation of profit will need to be outlined clearly to include any income based on production and separation of net income or expense beyond that.
2. The management of A/R as it is accrued and collected.
3. Management responsibilities and a clear understanding of who is responsible for the management of staffing issues, marketing, operations, and expenses.
4. The allocation and calculation of expenses, benefits, payment, and taxes.
5. Insurance needs to limit the liability of each individual should be explored and defined so that everyone is covered in case of any unforeseen events, including malpractice, death and disability.
6. Finally, as with any good partnership agreement, there should be a plan for dissolution so in a time of stress or conflict, the steps have already been clearly defined when everyone was cooperating at the beginning of the relationship.

Buying a Practice

Purchase agreements will have several formats and include a great deal of detail. The following are some of the general contents of a practice purchase agreement:

1. *Financial terms*: Although there are numerous articles and opinions about the financial terms and valuation of a practice opportunity, this topic is discussed especially in Chapters 4, 5, and 9, and we will not cover it in detail here. The important note here is that the financial terms of the transaction should be negotiated in advance and clearly included in the agreement to buy or buy into the practice. Such terms would include the price, what is included in the price, and when and how it will be paid.
2. *Purchase price and breakdown*: This breakdown includes such items as equipment, A/R, supplies, furniture and fixtures, covenant not to compete, charts, tenant improvements, and goodwill. The important note here is that as you negotiate this breakdown of price, *both parties should have the input of their tax advisors*. The seller will generally want to place more value in items that will produce long-term

capital gain and therefore be taxed at a lower rate, such as goodwill. The alternative for the seller is to pay tax on the items as ordinary income, which will be at a much higher rate, double, from 15% to nearly 40%. The buyer, on the other hand, wants to have as much as possible in items that will be depreciated faster on his or her tax return such as supplies, instruments, and A/R that are often deducted in 1 year. The other options would be to depreciate the item over a longer period, such as equipment that would depreciate over 5 years or goodwill and covenants not to compete that depreciate over 15 years. Again, please *consult your tax advisor*, as these are only generalizations.

3. *Assets/warranties*: This section describes the assets being sold and any warranties made in relation to those assets. Usually all of the existing furniture, fixtures, and equipment will be included in this section.

4. *A/R*: This section covers whether or not the A/R are being purchased and for how much they will be purchased. For example, will you be paying 80 cents on the dollar or some other discounted rate due to the aging of the accounts? If you are not buying the A/R, then are you going to have a nominal collection charge that you will charge the seller for the resources used to make that collection?

5. *Re-treatment*: This section describes the way to handle any treatment completed recently by the selling doctor that the buyer would need to replace. Details of this should include time since placement, types of procedures, how the costs for replacement will be recovered, and other such related items.

6. *Insurance*: This section of the contract addresses any insurance-related matters such as how each party would include the other in malpractice insurance as appropriate. Chapter 25 of this book provides a discussion on insurances.

7. *Custodian of records*: This portion of the contract commonly identifies the buyer as the custodian of records for the seller, defines the records, and stipulates the length of time that he or she would need to retain those records.

8. *Hold harmless*: This section outlines the manner and extent to which each party would hold the other harmless in the event of any future action.

9. *Contingencies*: This section could cover any contingency on the contract from either party that would keep the contract from being completed and not place the individual in breach of contract.

These are some general comments on the more common aspects of a purchase contract and do not serve as legal advice.

Another contract that you will see often in a purchase transaction is the *lease agreement*. These agreements usually include some of the following sections:

1. *Square feet and terms*: This section describes the total square feet of space that you will be renting and the general terms.

2. *Additional costs/NNN [triple net, which commonly includes property tax, insurance, and maintenance]*: Any additional cost or NNN fees that you will be responsible for such as common area maintenance will be outlined in this section.

3. *Usable versus rentable square feet*: There may be a difference between the space you are paying for and what you actually have access to use.

4. *As is or TI (tenant improvement) allowance*: This section describes the allowance, if any, the landlord will give or has given for leasehold or tenant improvements.

5. *Options*: This is an important section to understand when going through a purchase agreement since you will want to have some options to renew your

lease so you are not stuck having to pay for a move if the lease is due to expire soon. Many lenders will also require that the term of the lease and options will cover the length of the loan.

6. *First right of refusal*: This section will give you the right of refusal either for other dentists entering the building or for the first right to choose to purchase the building if it is going up for sale.

We hope that after reviewing this material, you are better prepared to make an informed decision on where you would like to work, what type of practice you will enter, and what you need to review and prepare before deciding to buy or buy into a dental practice. Practice purchase is one of the most important decisions you will make, and we wish you the best of preparation and opportunities.

Key Points

- Reviewing all variables when considering where to practice is essential to work/life balance and satisfaction.
- Every practice and every practice purchase transaction is unique—due diligence is critical to buying or buying into a practice
- Drawing on a team professionals, such as practice brokers, accountants, and attorneys, to assist you in this milestone transaction is fundamentally important to protect your interests.

References and Additional Resources

ADA Division of Legal Affairs. 2005. Business format guidelines for buying a practice. *J Mass Dent Soc* 54(1): 34–35.

Almonte, Peter. 2002. So you want to buy a dental practice. *NY State Dent J* 68(4): 20–23.

Baron, David P. 1996. *Business and Its Environments*, 2nd ed. Upper Saddle River, NJ: Prentice-Hall.

Conner, Vincent L. 2003. The due-diligence process of purchasing or buying into a dental practice. *Gen Dent* 51(6): 538–540.

Doran, George T. 1981. There's a S. M. A. R. T. way to write management's goals and objectives. *Manage Rev* 70(11): 35–36.

Gage, David. 2001. Choosing the right partner. *J Clin Ortho* 35(6): 365–368.

Johnson, Bruce A. 2002. Clean dealing: legal considerations for buy/sell agreements. *MGMA Connex* 2(10): 38–40.

Laing, Alan R. 2002. Practice transition tips for buyers and sellers. *J Mich Dent Assoc* 84(11): 38–41.

Lasky, Jeffrey I. 2003. Shall we dance? Taking a partner into your practice. *NY State Dent J* 69(4): 28–29.

Mattler, Martin G., and Mattler, Rise B. 2002. The ABCs of buying or selling a dental practice. *J N J Dent Assoc* 73 (1–2): 13, 15–17.

Rosen, Gerald. 2001. Twenty things you must know before you buy or sell a practice. *Alpha Omegan* 94(3): 14–18.

Rosen, Larry. 2005. What are the tax issues in acquiring a dental practice? *J Mass Dent Soc* 54(1): 36.

Ross, Stephen A., Westerfield, Randolph W., and Jordan, Brandford D. 1996. *Essentials of Corporate Finance*. Boston: Richard D. Irwin.

Schumann, Theodore C. 2006. The basics of due diligence for buyers. *J Mich Dent Assoc* 88(4): 16–17.

Simon, Risa, and Wilkinson, Shurli. 2005. Buyer beware: practice value drops without team buy-in. *J Mass Dent Soc* 54(1): 18–20.

Spiegelman, Randa. 2015. *Taxes: what's new for 2015?* Charles Schwab. Available at http://www.schwab.com/public/schwab/nn/articles/Taxes-Whats-New (accessed July 23, 2015)

Stockton, H. Jack. 1992. The dental practice purchase/sale: creating a win-win transaction. *J Can Dent Assoc* 58(8): 637–641.

———. 1997. Dental practice transitions: potential problems and possible solutions. *J Can Dent Assoc* 63(7): 539–541.

Tabak, Lawrence. 1996/1997. *If your goal is success, don't consult these gurus.* Available at http://www.fastcompany.com/27953/if-your-goal-success-dont-consult-these-gurus (accessed July 26, 2015).

Winter, Lois. 1996. Associateship/partnership: can it work for you? *NY State Dent J* 62(3): 38–41.

Wood, Patrick J., and Wood, Jason P. 2006. Why an attorney cannot represent both sides of a practice sale. *J Calif Dent Assoc* 34(5): 371–373.

U.S. Internal Revenue Service, Independent Contractor or Employee. Available at http://www.irs.gov/pub/irs-pdf/p1779.pdf (accessed July 23, 2015).

Learning Exercises

1. Identify the following as fixed or variable costs:
   A. Dental laboratory
   B. Staff salaries
   C. Credit card processing fees
   D. Rent
   E. Telephone
   F. Dental supplies

2. Calculate the net income for this practice (Table 7.8) and comment on how interested you would be in pursuing this opportunity to purchase the practice.

Table 7.8 Calculation of net income.

	2016	2015	2014	2013	2012
Revenue ($)	459,356	567,000	588,110	583,000	525,000
Expenses ($)	422,560	438,250	489,325	425,500	370,000
Net Income					

3. Please identify the following as components of a lease contract or a purchase agreement:
   A. Tenant improvements
   B. Accounts receivable
   C. NNN costs
   D. Covenant not to compete
   E. Custodian of records
   F. Options to renew

Answers

1. A, C, and F are variable costs. B, D, and E are fixed costs.
2. See Table 7.9.

Table 7.9 Answers for calculation of net income.

	2014	2013	2012	2011	2010
Revenue ($)	459,356	567,000	588,110	583,000	525,000
Expenses ($)	422,560	438,250	489,325	425,500	370,000
Net Income ($)	36,796	128,750	98,785	157,500	155,000

   This would not be an attractive practice because there is unstable income that trends down over the last 3 years of data and the expenses have not been controlled. There may be an opportunity here to make the practice more efficient, but it is a risky proposition.
3. A, C, and F are lease contract items. B, D, and E are purchase contract items.

Chapter 8
Starting a Dental Practice

David G. Dunning, Bradley Alderman, and Tyler Smith

> The link between my experience as an entrepreneur and that of a politician is all in one word: freedom.
>
> Silvio Berlusconi

This chapter describes some of the critical variables and steps related to starting a dental practice. While the chapter certainly does not cover every detail of a practice start-up, you will find that most of the issues are presented, including specific step-by-step do-lists for starting a practice. With the somewhat tarnished platinum age of dentistry described in Chapter 1, fewer dental graduates are starting or buying practices immediately upon graduation. Still, from our colleagues throughout the nation, anecdotal evidence suggests that most dental students eventually would like to own or co-own their own dental practices. And so a chapter on starting a dental practice remains relevant today.

"I Want to Be My Own Boss"

Applicants for dental college are routinely asked, "So, why do you want to be a dentist?" or a similar variation of this question. Answers to this query often embrace references to caring for people and to "lifestyle" (a code of sorts referring to a relatively high income and freedom of work schedule). Another commonly heard and honest reply is, "I want to be my own boss." The truth is that dentists tend as a group to be very independent people who enjoy calling the shots (no pun intended). This tendency often does not lend itself to being told what to do by others or to being an ideal employee who spontaneously abides by the wishes of an employer. Clearly, some individuals take the path of a practice start-up (or a practice buyout) simply because they are wired to be their own bosses. This "I want to be my own boss" mentality may also reflect in some dentists a more deeply abiding spirit of entrepreneurship.

Dental Practice Transition: A Practical Guide to Management, Second Edition.
Edited by David G. Dunning and Brian M. Lange.
© 2016 John Wiley & Sons, Inc. Published 2016 by John Wiley & Sons, Inc.
Companion Website: www.wiley.com/go/dunning/transition

Are You an Entrepreneur?

Exactly what is an entrepreneur? The Online Etymology Dictionary indicates that this concept originated from the French language, defining entrepreneur as "one who undertakes or manages." Chad Brooks (2015) offers a simple and insightful definition of entrepreneurship: "The development of a business from the ground up—coming up with the idea and turning it into a profitable business."

Historically, entrepreneurship, like leadership, has been understood in terms of personal characteristics and skills. Here is an incomplete list of entrepreneurial traits: money-conscious, competitive, risk-taking, professional, self-control, self-confident, a sense of urgency, ability to comprehend complexity, realism, emotional stability, social networker, a high need to achieve, positive "can-do" attitude, ability to anticipate developments, results-oriented, technical knowledge, a hard worker, disciplined, a focus on profits, total commitment. Other lists of entrepreneurial characteristics can be found in various resources, including Bowser (2015), Resnick (2014), Robinson (2014), and Stephenson (2015).

You can measure your entrepreneurial tendencies by doing an internet search for "entrepreneur quiz" and "entrepreneur test." Several sites as of this writing include allthetests.com, www.wesst.org/business-toolkit/entrepreneuer-quiz/izmove.com, www.bizmove.com and www.entrepreneur.com, among others. Interpret these and other assessments with caution—the results may not be accurate for you, although you will likely get a sense of your inclination toward being an entrepreneur.

In addition, those interested in entrepreneurship in dental practice may learn insights by listening to Dr. Mark Costes' The "Dentalpreneur" Podcast at http://truedentalsuccess.com/blog/category/podcast/.

Your Sense of Efficacy: Do You Believe?

Standardized (that is, scientific), multidimensional measures of entrepreneurship self-efficacy have also been developed through research: McGee et al. (2009) and Moberg (2013). We suggest contacting the researchers regarding the availability of these instruments for personal use.

So, what do the definition of entrepreneur/entrepreneurship, the admittedly incomplete list of entrepreneur characteristics, and the concept of entrepreneurial self-efficacy have to do with you? *Simply this: you are like the little engine in the children's classic story that "thought it could." If you think you can, you are much more likely to succeed. If you think you cannot, you are much more likely to be unsuccessful.* As applied to starting a dental practice, you really have to do a major "gut check." Even though you may have some doubt, you better believe deep down in your soul that you "can" do this before launching this adventure.

What Special Competitive Advantage Can You Leverage?

We are now going to contradict ourselves, at least partially. The definition cited previously about entrepreneurship included, "creating or seizing an opportunity and pursuing it *regardless of the resources currently controlled*" (italics added). It has been our experience that most successful dental practice start-ups involve some special resource. The entrepreneur leverages this resource in order to make the practice start successful (namely, profitable) in a relatively short amount of time, perhaps weeks or months. Here is an incomplete but representative list of these types of resources: having an incredible level of energy to work 80–100 hours a week (this seems a bit more than being a hard worker from the earlier list); benefiting from the sage wisdom of a relative (grandfather/grandmother, parent, sibling, cousin, etc.) with business experience, particularly in dentistry; enjoying the obvious benefits of a parent who is a general contractor and who will build-out lease space or build a gorgeous facility at or near cost; locating the practice in an area in which you have unparalleled strategic and/or financial advantage. Examples of the last scenario would include a rural area with a population of 3,500 and no competing dentist within 25 miles; and start-up incentives from state or local government or community programs that might involve no or low-interest loans, property tax waivers, student loan forgiveness programs for practicing in designated shortage areas, and so on. Some of these unique leveraging opportunities might be able to be "stacked" or added on top of each other by creative entrepreneurs.

We, of course, are not saying it is impossible to start a practice from scratch without a competitive advantage such as those listed above. We are saying that such resources offer incredible assistance in launching a practice.

Other Considerations

Special Marketing Ideas

For a much more thorough treatment of marketing issues, please refer to the chapters on internal marketing/customer service (Chapter 18) and external marketing (Chapter 17). Our purpose here is, obviously, not to review the discipline of marketing but, rather, to convey a couple of successful approaches to marketing used by people who have started dental practices. Ted Turner is quoted as saying, "Early to bed, early to rise, work like hell and advertise" (Shapiro 2004). This aphorism has some application for practice start-ups. One of the coauthors of this chapter went literally from door-to-door in the surrounding neighborhoods to market himself and his practice. While a unique approach, especially for a professional services business, meeting and greeting hundreds if not thousands of potential patients provided a direct method for communicating with the public.

Another dentist we know opened a practice in a small town in the Midwest and utilized an existing facility from a previous dentist. His advertising strategy included a distinctive series of black and white contrast newspaper ads. He purchased a portion of a page that featured a simple image of a molar. Beginning with a small molar, the tooth "grew" with each weekly issue of the paper. After several weeks, with the community talking about what in the world the tooth was all about, the dentist then utilized the same page space and announced the opening of his practice and the availability to schedule appointments. The simple and relatively inexpensive strategy worked effectively. In this age of internet and social media, clearly any new start-up should have a quality web presence since most people research through the internet to make decisions.

Special Real Estate Issues

A practice start-up raises concerns related to buying or leasing a practice facility. These parallel similar decision-making variables involved in buying/buying out a practice. However, with a start-up, the entrepreneurial dentist has no reliable patient cash flow and no accounts receivable. In all likelihood, a line of credit from a lender or some other revenue source (a spouse with steady and sufficient income) will have to fill the gap when the doors open in order to cover all the overhead expenses plus a minimal draw if needed as a living wage for the dentist.

Given this tenuous situation, the decision about buying or leasing a facility may be a sticky one. Monthly cash flow is one variable—that is, what it will cost to lease and what will be the monthly cost to make a mortgage payment plus insurance, real estate taxes, and upkeep. In most areas, it is more cost-effective to lease, especially when money is tight. This, however, is not always the case.

Dr. Eugene Heller (2012), national director of Sullivan-Schein's Transition Services, identifies three criteria in deciding to buy real estate for a dental office: (1) if replacement cost is 50–75% (or less) in comparing the building/office to new construction, (2) if the building is anticipated to be in a good location for 7–10 years or more, and (3) if the building is large enough for the practice or can be expanded to be large enough. So, in addition to issues of cash flow and affordability, these three criteria need to be examined in making the decision to lease or buy real estate for a dental practice.

In addition, some people have more of a "renter" mindset and prefer to avoid the hassles of "ownership" (leaky roofs and plumbing leaks, for example). It does not appear obvious to us that a person starting a practice from scratch would tend to side one way or the other on this particular issue. Still, it must also be considered. One entrepreneur might prefer to focus on producing dentistry instead of a building. Another with superhuman energy levels and construction skills might relish fixing roof and plumbing problems.

Financing is another issue related to real estate. Recent graduates may have to push the tolerances of lenders in starting a practice due to the expenses of building-out leasehold space and purchasing cabinets, chairs, equipment, technology, and supplies. While real estate in some sense involves less risk to a lender (given a building to resell if necessary), there may be limitations on the total amount to be borrowed in a more risky start-up venture. Thus, inability to get financing to purchase a practice facility may render moot the issue of buying a facility.

Finally, there exist some rare and lucrative opportunities, especially in rural areas, in which towns, cities, or owner-dentists may have some unique incentives involving real estate for practice start-ups. We know of situations where a student has purchased a practice, in essence, for only the cost of a building (with older but serviceable equipment considered part of the price of the building). Obviously, not having to pay for any goodwill or blue-sky could readily "tip" the scales and make the purchase of a building a smart business move.

Equipment Issues

Chapter 6 provides detailed information about equipment issues within the context of practice ownership. We simply would like to remind anyone who starts a dental practice to have any used equipment inspected and maintained. Further, it is vital to have a trustworthy relationship with someone who can readily make a service call for "down" equipment. A fledgling dental practice being sustained in part by cash flow can ill afford to have a compressor fail and lose the income that would have been produced for, potentially, several days.

It is also vital to pay fair market value for any used (or new) equipment purchases for a start-up. If necessary, an independent appraiser can inspect and value used equipment.

One other comment related to equipment is noteworthy here. As nationally acclaimed registered architect-dentist Dr. Mike Unthank warns (and this is a paraphrase), any piece of equipment that says "dentist" on it, literally or figuratively, will cost more money (Unthank 2015). This may particularly apply to cabinetry. So, as always, be a wise consumer of what you purchase.

Business Plans and Financing

We believe a metaphor is helpful in understanding the importance of business plans and financing in starting a dental practice: you have to build a bridge over the span of a river to reach the other side of profitability. The bridge consists of all of your business decisions, your skill-set, and your indispensable staff. The river to be spanned consists of all the market forces and overhead expenses with which you must contend in building a practice. Depending on the source with whom you talk, and depending on market forces and overhead expenses, it may take from a few months to a year or more to "span the river"/ build the bridge to profitability. In other words, it is likely to take months before you can pay for your overhead AND earn a profit. For the initial months of start-up, you will likely need a line of credit from which you can borrow to pay for your living expenses, unless you have some wonderful support (such as a spouse with a solid income).

Chapters 2, 3, 4, and 9 cover in detail financial statements, practice performance measures, business planning, and financing a practice. The bridge to profitability reinforces the vital importance of these topics for a start-up situation. Your business plan can be augmented by building upon software programs such as Business Plan Pro and Wells Fargo Practice Finance's Practice Success Series, which includes an interactive practice planner to help establish expense and income projections. Make sure that your business plan includes available loan money, probably a line of credit, for spanning the river.

As far as financing a start-up, our advice is to persevere, persevere, and persevere. The lending industry seems to ebb and flow in mysterious and unpredictable ways with market nuances. In other words, it is sometimes relatively easier and more difficult to obtain loans for start-ups. In any case, if you are turned down by one lender, especially a bank, we encourage you to go to another, and to another, and to another if necessary.

A Key Reference for your Additional Study

Dr. Gordon Osterhaus (2011) published an incredibly helpful book on opening or relocating a dental office. The book covers planning and players (including suppliers, architect/designer, contractors), coordinating and supervising (including engineering, installing equipment, and securing permits), making decisions about equipment, and detailed tips for non-profit organizations in establishing clinics. An accompanying appendix adds helpful resources such as worksheets and an overall flow chart.

Step-by-Step Process for Starting a Practice

> You cannot overestimate the need to plan and prepare. In most of the mistakes I have made, there has been this common theme of inadequate planning beforehand. You really cannot over-prepare in business!
>
> Chris Corrigan

Dr. Steve Jacobs of South Dakota with his wife, Trista, a certified public accountant, created the first start-up list (Table 8.1). Dates have been updated to correspond with

Table 8.1   Dr. Steve Jacobs's new dental practice start-up list and timeline.

Task	Time Frame (Years Updated from Original Dates to Coincide with the Publication of This Book)		Done by Steve (S) or Trista (T)
	Begin	End	
Develop overall marketing plan (see Chapters 17 and 18 for assistance with ideas)	10/1/2016	10/31/2016	S
Complete an annual projected budget of expenses	10/1/2016	10/31/2016	S
Decide whether to lease or buy building	10/1/2016	10/31/2016	S
Find a good attorney (network as needed for this)	10/1/2016	10/31/2016	S
Complete paperwork for business loan	10/1/2016	11/30/2016	S
Look at equipment in Brookings	10/1/2016	12/31/2016	S
Look at equipment from used dealer	10/1/2016	12/31/2016	S
Make a list of equipment to purchase new	10/1/2016	12/31/2016	S
Study and purchase disability insurance	10/1/2016	12/31/2016	S
Develop job description for each position	11/1/2016	1/31/2017	T
Create list of interview questions for each position	11/1/2016	1/31/2017	T
Research local rates of pay	11/1/2016	1/31/2017	S
Document salary/hourly rates and benefits to offer each position	11/1/2016	1/31/2017	T
Network for hiring staff	11/1/2016	5/31/2017	S
Hire receptionist	11/1/2016	5/31/2017	S
Hire assistant	11/1/2016	5/31/2017	S
Hire hygienist	11/1/2016	5/31/2017	S
Identify local major employers' insurance plans and decide whether to join them	12/1/2016	12/31/2016	S
Evaluate pros and cons of membership in managed care plans and decide which, if any, to join (capitation, PPOs, etc.)	12/1/2016	12/31/2016	S
Be aware that one in seven dentists is embezzled and have safeguards in place to discourage attempts	12/1/2016	12/31/2016	T
Possibly get special local license/permit	12/1/2016	12/31/2016	T
Make a due date list of all tax forms to be filed (payroll, income, sales, property)	12/1/2016	12/31/2016	T
Design office with supply representative (or architect)	12/1/2016	1/31/2017	S
Renovate facility	12/1/2016	3/31/2017	S
Obtain loan approval	1/1/2017	1/31/2017	T
Create consents	1/1/2017	1/31/2017	S
Have supplier representative appraise used equipment	1/1/2017	1/31/2017	S
Order equipment, office, and dental supplies	1/1/2017	4/30/2017	S
Post staff openings at schools	1/1/2017	5/31/2017	S
Place ads for staff openings on the internet and perhaps newspapers	1/1/2017	6/30/2017	S
Have systems in place to comply with OSHA and HIPAA guidelines and requirements	2/1/2017	2/28/2017	S

Table 8.1   (*Continued*)

Task	Time Frame (Years Updated from Original Dates to Coincide with the Publication of This Book)		Done by Steve (S) or Trista (T)
	Begin	End	
Arrange for equipment storage, if necessary	2/1/2017	2/28/2017	S
Start a list of patients to recruit (friends, neighbors, nearby businesses)	3/1/2017	3/31/2017	S
Make a policy on accepting insurance assignment benefits and whether to bill insurance for patients or not	3/1/2017	3/31/2017	S
Outline ideal day so that there will be a balance of small restorative, large procedures, new patient exams, and hygiene	3/1/2017	3/31/2017	S
Preblock a portion of daily schedule for significant treatment to meet production goals	3/1/2017	3/31/2017	S
Select dental software system	4/1/2017	4/30/2017	S
Write practice vision/mission statement identifying ideal patient, the quality of care to provide, and type of practice environment to create	4/1/2017	6/30/2017	S
Train on computer software	5/1/2017	5/31/2017	S, T
Get a telephone number (after becoming licensed)	5/1/2017	5/31/2017	T
Get business cards and plan for use	5/1/2017	5/31/2017	T
Develop procedures for daily data backup disks to be made with weekly updates to a disk set stored offsite	5/1/2017	5/31/2017	T
Arrange for payment options such as credit cards, healthcare credit cards, and ATM	5/1/2017	5/31/2017	T
Arrange to file electronic claims from office dental software	5/1/2017	5/31/2017	T
Have a manual or computer new patient log to track names, referral sources, amount diagnosed, amount accepted/appointed	5/1/2017	5/31/2017	T
Get DEA license from U.S. Department of Justice	5/1/2017	5/31/2017	T
Register with South Dakota Division of Public Health to prescribe controlled drugs	5/1/2017	5/31/2017	T
Order laboratory prescription pads from South Dakota Dental Association	5/1/2017	5/31/2017	T
Study and purchase malpractice insurance	5/1/2017	5/31/2017	T
Study and purchase workers' compensation insurance	5/1/2017	5/31/2017	T
Study and purchase general business liability insurance	5/1/2017	5/31/2017	T
Study and purchase personal property insurance	5/1/2017	6/30/2017	T
Get dental license	5/1/2017	7/31/2017	S
Have equipment delivered	6/1/2017	6/1/2017	S

Table 8.1 *(Continued)*

Task	Time Frame (Years Updated from Original Dates to Coincide with the Publication of This Book)		Done by Steve (S) or Trista (T)
	Begin	End	
Have personnel policies in writing and ready to be distributed to employees	6/1/2017	6/30/2017	T
Document standard operating procedures for my office (or buy off-the-shelf model)	6/1/2017	6/30/2017	T
Ensure that billing statements to patients list a specific due date	6/1/2017	6/30/2017	T
Develop cancellation policy with financial penalties for repeated appointment failures and sample patient warnings and dismissal letters	6/1/2017	6/30/2017	S
Have x-ray equipment examined and licensed by South Dakota Department of Health	6/1/2017	6/30/2017	T
Get South Dakota tax license	7/1/2017	7/31/2017	T
Get certificate of incorporation from South Dakota Secretary of State	7/1/2017	7/31/2017	T
Prepare to do hygiene until a full-time hygienist can be afforded	7/1/2017	7/31/2017	S
Draft articles of incorporation	7/1/2017	7/31/2017	T
Open bank account in corporation's name	7/1/2017	7/31/2017	T
Get Employer Identification Number	7/1/2017	7/31/2017	T
Obtain nitrous license	7/1/2017	7/31/2017	S
Network: physicians, pharmacists, nearby business owners, real estate agents, specialists, beauty/nail salons, plastic surgeons, community activities, sports teams, etc.	7/1/2017	7/31/2017	S
Develop a script for asking patients for referrals and plan to practice these skills with staff	7/1/2017	7/31/2017	S
Make bank deposits daily after checking a day sheet	7/1/2017	7/31/2017	S
Preappoint all hygiene patients for their next prophy	7/1/2017	7/31/2017	S
Reduce hygiene cancellations by use of reminder postcards as well as confirmation calls sent 2 days in advance	7/1/2017	7/31/2017	S
Develop system to track delayed or unaccepted treatment and actively urge patients to complete needed treatment now	7/1/2017	7/31/2017	S
Use computer or manual reports to track at least the following statistics: monthly/year-to-date production (dr. or hygiene), collections, new patient numbers, adjusted production due to managed care, total monthly expenses, and accounts receivable	7/1/2017	7/31/2017	T

the publication of this book. Dr. Jacobs' list was originally based mainly on the third checklist for start-ups summarized near the end of this chapter via a sampling from Wells Fargo Practice Finance. Accordingly, there may be some redundancy in comparing Dr. Jacobs's list and Wells Fargo Practice Finance's list. Dr. Brad Alderman then built upon Dr. Jacobs's detailed list (Table 8.2). Together, we believe that most of the critical steps you need to accomplish to start a dental practice are covered in the three lists. The lists have demonstrated their indispensable value over the years with many students.

Table 8.2 Journey to succeed: Dr. Brad Alderman's dental practice start-up guidelines.

X	Task
	Buy existing practice or start my own
	Visit other dental offices—ask questions!
	Complete paperwork for business loan
	Location, location, location—find the right one!
	Shop for business loans—start with local bank, be tough, and don't take "no" for an answer!
	Find an attorney
	Look early for used dental equipment—might find great deals
	Meet with dental equipment vendors—don't be oversold—you are the customer!
	Network for hiring staff—look to the dental community
	Start your office manual—be thorough but remember that it will change over time
	Research local rates of pay
	Hire staff—be picky—they represent you!
	Start a marketing plan—think outside the box!
	Decide whether or not to be a preferred provider for insurance companies, accept Medicaid, etc.—you do not have to be a PPO just because you're slow!
	Find accountant—call dentists in the area for suggestions
	Office design can be done by equipment representative or an architectural design group such as Unthank Design Group (www.unthank.com)
	Order equipment, office, dental supplies
	Start a list of patients to recruit
	Announce opening of dental office—I couldn't advertise my name without a license, but I hung a sign that said "Dental Office—Open June"
	Select dental software
	Train on dental software with all employees
	Obtain a telephone number—ask for a number that will be easy to remember (5555)
	Get business cards for myself and staff to use
	Think about financial policies for the office/put financial policies in writing—sign up with third-party financing (care credit), do not be a bank!
	Get DEA license from U.S. Department of Justice, www.dea.gov.
	Find malpractice insurance
	Find office overhead insurance
	Get dental license
	Develop cancellation policies for the office
	Have x-ray generating equipment licensed by Nebraska Department of Health
	Get Nebraska tax ID number
	Get articles of incorporation from attorney
	Walk through "typical" day with employees
	Advertise yourself—ask for referrals, carry business cards, beat the streets!
	Send W-9 to insurance companies so you can submit claims

Table 8.2   (*Continued*)

X	Task
	Develop continuing care systems
	Make sure every patient is scheduled for his or her next appointment prior to leaving
	Collect patient's entire portion of payment the day service is rendered
	Strive for portion of daily schedule to be used for productive treatment to meet production goals—tough to do when first starting out
	Excellent customer service training for all employees
	Employees trained on emergencies that could arise in the office

The lists provided by Drs. Jacobs and Alderman, combined with the comments by Dr. Smith, offer perspectives from different markets. The first market is a small city in the Midwest with relatively favorable demographics for a start-up. The second is a city in the Midwest with a relatively competitive market. The third is a very small town in the rural Midwest in desperate need of a dentist. It might be possible, though admittedly more challenging, to start a practice from scratch in a market more competitive than that entered by Dr. Alderman, as described below. Importantly, if you are considering a start-up in a larger metropolitan area, please study the same business plan detailed in Chapter 4.

The American Dental Association has also developed a "New Practice Checklist." It is available to members only at http://success.ada.org/en/practice/ownership-life-cycle/starting/starting-a-new-dental-practice-checklist. It lists major categories and related line-items to complete, detailing many of the key issues involved in opening a new practice. Categories include licensure, regulations, insurance, infection control and OSHA, and staffing.

It is critically important to recognize the value of other information in this book when reviewing/studying these lists for starting a dental practice. Virtually all of the other chapters inform, affect, or clarify these lists of steps, from Chapter 2 to Chapter 4, to Chapters 22–24 related to the dental team and staffing, to the chapters related to business and personal insurance (Chapter 25), and personal finance/investing (Chapter 26).

Dr. Jacobs's Steps for Opening a Practice

Dr. Jacobs refurbished an existing but unused dental office space in Brookings, South Dakota, a small city with a population of approximately 20,000 and a market area of approximately 25,000 patients. He opened his practice within weeks of graduation. This practice was not ideally located. Instead, alley access was necessary to enter the facility.

Dr. Brad Alderman's Additional Steps

Dr. Brad Alderman built out lease space in a very tight dental market in Lincoln, Nebraska, starting his practice in a location with few if any closely located competitors. Lincoln is a city of approximately two hundred fifty thousand and is perceived by many to have more dentists than it needs, in large part because the University of Nebraska Medical Center's College of Dentistry is located there. Like Dr. Jacobs, Dr. Alderman opened his dental practice within weeks of graduating from school (Figure 8.1). Dr. Alderman enjoyed so much success in starting a practice from scratch that, 3 years later, he helped his wife, Dr. Katherine Alderman, start a practice after graduation in another strategic location in Lincoln, Nebraska's competitive market (Figure 8.2).

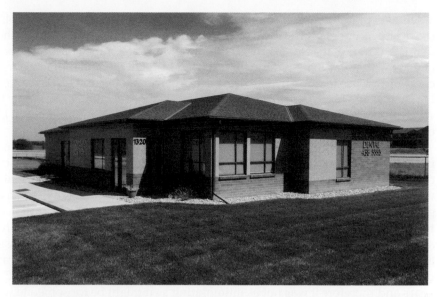

Figure 8.1.   Coddington Dental, Lincoln, Nebraska, started from scratch in 1994 by Dr. Brad Alderman.

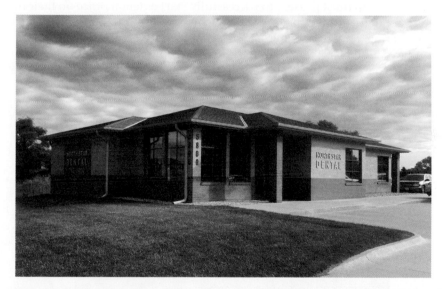

Figure 8.2.   Dr. Brad and Katherine Alderman's North Star practice in Lincoln, Nebraska.

Insights from Dr. Tyler Smith about Starting a Practice

Dr. Tyler Smith earned a Bachelor's degree in finance in 2000 and worked as an analyst at a large consumer finance company for 5 years. He became disenchanted with the corporate environment and sought to find a profession where he could utilize his entrepreneurial skills in a small business environment, working directly with people on a daily basis. Dr. Smith had always found dentistry a fascinating profession, thanks to a dental exploratory program in which he participated during high school. Fueled by the desire to find a professional life that better fit his skills, he joined 44 other aspiring dentists as part of the University of Nebraska Medical Center College of Dentistry class of 2009. Upon graduation, Dr. Smith started his general dental practice from scratch, choosing a lease location in a growing suburban area of southwest Omaha, Nebraska. He shares here his experiences and recommendations for some key points to consider when opening a dental office. See Figures 8.3 and 8.4 for photos of Dr. Smith's dental practice.

"At the start of my fourth year in dental school, a feeling slowly started to creep over me that soon I would leave this nice academic setting where your future is so nicely laid out in the form of a classroom syllabus. I was going to have to enter the real world and work for a living! I had ruled out specializing in a specific area of dentistry because I enjoyed the variety that general dentistry provided on any given day. That left me with two very simple choices: start beating the bushes to find an office to hire me as an associate dentist, or open a dental practice from scratch. In my prior professional life as a financial analyst, I knew the feeling of having a boss and the undesirable lack of decision-making that goes with it. Also, I had experienced the 'real world' for several years and therefore it was not as intimidating as it might be for someone who had not been in the workforce prior to graduate school. For these reasons, I chose to start a dental practice from scratch.

"Looking back – and I did not fully recognize it at the time – I think one of the key traits a person must possess to successfully start a dental office on their own (whether from scratch or utilizing a existing patient base from a different source) is an unwavering and undeniable sense of confidence. Not a sense of confidence that you have all the answers from the outset of your endeavor, but a sense of confidence that with hard work and determination you can *find* the answers as the questions arise.

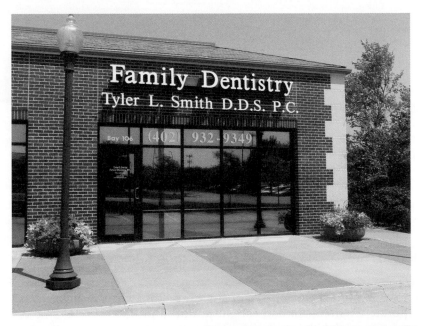

Figure 8.3. Front view of Tyler L. Smith Family Dentistry in Omaha, NE, opened within weeks of Dr. Smith's graduation from dental college in 2009.

No one, no matter the age or experience level, has all the answers. The key point is understanding that every successful entrepreneur has a sense of confidence that no matter the challenge or questions thrown at him, he can find an answer with some perseverance and a good amount of elbow grease.

"Armed with this confidence, I chose to open my dental office in a growing area of southwest Omaha, Nebraska. The beauty of a dental office is that you can open one anywhere you want to live. If you have a passion for skiing, head to a mountainous state; if you covet the open seas, head to a coastal state; if you like a year-round tan, head south. I chose my location because, having been raised in Omaha, I could stay close to family, and I knew it was an excellent place to raise children with the same values with which I was raised. More specifically, I was very familiar with the immediate surroundings of my office location because I had grown up less than five miles away. My available patient population included an abundance of young, married professionals with above average education and above average income. Although I could describe a myriad of other details that played in to a successful location, the key point is that I had an intimate understanding of my particular area of town from which I would seek to fill a patient base. I knew that I was right in the heart of growth and expansion in Omaha. I knew how close I was locating to other general dentists in the area. I understood the demographics of the population within a few miles radius of my office. I am certainly not saying you have to open a dental office in your childhood hometown. Rather, I would emphasize that if you choose to locate to an area because of some external factor (excellent hiking, year-round sun, abundant fishing), it would be wise to heavily research and even personally spend some time in that particular area to get a feel for the population that you will serve and the community with which you will likely be a part for many years to come.

"My choice of location has – thankfully – served me well over the past six years as I have steadily increased my patient base to near capacity for the lease space I occupy. Over the past six years, I have seen consistent themes play out in the success of my practice. I think that any dentist who follows these themes in a confident manner and who establishes a practice in a well-researched location can be very successful in the practice of dentistry. The themes are as follows:

Treat your patients as if they are family members. This may seem like an obvious and over-simplified statement, but it is amazing how many external forces will jump into your mind when making treatment decisions. You may be worried about how your patient will perceive you and what they will tell their neighbors as you explain the need for root canal treatment on a tooth. You may be worried about the new dishwasher that you just had to purchase in your home as you sit down to do an exam on a new patient. You may have the feeling that your patient does not have the means to follow through with the treatment you would like to recommend. Making treatment decisions is not a simple black and white process, and every dentist has a different level of aggressiveness when diagnosing dental problems. You will find your comfort zone. Regardless of where you fall on the treatment planning spectrum, if you talk to your patients and empathize with your patients as if they are your father, mother, brother, or sister, your patients can and will recognize your genuine concern for their oral health and the honesty in your treatment decisions. This is a special trust that your patients will hold with you, and no amount of 'selling' will ever be as effective as a genuine concern for their well-being. If you are honest and recommend what is best for your patients, they will intuitively recognize this and continue to support your business through their patronage.

Educate your patients. Just as a previous section in this chapter pointed out the importance of establishing a competitive advantage, I have discovered that providing a little extra dental information to my patients has given me a slight edge over my competitors. In my office, we utilize digital radiography and intra-oral digital photographs that can be displayed on a ceiling-mounted television easily seen by a patient seated in the dental chair. We have drafted take-home pamphlets with detailed explanation of treatment options. Most importantly, I purposely spend an extra minute or two talking to my patients about the evidence that supports my treatment recommendations. Patients often cannot see what we as dentists see when looking in their mouth. As previously discussed, the patient must rely on a trust factor to agree with and follow through with our recommended treatment. A great way to increase this trust and give patients a better sense of comfort with your diagnoses is to explain why we are recommending a particular treatment plan. I do this from the very first time a patient walks into my office and continue with a healthy dose of education any time something arises that is out of the ordinary. Your patients will appreciate the extra time you spend with them, and everyone feels more comfortable when they have a brief explanation of the 'why' behind a particular recommendation.

Build an outstanding team! Although much easier said than done, the establishment of a great group of staff (your team) is of paramount importance. I believe many factors have to line up just right to establish your dream team, and therefore it may take many years to accomplish this goal. In fact, it is likely that many dentists may never have a true dream team, and if they do it may only be for a short time period. The employer/employee relationship has changed over the past several decades as it shifts away from the loyalty-based model to that of the grass-is-greener-on-the-other-side model. Gone are the days of employees routinely sticking with the same employer for 20 to 30 years. Instead, you are much more likely to experience a high rate of turnover in your dental practice than if you lived a generation ago. This can be extremely frustrating, as it often happens that you will just be reaching the point where you are starting to fully trust a team member and the training process has finally slowed down; then, this person will come to you and announce their departure from the practice. The reasons people leave dental offices are endless, but the point is that you *must not* let your employee turnover sway you from a relentless pursuit of finding and building a great team. Your patients spend far more time with your hygienist, front desk, and even your chair side assistant than with you. The impression your team makes on your patients makes a monumental positive influence (or, potentially, negative influence!) on their desire to return to your office for future treatment. Have you ever left a medical office with a bad taste in your mouth because the last person with whom you had contact – usually the front desk employee – was rude, unfriendly, or dismissive? Do not let this happen in your own dental practice. Despite the constant frustrations you will encounter when building your dream team, it is worth every ounce of energy ten times over.

Be smart with your cash flow. During my senior year in college, nearing the completion of my Bachelor of Business Administration degree, I had the opportunity to interview with a successful financial services company for an entry-level position. Within the first minute, the interviewer asked me to describe the concept of 'cash flow' and its importance to a business' well-being. Somehow, despite countless hours of time spent in business school classrooms, I had missed this point. My blank stare effectively ended the interview on the spot.

This humbling lesson impressed upon me the need to have a firm grasp on the concept of cash flow if ever I was to venture into the business world. It is not that cash flow – specifically *positive* cash flow – is a difficult concept to understand; rather, it is a difficult concept to have the discipline to follow. Far too many business owners see their checking account balance grow and think they can immediately withdraw the money and spend it on a down payment for their dream car. They forget that payroll must be funded in a few days, and next week supplies must be ordered, and in a couple of months they will likely need to fund a repair of an old high-speed handpiece. The timing of patients paying you for your work does not always coincide with bills that come due. You must build a cushion in your checking account that allows for inflows and outflows of money without sweating over a possible overdraft fee. Spend less than you make and generally cash flow will be the least of your worries. Research your purchases, look skeptically upon the latest-and-greatest product that your dental sales representative is touting, and if in doubt, remember that excellent dental work can be done without spending excessive sums of money on supplies and equipment.

Avoid burnout. The best two strategies I have found to avoid getting burnt out on the daily grind of dentistry are to take time away from the office and to stay thirsty for additional dental knowledge. Taking time to physically step away from your dental practice (and I mean more than just weekends and holidays!) may mean going on vacation, traveling to another city for a dental continuing education course, or spending a day at home with your family. Whatever the reason, the ability to break up the routine at your sole discretion is one of the big perks of owning your own business. I would advise against abusing this privilege, as excessive work absences will not only negatively influence your team's morale but will also likely leave an unfavorable opinion of your work ethic with your patients. However, with careful planning, you can step away from your practice to give yourself a mental and physical break.

Breaking out of the confines of your 2000 square foot office space will open your mind to new ideas, may allow for interaction amongst your fellow dentists, and force you to step back from the daily minutia and think strategically about the direction in which your practice is headed. As you briefly step aside from the daily routine, I believe it is essential to have an eagerness to continue your education. Reading periodicals, attending live courses or watching online webinars, interacting with your colleagues through a study club, and any other form of out-of-office study will have a profound impact on your ability to stay excited about the profession. Personally, I make it a point to attend at least one out of town continuing education course each year. Although more expensive than an in-town course sponsored by a local dental specialist, a course to which you must travel almost always results in greater educational dividends. When it comes to dental continuing education, you usually get what you pay for. I also make time to read Dr. Gordon Christensen's monthly *Clinician's Report* newsletter. This is a completely independent and unbiased (no research funding accepted from dental supply or equipment companies) report on the products and equipment you use in your office from one of the foremost educators in general dentistry. Reading this report will improve your clinical techniques and lower your clinical expenses. Lastly, I would recommend continuing your education in disciplines other than dentistry. You will find that taking your

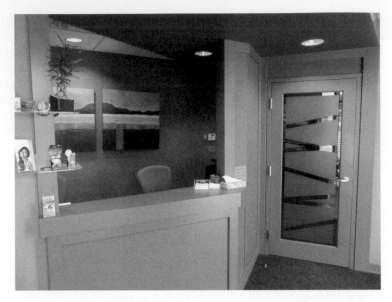

Figure 8.4.   Reception/front desk in Tyler L. Smith Family Dentistry in Omaha, NE.

mind off teeth through the study of music, history, gardening, athletic competition, or any other form of extracurricular activity makes you have a healthier appreciation and higher energy level for the practice of dentistry. One area in which I have chosen to research and become proficient is that of investing and personal finance. If you also have this interest, I would highly recommend a short book entitled *The White Coat Investor* by James M. Dahle, MD. Dr. Dahle demystifies the world of investing and financial planning to the point where you can manage your financial matters just as proficiently as managing your dental practice.

Starting a dental practice is an extremely challenging and infinitely rewarding experience. You will have days where you cannot imagine yourself in any other situation, and you will have days when you question your sanity in choosing to fly solo. In the end, I believe the advantages far outweigh the brief periods of setback as long as you keep proper perspective and continue to have an unwavering sense of confidence. I wish you the best of luck!" (Figures 8.4)

A Summary of the Practice Start-up Checklist from Wells Fargo Practice Finance

Wells Fargo Practice Finance has created a detailed practice start-up checklist. The checklist includes the major sections and sample line-items below. You may request the complete list by contacting Wells Fargo Practice Finance at 888-937-2321 or wellsfargo. com/newdentist.

"Location & accessibility

- I have researched the population in the area around the location where I wish to start my practice and confirmed it is compatible with my practice objectives.

Technology

- I have selected a dental practice management software system and plan to complete training to operate it.

Staffing

- I have developed job descriptions for each position I plan to hire

Marketing

- I have a policy for accepting insurance assigned benefits and have determined whether I will bill insurance for patient services.

Appointment Scheduling

- I have outlined my ideal day so that there is a balance between small restorative procedures, large procedures, new patient exams, and hygiene appointments.

Embezzlement Safeguards

- I am aware that one in four dentists [or more] is a victim of embezzlement and understand how to put safeguards in place to protect my practice [see Chapter 16 for a detailed discussion on embezzlement issues].

Continuing Care

- I have procedures in place to pre-appoint all hygiene patients for their next hygiene appointment.

Results Tracking

- I am prepared to maintain a computerized new patient log to track names, referral sources, amount of treatment diagnosed, and amount of treatment accepted/appointed, using either practice management software or a self-generated spreadsheet

OSHA Guidelines

- I have a job description in place to assign OSHA officer duties to one of my staff members"

References and Additional Resources

Bowser, Jason. 2015. *8 traits of successful entrepreneurs: do you have what it takes?* www.mdba.gov.

Brooks, Chad. 2015. *What is entrepreneurship?* Available at http://www.businessnewsdaily.com.

Business Plan Pro. www.businessplanpro.com.

Costes, Mark. 2013. *Pillars of Dental Success*. North Charleston, SC: CreateSpace Independent Publisher Platform.

Dahle, James M. 2014. *The White Coat Investor: A Doctor's Guide to Personal Finance and Investing*. The White Coat Investor LLC.

Heller, Eugene W. 2012. Lecture comments, "Becoming a Practice Owner." University of Nebraska Medical Center, College of Dentistry, Lincoln, NE, September.

McGee, J. E., Peterson, M., Mueller, S. L., and Sequeira, J. M. 2009. Entrepreneurial self-efficacy: refining the measure. *Entrep Theory Prac* **33** (1): 965–988.

Moberg, Kåre. 2013. An entrepreneurial self-efficacy scale with neutral wording. In: Fayolle, Alain et al. (Eds.), *Conceptual Richness and Methodological Diversity in Entrepreneurship Research*, Entrepreneurship Research in Europe. Northampton, MA: E. Edgar, pp. 67–94.

Osterhaus, Gordon F., Jr. 2011. In: K. Curtis, Eric (Ed.), *How to Open a New Dental Office or Relocate Your Current One*. Phoenix, AZ: GFO Publishing.

Resnick, Nathan. 2014. *5 key characteristics every entrepreneur should have*. Available at www.entrepreneur.com.

Robinson, Joe. 2014. *7 traits of successful entrepreneurs*. Available at www.entrepreneur.com.

Shapiro, Gary. 2004. Turning into Ted Turner at the Y. *The New York Sun*, September 30.

Stephenson, James. 2015. *25 common characteristics of successful entrepreneurs*. Available at www.entrepreneur.com.

Unthank, Michael. 2015. Lecture comments, "Dental Office Design," University of Nebraska Medical Center, College of Dentistry, Lincoln, NE, February.

Learning Exercises

Practice Start-Up Case #1: Rural Midwest

You grew up in the rural Midwest and are considering starting a practice from scratch in a county that the state has designated as a "shortage" area. The small town you have your eye on has a population of 1,100 and the county a total population of 2,000. The nearest dentist is a 30-mile drive from the town in another county. The total population of the four adjacent counties is 6,000 with three dentists, one of whom is 70 years of age and practices about 20 hours a week.

As you contemplate this possibility in the spring of your D-3/junior year of dental school, what are some of the key variables that need to be considered/managed?

Some Key Variables and Questions to Consider

Do you have an inclination toward being an entrepreneur? Do you have entrepreneurial self-efficacy?

Do you anticipate anyone else competing in this larger market in the next several years?

What resource can you leverage to maximize your chances of success?

Will the community, county, or state provide any special financial assistance?

What strings are attached to any such assistance?

What is the general and projected health of the local economy?

Are there any major employers in the area?

What is the income profile of the population? What is the dental IQ of the population?

Is there any insurance coverage for some of the population?

What are the reimbursement rates?

What space is available to renovate? Building a new facility may be a challenge financially and practically.

What assistance can a dental supplier provide for you?

What kind of advisors will you need, and when?

What will it cost to renovate space and to buy needed equipment and supplies?

What kind of financing will you seek? What kind of a business plan will you need to develop, and how will you develop it?

Are qualified staff available to be hired? Are you willing to practice for a time without a hygienist? It may be difficult to recruit one to the area.

Practice Start-Up Case #2: Front Mountain Range of Colorado

You grew up in Quite Lovely, Colorado, and would like to start a practice from scratch there. Quite Lovely's population is growing at about 5% per year and currently is 80,000. Other growing communities are within 15 miles of Quite Lovely, but you anticipate that nearly 100% of your patients live in or very near Quite Lovely.

There are thirty-five general dentists in Quite Lovely, eight of whom are over 65 years of age and could possibly retire in the next 5 years or so. The practicing community appears to be quite "closed," meaning that practitioners seem reluctant to share information about their practices and are somewhat skeptical about the need for another dentist. In fact, even your childhood family dentist told you, "I'm not sure you can start a practice from scratch here and succeed. I'm not sure we need another dentist right now."

As you contemplate this possibility in the spring of your D-3/junior year of dental school, what are some of the key variables that need to be considered/managed?

Some Key Variables and Questions to Consider

Is your family dentist correct about the need for another dentist? How confident are you about the market and the need?

Is there someone looking to sell an existing practice or perhaps would be interested in an associate-to-buyer transition in the next 2 years?

How might you try to discover such opportunities?

Do you have an inclination toward being an entrepreneur? Do you have entrepreneurial self-efficacy?

Do you anticipate anyone else competing in this market in the next several years?

What resource can you leverage to maximize your chances of success?

What is the general and projected health of the local economy?

Are there any major employers in the area?

What is the income profile of the population? What is the dental IQ of the population?

Is there any insurance coverage for some of the population?

What are the reimbursement rates?

What space is available to renovate? Building a new facility may be a challenge financially and practically.

What assistance can a dental supplier provide for you?

What kind of advisors will you need, and when?

What will it cost to renovate space and to buy needed equipment and supplies?

What kind of financing will you seek? What kind of a business plan will you need to develop, and how will you develop it?

Chapter 9
Financing a Practice
Gavin Shea

Introduction

Many new dentists worry about obtaining essential first-time financing through a commercial loan. Although most have acquired a student loan, many new doctors are not prepared to approach a commercial lender. They are understandably concerned that they will not meet the basic requirements for approval. This chapter seeks to demystify the lending process in dental acquisition.

Financing Dental Transitions: The State of the Industry

In today's commercial lending environment, dental transition financing can cover up to 100% of the purchase price and include additional working capital. Serious lender candidates will meet underwriting criteria specific for dentistry and may have a portfolio or group of past loans from which inferences can be drawn and risk mitigated.

Other sources of lending for new dentists include seller financing, local or community bank financing, and loans secured by the U.S. Small Business Administration (SBA), in association with another lender. In general, all lenders are looking for borrowers with demonstrated ability to manage debt, as evidenced by a satisfactory review of personal credit. Chapter 26 discusses important concepts in personal finance.

Few other start-up small businesses have access to this type of 100% financing. Dentists have an attractive record of paying their commercial loans in full and on time. Their default rate is low. Whether this is due to favorable demographics, ethical character and professionalism, or the general success of the industry, lenders do favor doctors with good personal credit and typically allow them to finance a qualified practice at 100% with favorable terms. The specifics of achieving such financing will be explored throughout this chapter.

Dental Practice Transition: A Practical Guide to Management, Second Edition.
Edited by David G. Dunning and Brian M. Lange.
© 2016 John Wiley & Sons, Inc. Published 2016 by John Wiley & Sons, Inc.
Companion Website: www.wiley.com/go/dunning/transition

Historical Perspective

Only as recently as the 1980s did the dental industry recognize that practices had a value beyond their equipment that was transferrable. Most doctors in the 1970s had only the options of working for another doctor (which few did), or "hanging out a shingle" and starting from scratch, as retiring dentists tended to close their practices rather than attempt to sell them.

When appraisal and evaluation of *goodwill* were introduced, few lenders were comfortable with such *blue-sky* transactions. When a practice was sold, the primary option for financing available to the new doctor was typically a loan from the seller.

Many of these internally financed loans had their pitfalls. Sometimes the loan hinged on the seller's staying on as an employee, making it difficult if not impossible to fire the practice "banker" if the relationship did not work out. Some of these transactions lacked the *due diligence* necessary to determine whether the buyer could afford or had sufficient cash flow to take on the practice loan. Without the lender's objective perspective, such analysis never occurred. Without the analysis, the buyer did not know if the practice's cash flow would support his or her lifestyle. The results could be painful.

Sellers also disliked the risks associated with being the bank for their buyers. At a time in their lives when they were trying to leave dental practice responsibilities behind, sellers found themselves still bound to the practice for income.

As a result of these problems and the availability today of external financing through specialty lenders, very few transactions now involve seller financing.

Preparing for a Practice Acquisition Loan

Commercial Loan versus Consumer Loan

Banks make a distinction between commercial and retail (that is, consumer) products. Frequently, commercial and retail loans are handled by different banking departments. Some banks focus on retail lending and have few resources devoted to commercial lending. Student loans, home mortgages, car loans, and personal credit cards are considered retail lending. New doctors who seek commercial financing are venturing, usually for the first time, into the commercial departments of the bank.

In general, commercial loans are granted based on the financial strength of the borrower and the business opportunity he or she represents. Loans are typically secured by the assets of the borrower, including the business. The typical business loan is structured over a 5–10-year period. Interest rates may be fixed or floating, and there may be conditions that relate to the business (for example, a lease on the property where the business will reside) and to the borrower (for example, insurance requirements such as disability and life insurance, or a personal guarantee). Of primary importance is the doctor's personal credit profile.

Assessing the Borrower's Personal Credit

The first step in preparing for practice ownership is maintaining good personal credit. Lenders and other vendors access personal credit information by requesting a credit report from at least one of the three nationwide credit agencies: TransUnion, Equifax, and Experian. These bureaus gather data on each consumer and provide a report that includes a list of accounts, timeliness of payment, and public information such as tax liens or judgments. The bureaus also employ statistical modeling of these data to create a credit score on each consumer based on past performance. This score helps lenders evaluate how likely the borrower is to repay the loan promptly. Credit scores range from 300 to 850, with higher scores indicating lower risk for the lender.

A credit score over 750 is considered excellent and will garner the borrower the best rates and terms available. Scores below 665 will significantly narrow the number of commercial lenders interested in a financing project. If such projects can be approved at all, a low score will result in a higher rate and more rigid terms.

Credit scores are influenced by the following factors (by priority):

- Timeliness of monthly payments
- Amount of debt
- Type of debt
- Inquiries from outside vendors

Experian, one of the major consumer credit bureaus, advises consumers to maintain good credit by paying bills on time, seeking out credit only as needed, and monitoring credit annually to guard against errors and identity theft.

The Federal Trade Commission (http://www.consumer.ftc.gov/topics/money-creditwww.ftc.gov) has excellent information on managing personal credit. The FTC advises consumers to check their credit rating through a website set up through the Fair Credit Reporting Act—www.annualcreditreport.com—mandating that all three bureaus give consumers access to a free credit report annually.

Years of experience in evaluating the credit reports of new doctors have revealed several common but easily avoided problems.

- Sometimes student loans that are in deferment show up on the credit report as late payments. These "late pays" can and should be disputed and eventually removed from the report.
- Similarly, small medical bills, unknown to the student, are reported as collections accounts. Since students move frequently, a delayed medical bill may be sent to a past address. The young doctor may have no knowledge of the tardy bill, but it ends up in their credit report as a collection account—generating evidence against the doctor's claim of a prompt payment history.

Although these accounts cannot be disputed, they can be neutralized over time. Annual credit reviews or credit reporting services that report changes as they happen can alert borrowers to these oversights, allowing quick payment and resolution. After such bills have been paid, the credit score may have time to recover, minimizing the negative effect of late payments.

Assessing Your Income Requirements

Before buying a practice and applying for a business loan, it is essential to know the amount of money you will need to run your household—otherwise known as a personal or family budget. Income requirements are a key part of the basic information that every doctor should know before considering a particular practice purchase.

Although there are many ways of estimating personal income requirements, one proven method, shown in Table 9.1, is to determine your monthly expenses based on a

Table 9.1   Estimating personal income (example).

Expenses		Commitment	Outstanding	Mo Pmt
Housing	1st mortgage	$200,000	$157,936	$1,385
	2nd mortgage	$0	$0	$0
	Cost of home	$240,000		$0
	Mkt val home	$0		$0
Total Housing		$200,000	$157,936	$1,385
Installment Loans		Commitment	Outstanding	Mo Pmt
1	Car payment 1	$19,885	$7,155	$250
2	Car payment 2			
3		$0	$0	$0
4		$0	$0	$0
Total Installment Loans:		$19,885	$7,155	$250
Credit Cards/Revolving:		Commitment	Outstanding	Mo Pmt
1	Chase	$5,000	$1,000	$200
2	Capital One	$2,000	$400	$40
3	Wells Fargo	$5,000	$500	$60
Total Credit Card:		$10,000	$1,900	$300
Student Loans:		Commitment	Outstanding	Mo Pmt
1		$100,000	$84,153	$631
2		$0	$0	$0
3		$0	$0	$0
Total Student Loans:		$100,000	$84,153	$631
TOTAL REVOLVING		$10,000	$1,900	$300
TOTAL INSTALLMENT (car/student)		$119,885	$91,308	$881
Total Monthly Obligations:				$2,566
Total Loan Outstanding:		$329,885		
Living Expense $300 a Month Per Family Member				$1,200
Total Monthly Expenditures				$3,766
20% "Hedge"				$753
Total Income Requirements				$4,519

review of monthly obligations combined with a monthly expense allotment per family member. Chapter 26 includes an alternative format for a personal or family budget.

List your mortgage debt (or rent payment) as well as installment debt (usually automobile debt, but it could be any installment debt that is unrelated to school debts). Next, account for credit cards and lines of credit. (Minimum payments on credit cards are used as the monthly expense in this exercise.) Finally, list student debt payments.

Expenses other than monthly debt obligations can be estimated by multiplying the number of family members by $300. This accounts for most day-to-day expenses. In this example the doctor needs a bare minimum of $1,200 a month to cover basic living expenses for a family of four. Unusual or other specific obligations (that is, alimony, child support, special investments) should be accounted for and added to monthly obligations.

In looking at income requirements, many doctors ask if it is appropriate to include an accounting of spousal income. If the doctor's income is insufficient to make the deal viable, many lenders will in fact ask for additional income support, often provided in the form of the spouse's income and personal guaranty. If the practice cash flow is sufficient without the spouse's income, then the lender may not ask for additional income and guaranty.

Once a doctor has a good understanding of his or her family expenses, projecting income requirements becomes easy. It is recommended that you take these basic expenses, add a small hedge of about 20% on top, and use this final number as a monthly income requirement. In Table 9.1 the doctor in question needs $4,519 per month to comfortably continue his or her lifestyle after the practice purchase.

This is an appropriate place to acknowledge the reality of rising dental student debt. Note the impact if the student debt rises in Table 9.1 from $100,000 to $250,000, an increasingly common scenario given that the average currently hovers around ~$225,000 and continues to increase every year. Instead of a monthly student loan payment of $631, the payment grows to $1,578; the "Total Monthly Expenditures" reaches $4,713 (vs. $3,766). Adding in the 20% hedge ($4,713 × 1.2), the "Total Income Requirements" become $5,666 instead of $4,519. Similarly, differences in other variables such as a housing market twice more expensive than listed in Table 9.1 would have significant increases in the needed total monthly income requirements.

Preparing Your File for a Commercial Lender

An easy task to be done ahead of time is to prepare a file of financial information for the lender. It is recommended that a potential borrower have the items below handy when applying for a loan. All lenders will require the first three items. The additional items are useful in telling your story and positioning you for a positive outcome. Start immediately to gather this information, as it will eliminate much of the stress associated with applying for a commercial loan:

- 2 years of personal tax returns
- CV (curriculum vitae) or résumé
- Dental license
- Production reports from current associateship (if available)
- Life insurance and disability policies (if available)
- Personal financial statement (list of assets and debts)—see Table 9.1 for an example
- Income requirements (personal budget)
- Copy of self-obtained credit report
- Any appropriate references (especially if you have a short work history)

Understanding the Commercial Lender

Many doctors are confused at the array of commercial lenders who seem interested in doing business with them. In this section we explore the two overarching credit philosophies that are used in making credit decisions. We also examine the types of lenders available and the benefits and challenges of each.

Two Credit Philosophies

In general, lenders can be divided into two categories: asset-based and cash-flow-driven. As the term implies, an *asset-based lender* looks first at the collateral or hard assets of the business to secure the loan. Equipment, furnishings, inventory, and work in progress are examples of hard assets. Most community banks and large, non-specialized banks would look to cover most of the loan proceeds with this kind of asset base. Dental practices as a rule do not have this collateral base. The sale of a dental practice most commonly does not at least initially include real estate or land—only the dental practice business.

Cash-flow-driven lenders tend to be specialty oriented. These lenders make their decisions based on the historical performance of the business—that is, its ability to generate enough profit to fund the debt while allowing the owner to maintain his or her lifestyle. These lenders do not typically expect personal or business collateral (assets) to protect the loan. Rather, they base loan approval on sufficient practice cash flow and their understanding of the dental industry.

Therefore, doctors who approach only community banks or large banks with little dental experience for a practice acquisition loan may be frustrated by these lenders. There may be exceptions, however. Occasionally, a local or a regional bank will choose not to follow its asset-based lending approach and provide instead a loan program that resembles that of a specialty lender. It is more common, however, for the local bank to proceed within its traditional philosophy and use other methods to shore up its collateral coverage (discussed below).

Types of Lenders

Understanding how each type of lender is prone to respond to practice purchase applications empowers loan seekers to find the right lender for their project. It will also help identify exceptionally good "deals."

Potential lenders for a practice acquisition can include the seller, the local bank, the SBA, the specialty lender, and the loan broker. The benefits and challenges of each will be discussed.

Seller Financing

As discussed earlier, seller financing historically was much more common and potentially could still offer the buyer some advantages. The seller may offer more favorable terms than the commercial lender. In the event that the buyer is unable to get outside financing (for example, due to a poor credit history), seller financing may be the only option available. If the transaction has a particular challenge—such as a large practice being bought by a new, financially unproven dentist who needs mentoring—the seller might be willing to carry a small loan for the buyer to augment outside financing. In this manner, the seller in effect shares some of the risk in the transition.

The biggest challenge of seller financing is that it simply may not be available. After all, sellers do not necessarily have to provide financing in order to sell their practices. In a competitive situation, holding out for a seller-financed loan can result in failure to purchase the practice.

If seller financing is available, the relationship pitfalls mentioned earlier *must be* avoided. It is important for the buyer to ensure he has a competent and experienced dental-focused advisor who can thoroughly review the transaction. The seller-financier for the practice purchase obviously has a conflict of interest. She or he may be unable to provide objective analysis about the true cash flow with the aim of protecting the buyer, plus she or he could potentially even avoid disclosing key financial information that another lender would probably detect.

Local Bank

As mentioned previously, local commercial lenders tend to be generalists with asset-based lending philosophies. However, some local lenders can, at times, vary their offering for dentists in some markets. The benefits are that the borrowing dentist can centralize his or her banking in one institution. Rates are usually favorable and might be 0.5–1% lower than some specialty lenders.

Typically, however, local banks have difficulty offering 100% financing. They may require a co-signer for the loan or look for liens on personal residences to shore up their collateral position (mitigate risk). Frequently, a local lender will require the practice to maintain a business account and sometimes to agree to a minimum balance in that account.

This type of lender may have trouble finalizing a loan decision because the loan request is unusual. The borrower may not meet the lending criteria. So the bank may ask for a co-signer or guarantor on the note (for example, a parent with a positive balance sheet). More often than not, a local bank or large, nonspecialized lender will offer a young doctor an acquisition loan that uses the SBA guarantee to shore up its collateral position.

In some unique transition situations, unique financial support for a practice purchase might be available through state agencies or local community organizations, especially in areas in great need of dentists.

SBA Loans

The Small Business Administration was established in 1954 with the mission of helping small businesses flourish in the United States. Since 1991, the SBA program has guaranteed small business loans totaling $94.6 billion.

An SBA loan is a term loan offered by a bank or commercial lending institution according to SBA guidelines, with the loan partially guaranteed by the Small Business Administration. The lending institution provides the funds and loan terms, while the SBA guarantees as much as 85% of the loan principal on loans of up to $150,000 and 75% on loans of more than $150,000. This allows traditional, asset-based lenders a significant collateral position.

The SBA loan program is known for its favorable terms. While conventional business financing often requires a large down payment of 20–30% or more, the down payment for an SBA loan can be as low as 10% amortized over 25 years. In addition, interest rates may be comparable or lower than those for conventional loans. However, the loan also incorporates a fee that usually averages to around 2.6% of the total loan amount, depending on the size of the loan. Furthermore, even a 10% down payment may be difficult for many early-career dentists.

The SBA loan is what many local, nonspecialty lenders will offer dentists seeking to buy a practice. The most popular and heavily utilized SBA programs are the 7(a) and 504 loans, particularly for transactions involving commercial real estate. In fact, this type of loan is particularly beneficial when real property is being purchased, as virtually all commercial real estate loans from traditional lenders require a 20% down payment. Thousands of small business owners successfully take advantage of SBA loans every year to finance owner-occupied commercial real estate purchases—from existing facilities to raw land and building development.

Specialty Lenders

Historically, specialty lenders in the dental industry were privately owned. While they offered 100% fixed-rate financing, their rates were significantly higher than local banks and had restrictive terms including significant prepayment penalties. Today there are several large banks that have dental specialty lending divisions. They and some regional lenders make up the majority of specialty lending in the dental industry. They benefit doctors by providing 100% fixed-rate financing, usually with minimal fees and flexible terms for prepayment. A specialty lender can usually tailor the loan package to meet the buyer's specific budget and circumstances, and may also be able to provide a broader range of loan options, from short-term fixed rate loans to low variable rate mortgages.

Specialty lenders often have complementary services that help facilitate the practice purchase and/or assist the doctor should problems arise in the practice. Although these services in no way take the place of competent advisors (that is, the accountant, lawyer, and practice management consultant), they do augment more traditional advisory resources and help make the lender an informed member of the doctor's team.

Loan Brokers

Loan brokers bring borrowers and lenders together, but it is important to know that they do not underwrite the loan or keep the loan long term. Also, brokers do not add value in a market where lenders are already present and active. However, brokers can be of great value in situations when a loan is difficult to place. They can streamline the process for the borrower and find a "home" for a difficult loan.

Brokers are likely to be the most costly loan source in the market, since the broker must be paid in some fashion, either by fees or increased interest rates. Finally, since the broker is not the underwriter, he or she cannot provide other services to remedy problems the doctor may experience along the way.

Questions to Ask Potential Lenders

Frequently, doctors do not realize that they are not working with the primary lending source until the loan is already in progress. By that time, they may feel it is too difficult to start the underwriting process over again and thus settle for a lender they know little about. If you ask the right questions up front, it is definitely possible to avoid this problem.

The following questions will help you understand if a prospective lender is truly interested in helping you, has comprehensive knowledge of practice acquisition lending, and is the primary lender for the loan.

- What markets does your bank serve?
- Does your bank provide commercial loans for new professional practices?
- Do you offer 100% financing for business loans?
- Do you have other dental clients? May I speak with one of them?
- How does the loan decision get made? How long does it usually take to get a decision?
- Who will fund the actual loan?
- Who will service the loan long-term?
- If I have problems, whom do I call?

Analysis of the Buyer

When a lender prepares to evaluate the loan applicant's credit in connection with a practice acquisition, the process involves an analysis of the buyer's situation, the practice, and the deal itself. The evaluation is based on the parameters discussed earlier in this chapter.

First and foremost, the lender will assess whether the buyer's personal credit history indicates an ability to secure and manage credit. If the buyer has prepared well for a loan application by reviewing and improving his or her credit standing, the analysis should be easy for the lender and result in optimal financing terms.

Similarly, the lender will review the buyer's personal assets and liabilities to clarify current cash flow. Income requirements will be another key consideration for the lender (remember the importance of your personal/family budget). Those buyers with modest income requirements are better positioned to "afford" the practice.

Beyond financial analysis, the lender will evaluate the practical work experience of the doctor. A lender familiar with the dental industry will be concerned that the clinical skills and interests of the buyer match the practice environment. For example, if the doctor is relatively new in practice but has a history of being able to generate strong production, a favorable production report from an associate position held by the doctor would bolster the lender's belief that the operation will succeed. Perhaps the practice currently outsources all in-house endodontic or oral surgery procedures, but the buyer can bring the advantage of that expertise into the new acquisition. This type of subjective information can aid in the analysis and help support the buyer's case.

Lenders may seek other subjective information that helps evaluate the buyer's risk potential. For instance, if the doctor plans to be somewhat involved in the community, that seems to predict some measure of success. Dentistry is a community-based business. Doctors who live in and are invested in the particular area in which their practice resides tend to do better than doctors who buy a practice simply because it is a "job" with no community connection. The doctor's plans for marketing, staffing, and other business planning issues are important and weigh on the lender analysis of the opportunity.

Analysis of the Practice

Regardless of other analyses done by appraisers or other advisors, all lenders must and will insist on performing their own analysis of the practice's cash flow. Insufficient cash flow will prevent loan approval. Remember the vital importance of "cash flow, cash flow, cash flow" made in Chapter 7 about buying–buying into a practice.

Specialty lenders commonly ask for 2 years of corporate tax returns (or Schedule C and expenses, if the owner is sole proprietor) and current-year profit and loss statements as essential for analyzing a practice. Other lenders typically require 3–5 years of tax returns in evaluating a potential practice purchase opportunity, paralleling time parameters discussed in Chapters 4 and 5 (business planning and practice valuation). The lender will evaluate previous years and the interim year (if that applies) to check for trends. For instance, a practice with a declining revenue base or profitability is likely to alarm the lender as a "red flag" that requires acceptable explanation.

The analysis is performed by taking the net income of the practice and "adding back" expenses that the new owner can eliminate or use to help cover debt and personal expenses. This is the same essential process described as *normalization* in Chapter 5. Examples of common "addbacks" include the following:

- Owner's compensation
- Pension relating specifically to the owner
- Associate's salary (if the buyer will be able to do that production without an associate)
- Depreciation expense
- Extraordinary expenses

If necessary and appropriate, the doctor can add back additional personal choice expenditures such as travel expenses, car expenses, and certain staffing positions to help improve cash flow.

After the objective analysis has convinced the lender that the buyer represents a reasonable risk, *subjective factors* become relevant. The lender will review the demographics of the area, the clinical makeup of the practice, staffing, marketing, and "payor mix" (a combination of preferred provider organizations, health maintenance organizations, private pay, and Medicaid). The lender will assess the size of the physical space, hours of operation, and availability of a suitable lease. Characteristics and factors that need to be carefully matched to the buyer's needs and abilities become obvious.

During Transition

Matching the subjective elements of the practice to the buyer is vital to long-term success and requires a transition plan. An experienced lender will be watching for obvious practical problems during transition to the new practice, and may ask the buyer to do further analysis to clarify and resolve any issues. Examples of problems the lender might ask the buyer to address include the purchase of a practice that emphasizes clinical competence that the buyer lacks, such as high-end cosmetic dentistry; a seller who is unwilling to sign a sufficient covenant not to compete; or a practice where the seller's spouse was the office manager, so that the transition, while successful, also involves filling this position. These problems can be managed, but must be recognized and handled as a part of the transition plan.

An example of a subjective factor that can actually work against loan approval is the inability to obtain a lease with renewal options that ensure the new buyer can depend on a place to practice for at least 5 years. It is helpful to remember that the buyer's key advisors (accountants and lawyers with expertise in dental transitions) would raise the same concerns about such issues as they are also invested in the success of the transition.

Loan Terms, Rates, and Typical Conditions

Terms, rates, and conditions will vary from time to time and from lender to lender. This section discusses terms as they exist as of this writing.

The Proposal Letter

The lender's proposal letter is designed to help the borrower assess what a lender is likely to offer in advance of the exhaustive underwriting process. Therefore, it is standard practice for the lender to draft a letter proposing rates, terms, and conditions for the loan transaction. The proposal might be issued after a simple review of personal credit, or sometimes after a more thorough evaluation. However, since a true in-depth analysis has yet to take place, such a proposal is not to be interpreted as the lender's approval. The proposal letter merely details the terms and conditions the lender can offer. It is not a commitment to do so.

The proposal letter should contain the following rate and term information:

- The name of the entity who is borrowing the money and the guarantor (the borrower).
- An outline of the purpose of the financing, such as an amount for purchasing the practice and an amount for working capital.
- The term of the loan (typically 7–10 years).
  - An experienced lender may provide a three-month deferral so that the borrower does not begin making payments until month #4.
- The interest rate of the financing.
  - This must be very clear. It could be fixed for the entire term of the note or variable (priced around prime). It may be fixed for a number of years and then "float" until the end of the term. Generally, 10-year fixed-rate financing is preferable.
- The expiration date of the offer.
  - Most proposal letters have a time limit or some way to increase or decrease rate over a period of time. Usually a lender can fix the proposal letter's rates and terms for 30 days.
- Fees that are clearly stated.
  - A small documentation fee (around $350) is common, but other fees and points may be included (points are fees amounting to 1% of the total loan amount). In

SBA financing, additional fees can be as high as 3%, or 3 points. If the loan amount is high, some fees might take the form of advance payments on the loan, increasing the real cost of financing. These should be noted.

The next section of the proposal letter should contain the standard approval conditions that will appear on the loan. At the proposal stage, it is too early for the lender to anticipate the necessity of adding more conditions. However, there are standard conditions that appear on every proposal letter, and it is reasonable for a lender to supply these. Sample conditions include but may not be limited to the following:

- Evidence of a professional license
- Evidence of a legal entity in good standing (corporation or partnership), if one exists
- Satisfactory review of a buy/sell agreement that includes a list of equipment and documented evidence that the buyer is protected from competition with the seller
- An office lease that shows the doctor can practice at the site for a minimum of 5 years
- A provision stating that the lender may secure a first security interest in the practice (blanket lien)
- Available funds to be used for business purposes

It should be noted that the SBA or banks without a dental specialty may ask for additional conditions such as a lien on a home, a parental guarantee, and so forth.

Other items in the proposal letter may relate to insurance requirements. At larger loan amounts ($300,000 and above), many lenders will ask the borrower to carry life insurance, disability, or business overhead insurance. All lenders will require property and hazard insurance. These insurances are prudent for any new business owner.

For some borrowers a prepayment requirement to comply with a lender's policies can pose a serious problem. For that reason, the lender's prepayment policies should be clearly stated in the proposal letter. Carefully review prepayment policies before proceeding with any lender to ensure you understand the terms. Prepayments are not always a negative and can sometimes help reduce rates.

Finally, the proposal letter should outline the next steps for submission into underwriting, where the credit decision will be made. At that time, the lender should request all outstanding documents or forms. To proceed to the next steps, the potential borrower should indicate acceptance of the terms and conditions in the proposed offer, sign the letter, pay any conditional fees, and submit everything to the lender.

The Commitment Letter

After the credit underwriting (analysis) is complete and the loan is approved, the lender will issue a commitment letter. In most respects, this letter should match the proposal letter. However, the commitment letter will also state that the application for the loan has been approved. Upon receipt, it is essential to have an advisor, such as your attorney, review the letter to confirm that the terms and conditions are clear and consistent with your needs. The loan rate, basic terms, insurance requirements, and prepayment policies should not have changed. Material changes to these factors may raise questions about the reliability of the lender.

There will be an easy explanation for some changes that appear in the commitment letter, however. Normal processing may result in a change to the loan's dollar amount and/or conditions. For example, cash-flow analysis may have indicated that the requested loan amount is unrealistic and cannot be supported. In these cases, the lender may return a counteroffer and approval of a reduced loan amount. In another example, cash-flow analysis may indicate that the lender must declare a maximum on the monthly lease amount. The lender may decide to require an additional guarantor, and such a condition would appear on the letter.

The commitment letter will also have an expiration date that must be heeded. Commitments can be withdrawn after this date, and rates can no longer be guaranteed.

Comparison of Lenders through Proposal and Commitment Letters

As indicated above, it is wise to retain an advisor to evaluate a lender's proposal and commitment letters. Some new borrowers make the mistake of focusing only on the rate in the proposal, not realizing that fees, advanced payments, and terms that may stunt the growth of the practice (five-year versus ten-year, for example) significantly change the offer in real terms. An advisor such as an accountant with experience in the dental industry can help arrive at an "apples to apples" comparison.

Due Diligence and Closing

After the commitment letter is signed, the closing process begins. At this time, the buyer and his/her team of advisors must perform the due diligence activities that will protect the new practice. A lien search will be performed to identify any creditors with a legal claim to property owned by the seller and buyer. All liens on the seller's practice must be cleared up, either with available funds or proceeds from the loan. Loan documents including a note, security agreement, personal guarantee, and corporate guarantee must be reviewed and signed. A competent lawyer versed in dental practice transitions is important to the buyer at this time. The lender will follow up for all the items requested as a condition (license, buy/sell agreement, evidence of insurance or that applications have been made, etc.). Wiring of payment instructions will be requested so that the funds are available on the day of the closing. Most lenders will not be present at closings; their work is done ahead of time.

How to Maintain an Excellent Relationship with a Lender

From the Borrower's Perspective

After the sale is complete and the loan is in place, the borrower should expect timely and accurate bills from the lender. A good service center should be available to handle problems and prevent errors. Should the borrower have additional lending needs, it is reasonable to expect the lender to provide advice and assistance. Specialty lenders also supply relevant data and assistance in operating the practice itself. For marketing information, referrals to other dental professionals in the industry should be available, as well as information on how the practice is doing vis-à-vis industry standards. These services are not usually supplied by general industry-based lenders.

From the Lender's Perspective

Lenders expect timely payments. This is essential to maintaining a good relationship with any lender. It follows that a new buyer who is having difficulty paying promptly must make a priority of informing the lender. There are valuable tools and resources available from experienced specialty lenders that can help you keep your new practice on track, but only if they have been informed of problems in a timely enough manner to actually put these tools to good use. Frequently, a good lender can help restore stability to the practice and resolve difficulties. However, the worst situation for the lender and for the buyer occurs when a bad situation is hidden until the practice is near default and time is growing short. At that point the lender has few alternatives and little flexibility to work with the doctor to save the practice.

Fortunately, events that threaten the life of the practice are rare in dentistry. An experienced lender and an educated borrower can develop successful transitions and keep practices healthy far into the future.

Assessing Your Future

Perhaps you are still weighing the alternatives of acquiring an existing practice or starting one yourself. While many of the factors are similar, there are a few differences. The design of your office is one example. If you are acquiring, then you will have to work with the existing footprint. If you are starting a new practice, you can design from the ground up. Below you will find examples of some of the questions you should consider when assessing your direction. Remember whichever path you take, good planning will help ensure success. And remember the complementary, foundational information provided especially in Chapter 2 (financial statements), Chapter 4 (business planning), Chapter 5 (practice valuation), Chapter 7 (buying–buying into a practice, and Chapter 8 (starting a practice).

Practice Acquisition

Location and Accessibility

1. How accessible is the office including parking, public transportation, and handicap requirements?
2. What is the competitive landscape? How many dentists are in the area already? What kind of services do they offer?

Office Layout and Design

1. What does a patient see and experience when they walk in the door?
2. Are the treatment rooms properly equipped for your style? What kind of updates will you need?
3. How does the division between public, treatment, and private areas match up to your needs?

Business Systems

1. Is the selling dentist's fee schedule compatible with yours?
2. What types of payment are accepted by the practice?
3. How are prescheduling, cancellations, and emergencies handled?
4. How well maintained are patient records?

Marketing

1. What types of advertising and/or promotion has been done to help acquire new patients?
2. What kind of a plan do you have to reach out to patients who are or become inactive?

Staff

1. What processes are already in place for personnel management?
2. How concerned, involved, or engaged is the staff in the overall success of the practice?

Practice Start-Up

Financial & Business Planning

1. What is your project budget? Does it support all of your needs and plans?
2. What types of insurance and payments will you accept?
3. Have you done a cash flow projection for your new practice? What is your plan to build positive cash flow and sustain practice growth?

Location and Accessibility

1. What are the local demographics? What kind of practice is best suited for this area? Does this match your vision?
2. What is the competitive landscape? How many dentists are in the area already? What kind of services do they offer?

Technology & Equipment

1. How will you handle the following:
    a. Scheduling; Appointments/cancellations?
    b. Financial record-keeping?
    c. Staffing and payroll?
2. What clinical technology do you need to have from the beginning? What do you plan to add later, as your practice grows?

Marketing

1. How will you develop and implement your marketing plan?
2. What types of outreach will you use to let people know about your new practice?

The questions above will help you get started on the road to practice ownership, but are by no means all you need to consider. There are many excellent resources available to help you figure out your plan. For example, Wells Fargo Practice Finance offers practice acquisition and start-up checklists, plus an easy-to-use business plan template that will help you build a solid foundation upon which to develop your practice. Other lenders and sources may also offer similarly helpful information. For more information, contact your regional financing specialist at 1-800-326-0376 or visit wellsfargo.com/contactpracticefinance. Wells Fargo Practice Finance is the only practice lender selected especially for ADA members and endorsed by ADA Business Resources.

References and Additional Resources

Federal Trade Commission. 2014. *Building a better credit report*. Available at http://www.consumer.ftc.gov/articles/pdf-0032-building-a-better-credit-report.pdf.

Lovelace, G. (n.d.). *For sale: one dental practice*. Dental Economics. Available at http://www.dentaleconomics.com/index.html.

Small Business Administration. www.sba.gov.

www.adabusinessresources.com/en/.

www.consumer.ftc.gov/topics/money-credit.

https://practicefinance.wellsfargo.com/dentists/dental-calculators/calc.html.

Learning Exercises

Complete the following exercises to help ensure your understanding of the information presented in this chapter:

1. What is the difference between a collateral-based lending philosophy and a cash-flow lending philosophy? Give examples of each.
2. Go online to annualcreditreport.com and do the following: (1) identify the three major credit bureaus; (2) select one bureau and order your credit report from that bureau; and (3) after reviewing your personal credit, identify if you have any delinquencies or "late payments."
3. What are the major advantages and disadvantages of a seller-financed practice acquisition loan?
4. Name four items that should be in the file you take to a commercial lender.
5. In evaluating a practice for purchase, what are some of the subjective factors to consider?
6. What are appropriate practice expenses that can be "added back" to net income to give a realistic assessment of cash flow?
7. How is a proposal letter different from a commitment letter?

Chapter 10
Business Entities
Arthur S. Wiederman and Ross L. Crist

Sole Proprietorship

Description

The sole proprietorship is the least complicated of the available business entity forms. As a sole proprietor a business is simply operated under an individual's name (e.g., John Smith, D.D.S.). A sole proprietorship may also use a specified title, or a "doing business as" name (or d.b.a.).

Necessary Documentation

Unlike the other entities to be discussed later in this chapter, with the sole proprietorship, other than one's professional license, there generally are only a few business application forms necessary for local, state, or federal government agencies to establish this business entity. Typically, the practitioner only needs to obtain a business license from the local jurisdiction (city, county, etc.), a state dental license, and federal and state drug prescription licenses. The owner sole proprietor will need to secure a federal tax ID number for employment tax purposes. Some states may also require a special tax license. Although a dentist may use his or her individual name and title (for example, John Q. Smith, D.D.S.), the business may also operate under a d.b.a. name. In the case of a d.b.a., John Q. Smith, D.D.S. could use as his d.b.a., Lincoln Avenue Dental. He may choose to do so for unique marketing and/or identification purposes because the practice is located on Lincoln Avenue. But in order to do this, Dr. Smith is typically required to post notice in the local newspaper for a period of time (usually a month or 2), or file the assumed name with the local county government prior to the opening of his business. This serves as legal notice to others who may have a similar name, to be made aware that Dr. Smith intends to use Lincoln Avenue Dental as his d.b.a. If others have a conflict with Dr. Smith's d.b.a., they have adequate time to legally contest the use of Dr. Smith's d.b.a. business name.

Dental Practice Transition: A Practical Guide to Management, Second Edition.
Edited by David G. Dunning and Brian M. Lange.
© 2016 John Wiley & Sons, Inc. Published 2016 by John Wiley & Sons, Inc.
Companion Website: www.wiley.com/go/dunning/transition

Operational and Management Aspects

To begin operating as a sole proprietorship, one needs to go to a bank (typically a local bank) and open a business bank account. Usually a checking account is the first account established. This account is opened under the name of John Smith, D.D.S., or his d.b.a. The account, even though used for business purposes, is treated as a personal account of Dr. Smith, and Dr. Smith is personally and legally responsible for all activity on the account, just as he would be for his personal checking account.

As the owner, all deposits or income of the dental practice are placed into this account and are used to pay office expenses. Additionally, the practitioner may also decide to open a business savings account for the practice. But again, the savings account, while used for business purposes, is still considered a personally guaranteed account of the practitioner. Personal income from the business to the dentist is usually taken from the business account in the form of a draw or check. This can be any amount and may be taken at any time, depending on available funds. While some dentists may choose to pay personal bills such as mortgage payments, home utility bills, and so forth from their business account, it is not recommended. If personal bills are paid from the business account, they must be treated as personal draw checks or personal income. This may create confusion regarding business expenses versus personal expenses in calculating true business overhead and in paying the correct taxes at year's end. Instead, most dentists take a periodic monthly draw, transfer it to their personal bank account, and use their personal account to pay personal bills. This allows clear delineation of business versus personal expenses. Draws taken from the business account will obviously depend on the cash flow, or income and expenses, of the business. As collections and overhead expenses in a dental practice vary from month to month, draw checks also vary as to amount and as to when they are taken for personal use.

Again, we do not recommend that you pay your personal bills from the business account. By taking a periodic and preferably a set monthly draw from the business, a personal as well as business "budget" can easily be established. This in turn will allow for the accumulation of more money both personally and in the practice, which over time can provide a means for larger equipment purchases, retirement planning, and so forth. Paying all personal bills through a business account makes it harder to save money and meet goals in both the business and in personal life. Chapter 26 discusses personal budgets and personal finance.

Income Tax Issues

As a sole proprietor, earnings from a dental practice are reported on the practitioner's individual income tax return. Business gross income and allowable business expenses are reported on Schedule C of Federal Form 1040. The net income of the practice is shown at the bottom of Schedule C and then is transferred to page 1 of Form 1040. Thus, business income is reported just like any other type of income on a personal tax return.

Example: Dr. Smith's dental practice collected $600,000 for the current tax year. His deductible business expenses (staff salaries, lab, supplies, depreciation, etc.) for the year were $400,000. Dr. Smith will report income on his individual income tax return of $200,000 for the year.

When starting dental practice, it is possible to incur a loss of income (and is most likely in the first few months or perhaps years of operation). This loss is tax deductible if the individual's personal investment in the practice is what is called "at risk." For example, if a practice that is started on October 1 collects a total of $40,000 for the months of October, November, and December, and during that same period the expenses of the practice are $55,000, there would be an operational loss of $15,000. If money to fund the $15,000 loss is borrowed from the bank and the dentist is personally liable for the loan (which is typically the case with bank loans), then the dentist is considered "at risk" for the $15,000 loan and is permitted to deduct the loss on his or her personal tax return.

For purposes of allowable tax deductions, now is a good time to discuss the concept of *depreciation*. As a dentist, the sole proprietor typically operates on what is referred to as the cash basis of accounting. This requires the practitioner to report receipts (income) as collected and deduct all expenses as paid. The one exception is for fixed assets (like equipment, furnishings, or fixtures) purchased for the business. For tax deduction purposes, fixed assets are allowed to be depreciated, or expensed to offset taxes, over time. This means that instead of taking a full tax deduction the same year equipment is purchased, the individual is allowed to depreciate or deduct a portion of the cost of that equipment over a period of several years.

Example: Assume Dr. Smith buys $100,000 of dental equipment. Federal tax law says that he can depreciate dental equipment over a period of 5 years; however, it takes 6 calendar years to fully depreciate a 5 year asset. So the doctor's allowable tax deduction each year for this purchase equipment, according to current tax law, is as follows:

Year 1 (20%)	$20,000
Year 2 (32%)	$32,000
Year 3 (19.2%)	$19,200
Year 4 (11.52%)	$11,520
Year 5 (11.52%)	$11,520
Year 6 (5.76%)	$5,760
Total depreciation	$100,000

Note: There is an exception or provision that was put into law several years ago regarding the depreciation of newly purchased fixed assets. This tax law provision is referred to as Internal Revenue Code *Section 179* and allows for the *full deduction* of expenses for equipment purchased in the same year it is placed into service up to specified total or maximum. The Consolidated Appropriations Act (2016) made Section 179's $500,000 maximum total "permanent" and added some inflation adjustments for the future. You and your advisory team should continue to analyze Section 179's generous depreciation opportunities and any associated limitations going forward. This tax provision has been created as an incentive for small business owners to expand their businesses. This in turn is intended to help stimulate the U.S. economy. So with the Section 179 provision, a small business like Dr. Smith's is allowed to expense or deduct the cost of all the equipment in 1 year instead of depreciating it over a 5-year period as shown in the example above. There are no restrictions for the sole proprietor, other than the total amount per year, in taking this deduction; and this deduction can create a loss on the practitioner's Schedule C for the year, as long as the individual is "at risk" (as previously discussed) in the investment or cost of that equipment. Remember, no matter how the equipment is paid for, whether through a bank loan, dental specialty lender, or from private resources, such as a family loan, and regardless of when the loan is paid off, the cost of equipment is deductible in the year it is *placed in service*.

Example: Dr. Smith opens a new dental office the first day of October. He has worked the first 9 months of the year, earning $100,000 as an associate in another office, where he intends to continue to work a few days a week as an associate until his new practice is busy enough for him to quit the associate position. He will earn an additional $20,000 for the last 3 months of the year as an associate; thus, he will have total income from the associate position of $120,000.

For the first 3 months (October, November, and December) of his new practice, Dr. Smith's office collections are $40,000, while the operational expenses (before depreciation) are $55,000, leaving a loss of $15,000. Assuming Dr. Smith purchased $100,000 of equipment and furnishings to start the new office, and that these were placed in service on October 1, the day he opened the office, he can elect to use Section 179 to deduct all or any part of the $100,000 equipment and furnishings (assuming Congress increases the Section 179 deduction to a level at or above $100,000) purchased and can increase his deductible loss on Schedule C to as much as $115,000 ($15,000 operating loss plus $100,000 Section 179 equipment expense). This $115,000 loss would almost totally offset the $120,000 in salary from his associate position and would result in Dr. Smith paying little or no taxes for the year.

As you can see, there is significant tax planning that should be done, especially in the first year of a new dental practice. Again, consultation with an accountant experienced in this area is critical.

With regard to payroll taxes, all persons who work as employees and receive W-2 wages not only pay income taxes but are required to pay into both the Social Security and Medicare systems. An employee, like a dental assistant, pays 6.2% of wages up to an annual limit in Social Security tax, and the employer matches this amount. The employee will also pay 1.45% of wages in Medicare tax (there is no income limit on Medicare withholding), which is again matched by the employer.

As a sole proprietor, the owner is liable not only for employer taxes on employee wages (Social Security and Medicare as mentioned above) but also for what is known as the self-employment tax for the practitioner's earnings. Because a sole proprietor is earning income (draws) and thus is not likely receiving a true payroll check, the government created the self-employment tax, which is computed on an individual's tax Form 1040 (Schedule SE) each year. A sole proprietor is in essence both the employer and employee and must pay both halves of the Social Security and Medicare tax as well as income tax each year based on calculations from the tax Form 1040 Schedule C profit. Combined, the two halves of Social Security and Medicare taxes reach 15.3% (with Social Security tax ending once an annual income limit is reached). Thus, great care must be taken into account in planning tax liability. Self-employment tax can and often does run into five figures annually, and without proper advanced tax planning, many sole proprietors find themselves financially challenged when it is time to pay their self-employment taxes in addition to their income taxes.

Finally, the sole proprietor is not allowed some of the same tax deductions that a C corporation is allowed. These include items such as deduction of long-term disability insurance premiums, medical reimbursement plan contributions, child care plan contributions, cafeteria plan contributions, and so forth. This will be discussed further in the corporation portion of this chapter.

Liability Issues

One of the disadvantages of operating a business as a sole proprietorship is that the practitioner's personal assets are subject to creditor claims in the event of a lawsuit stemming from the operation of the business. Other types of business entities, yet to be discussed, can provide personal liability protection against such suits. In the event of a lawsuit against a sole proprietorship, creditors can seek compensation in the form of personal property–that is, real estate, vehicles, and even personal investment accounts. However, insurance can protect against general and professional liability judgments.

Example: Dr. Smith operates his business as a sole proprietorship. He owns a home and three pieces of rental real estate and has personal investment accounts. In his third year of business, he terminates the employment of the front office manager, Julie, who in turn sues Dr. Smith and wins a civil judgment in court for $75,000 for wrongful termination. Because he is operating the business as a sole proprietor, Dr. Smith is personally liable for this $75,000 judgment to the former employee. If he does not have the cash to pay this former employee, she can go after his home, real estate, and investment accounts to secure and settle her judgment against Dr. Smith's business.

Again, consultation with an attorney who works with dentists in the matter of liability of a sole proprietorship is absolutely critical before choosing this business model.

Advantages

The advantages of operating as a sole proprietor begin with the simplicity of this form of doing business. There are few government submission requirements, no need for the owner to take salary and withhold taxes (sole proprietors, however, usually plan for and pay their income taxes using quarterly estimated tax vouchers), and no annual state or federal filings that are commonly required of corporations, partnerships, or limited liability company (LLC). It is simply the least complex business entity for operating a business.

Disadvantages

There are two major disadvantages to operating as a sole proprietor. First, the liability issue as discussed above (this issue alone in many cases steers the decision of business entity away from the sole proprietorship). Second, experience shows that Schedule C sole proprietorships have a higher rate of being selected for IRS tax return audit than do corporations, partnerships, or LLCs.

Corporations

An Overview

For dentists entering practice ownership, forming a corporation has many advantages and a few disadvantages that will be discussed. As mentioned in discussing sole proprietorships, business owners are strongly motivated to form corporations for the liability protection it offers for their personal assets. Done correctly, forming a corporation will in most cases protects personal assets, such as homes, cars, and investments.

However, incorporating requires that the business owner follow certain formalities. These include taking income or salary just like other employees (paying regular income taxes through payroll deduction vs. self-employment tax) and having to file required government forms throughout the year. While providing a method of insurance against personal liability, the corporation can also provide certain income tax benefits. Characteristic differences between C corporations and S corporations will be delineated and are generally differences in taxation.

Description and Necessary Documentation

A corporation is a legal entity typically formed by submitting a fee and a state specific application. The business owner typically creates the corporation when he or she transfers money or other property (that property being dental equipment, furniture, fixtures, and other practice assets) to pay for, or in exchange for, stock in the corporation. In dentistry, most corporations are typically started for a transfer or cost (known as capitalization) of between $1,000 and $5,000.

It is strongly recommended that an attorney be employed to submit the necessary paperwork, such as articles of incorporation and bylaws, to the secretary of state or other agency responsible for forming corporations in the state in which the corporation is to be formed. Following the legal formalities to form a corporation is critical. If a corporation is not formed correctly, and thus is not in good standing with the state, another party could "pierce the corporate liability veil" if a lawsuit occurs. A lawsuit can be catastrophic to the stockholder if the corporation is found to not be a legal entity. In such case the shareholder is personally liable for the lawsuit judgment (just like the sole proprietor).

Once the state approves and returns the articles of incorporation and bylaws, a corporate seal or stamp is created. This seal may be created by the state or may need to be done with the assistance of an attorney. Next, with the help of a local bank, a corporate bank account can be created. For legal purposes, banks will often require copies of the articles of incorporation, the bylaws, and the corporate seal in order to establish a corporate business account. In addition, the corporation will need to obtain a federal employer number or tax identification number, also known as a TIN. This number is needed to file corporate tax returns and to send claims to insurance companies for the dental services provided to patients of the practice.

Dentists desiring to operate their business entity in the form of a corporation, whether at the start of a new practice or when purchasing an existing practice, will normally transfer some cash to the corporate account to purchase the stock, and also to provide working capital to the corporation. The dentist/shareholder can then acquire a loan from a bank or a specialty dental lender in the name of the corporation. For example, say Dr. Susan Jones is operating her dental practice as a corporate entity (Susan Jones, D.D.S., P.C.) and decides to borrow the funds to buy another existing practice that costs $400,000. In purchasing the existing practice, the assets of that business are allocated among equipment, furnishings, supplies, goodwill, and probably a covenant not to compete. All of these assets will become assets of her corporation. The corporation is actually buying the practice and will be liable for the debt. So the corporation will have $400,000 in assets and $400,000 in bank debt. Dr. Jones is simply the stockholder of the corporation.

However, issues are much more complex for a dentist who has operated his or her practice as a sole proprietor for many years and then decides to incorporate. Before incorporating, it is very important to consult with an accountant to determine how much in assets and liabilities the sole proprietor has immediately preceding the proposed incorporation. This determination is critical due to the potentially onerous tax provisions of Internal Revenue Code Section 357.

When a sole proprietor incorporates, if the sole proprietor transfers liabilities (what is owed) in excess of the basis (original cost) of assets to the newly formed corporation, the excess, or difference, of liabilities over assets is considered taxable income to the dentist (that is, the sole proprietor "on paper" is gaining income from forming the corporation). Accounts receivable (what is owed to the business) and accounts payable (bills the business needs to pay) are excluded from this calculation.

Example: Dr. Jones has been operating her sole proprietorship for 4 years. She decides to incorporate as of January 1. The assets of her practice have an original cost of $250,000, and due to accelerated depreciation and Section 179 deductions (discussed earlier in this chapter), Dr. Jones has taken $200,000 in depreciation as a sole proprietor. For this reason, her depreciable basis in her assets is the original cost of $250,000 less accumulated depreciation of $200,000, or $50,000. At this same time, she still owes the bank $200,000 for the original build-out expense of the office. If Dr. Jones incorporates, she has $150,000 of taxable income (which is the $50,000 of basis of assets less the $200,000 of debt transferred to the corporation).

The reasoning behind this rule in the example above has to do with the fact that Dr. Jones has received income tax deductions of $200,000 in depreciation as a sole proprietor but has only paid off $50,000 of her debt. So she has really received $150,000 in tax deductions without having to pay cash out. Thus, when the assets and liabilities are transferred to the corporation, the theory is that Dr. Jones is being relieved of personal debt of $150,000 (indirectly receiving income).

There are three ways of avoiding this tax while still incorporating:

- First, Dr. Jones can transfer up to $50,000 of her bank debt to the corporation and not transfer the other $150,000 of debt to the corporation. This would mean that she will transfer assets of $50,000 and liabilities of $50,000 to the corporation, so there is no debt forgiveness or taxable income to her personally. Under these circumstances, Dr. Jones has to pay off the $150,000 personally to the bank, with after-tax dollars. This may make more sense than incurring a taxable gain of $150,000, since she has already received personal tax benefits, from accelerated depreciation, as a sole proprietor. However, the bank may have difficulty agreeing to split the total $200,000 debt between the corporation and the individual and still may require a personal guarantee.
- Second, Dr. Jones can transfer the $50,000 of net assets and the $200,000 in debt to the corporation. In so doing, she then can execute a promissory note to the corporation for $150,000 and pay it back to the corporation with a fair rate of interest. This loan must be a bona fide loan over a reasonable period of time. This will allow her to pay back the corporation with after-tax dollars.
- A third way to handle this is for Dr. Jones to keep the equipment in her name, retaining the title to the capital equipment personally and then to lease the equipment to the corporation. She will receive lease payments as an individual and file a Schedule C for the leasing income and pay the debt from this income.

In the authors' experience, these types of taxable-event issues occur often and are *often overlooked* in establishing corporations. If a sole proprietor dentist changes his or her business entity to a corporation without proper income reporting and then is audited by the IRS, not reporting income correctly can create a significant amount of taxes, interest, and penalties.

Operation and Management

Once a corporation is set up and a bank account is established, the business essentially operates in a similar fashion to the sole proprietorship.

The major difference between operating a business as a sole proprietorship and as a corporation is that, as a sole proprietor, the owner is not an employee of the business. As a sole proprietor, the collections minus the deductible expenses is the net amount of what the individual (owner) pays personal income taxes on. When the business is incorporated, the dentist becomes an employee of the corporation and will usually take a regular salary, with regular income tax deductions. His or her salary is reported on a W-2 form issued by the corporation at the end of the year, just as it is for other employees or staff. Income taxes are paid based on the salary received and are reported on the individual's income tax return. As a corporation, how the doctor's salary is, or should be, taken depends on whether the business is a C corporation or an S corporation. We provide more detail about C and S corporations, in this regard, later in this section.

Liability Issues

One of the biggest advantages to forming a corporation is what is known as limited liability. The corporation can be sued, but the personal assets of the stockholder are protected from the suit. In a sole proprietorship and in a partnership, if the owner or partner is sued, his or her personal assets are at risk, as discussed earlier under sole proprietorships. The plaintiff (person suing) can win a judgment against the sole proprietor in court and then collect by procuring the dentist's personal assets. However, as a corporation, the stockholder/owner's personal assets are generally protected from a liability judgment.

When it comes to malpractice suits, dentists are not typically protected by the corporation entity. Since the malpractice suit is based on a contractual agreement between the dentist performing services and the patient receiving those services, that agreement is considered a personal contract with the dentist, and thus the corporate veil generally does not protect the individual dentist. However, dentists should have trustworthy malpractice insurance that protects against malpractice judgments. See Chapter 25 for more information on malpractice insurance.

Obviously, different states can and do have different laws, so it is critical to discuss the liability as well as malpractice protection issues with a qualified attorney.

Tax Issues

There are two different types of corporations: C corporations and S corporations. The differences between C corporations and S corporations are strictly tax related.

C Corporations

All corporations when formed are automatically C corporations. To become an S corporation an election must be made (see later). The C corporation is a taxable entity, and the owner of a C corporation annually files a Federal Form 1120 reporting the gross receipts and expenses. In a C corporation, if the gross receipts of the corporation exceed the deductible expenses, the corporation will have a taxable profit and will pay a corporate or business tax. The corporation is allowed to deduct a reasonable salary to the owner.

Many years ago, Congress required that any taxable income of a C corporation deemed to be a "personal service corporation" is to be taxed at the highest maximum tax rate from the first dollar of income. As of this writing, this currently is 39.6%. Dental corporations are personal service corporations. This can be very expensive for the C corporation owner.

Example: Dr. Jones collected $600,000 in her dental practice in the current calendar year. Her deductible expenses for the year, including a $150,000 salary to Dr. Jones, were $580,000. Therefore, Dr. Jones's C corporation has a taxable income of $20,000. Since she is a C corporation, she has a corporate tax due of $7,920 ($20,000 corporate profit × 39.6% tax rate). This is compounded by the fact that the $7,920 when paid is not deductible to the corporation. Because it is not deductible, $7,920 of "phantom" taxable income for the next tax year is created when she again pays tax. This can cause additional and compounding tax problems going forward in the following years.

Once the shareholder pays the corporate tax, he or she then also has to pay a second tax when taking the remaining corporate profit. So in the example above, Dr. Jones had a profit of $12,080 (left after paying the $7,920 corporate tax on the $20,000 profit left in the corporation). When she takes out the remaining $12,080 in profit, she will pay personal tax at her personal tax rate. This is called *double taxation* and is a huge disadvantage of a C corporation.

For this reason, it is imperative that the C corporation owner "zero out" the corporation each year. This requires detailed annual planning to ensure that the C corporation owner pays additional business expenses at the end of the year, such as taking a salary bonus or contributing the year-end corporate profit to a qualified corporate retirement plan, so that no profit is left in the corporation that would be subject to tax.

Example: In the above illustration, Dr. Jones could have used the $20,000 profit to either pay bills at the end of the year (such as January's rent, or lab and supply bills that she owes on December production, etc.), she could take a $20,000 salary bonus, or she could contribute $20,000 to the company retirement plan. By doing so, there is no end-of-year profit left in the corporation, as it is "zeroed out" for the year and owes no taxes.

In general, C corporation owners take a "reasonable" salary from the corporation to pay their personal expenses, and it is this salary that offsets profit from the corporation. In the example above, Dr. Jones is taking a salary of $150,000, which represents most of the business profit for the year. Dr. Jones will pay Social Security and Medicare tax on this salary like any other employee. If the corporation were to have an extra $75,000 of profit at the end of the year, she could then take a year-end bonus, or she could contribute this amount to the company retirement plan to "zero out" the corporation. As we show later in this chapter when we discuss S corporations, there also may be a Medicare tax saving opportunity for dentists earning higher net incomes by operating their practice as a corporation.

One potential disadvantage of operating as a C corporation is a new provision brought into the law as part of the Affordable Care Act. Any salary taken by the C corporation shareholder that brings his or her total salary over $250,000 would subject the dentist/shareholder to an additional 0.9% in Medicare tax. This $250,000 is the limit for taxpayers who are married and file jointly with their spouses and includes the wages or self-employment income of both spouses. The threshold amount for a single taxpayer or a taxpayer who files as unmarried head of household is $200,000.

For example, assume Dr. Jones is incorporated and operates as a C corporation. As a C corporation, Dr. Jones needs to zero out his corporation. If he earns $400,000 as W-2 salary and he is married filing a joint return, assuming his spouse has no W-2 or other self-employment income, he and his spouse will pay additional Medicare taxes of $1,350. This is 0.9% of the $150,000 Dr. Jones earned in excess of the $250,000 limitation. As will be discussed later, this tax can be avoided by operating as an S corporation.

C corporations also benefit from certain income tax deductions that sole proprietorships, S corporations, partnerships, and LLCs cannot.

C corporations are the only business entities that are permitted to deduct long-term disability insurance premiums of their owners. For an owner age 50 or older, this can be a significant deduction. Importantly, however, the major disadvantage of paying long-term disability premiums through the corporation is that if the owner becomes disabled and receives benefits from the policy, the benefits are *taxable* to the recipient as an individual. We generally recommend that long-term disability premiums be paid personally, so that benefits are not taxable when received.

C corporation owners can also establish medical expense reimbursement plans, or MERPs. These are written plans established to pay for medical expenses that are not covered by the corporation's medical insurance policy, such as deductibles, copayments, excluded procedures, and perhaps prescriptions. A medical expense reimbursement plan, however, must be provided on a nondiscriminatory basis to all employees of a dental practice. If it is not, the benefits are considered a dividend to the owner and, while not taxable to the owner, are nondeductible to the corporation.

The corporation can also include the C corporation owner in a "cafeteria plan" of the corporation. This is a plan that provides a series of personal expense benefits (such as medical, child care, group legal, etc.) to the participant (hence the name "cafeteria"). Here again, the cafeteria plan must be made available to qualified employees.

As far as insurance is concerned, the C corporation can pay for the owner's health insurance (again, the corporation must provide insurance to eligible employees of the practice), as well as long-term care insurance. The C corporation does not have to provide long-term care insurance for employees—this is an exception to the general rule that employees have to be included as part of benefit programs.

Finally, one significant disadvantage of the C corporation is double taxation upon liquidation. Prior to 1986, Internal Revenue Code Section 337 allowed for a corporation to sell the business, distribute the cash to the shareholder, and pay one capital gains tax on the sale.

The Section 337 provision, known as the General Utilities Doctrine, after the court case that upheld this tax treatment, was repealed in 1986. Now, upon the sale of corporate assets, the shareholder not only has to pay the corporate tax but also has to then pay personal income tax when any remaining cash of the corporation is distributed.

Example: Dr. Jones sells her practice for $300,000. The basis in her stock is $1,000. She pays a corporate tax on $299,000 that is approximately $100,000, leaving $200,000 for distribution to Dr. Jones. She then pays personal income tax on the $200,000, so she essentially, as the stockholder, pays double tax.

A recent U.S. Tax Court case, *Norwalk v. Commissioner of Internal Revenue Service*, gives dentists a way around the double taxation issue by providing that the goodwill portion of a dental practice is actually owned by the dentist as an individual and not by the corporation. This removes a large part of the sales proceeds from the corporation and, in turn, allows for the more favorable single capital gains tax treatment on the goodwill portion.

Therefore, a dentist operating as a corporation needs to discuss this case as a reference authority with his or her professional advisor when selling an incorporated dental practice.

S Corporations

The biggest difference between the C corporation and the S corporation is this: while the C corporation is a taxable entity and pays tax on any profit left inside of it, the profit of the S corporation is allowed to "flow through" directly to the shareholder's personal tax return. As an S corporation, it is not necessary to "zero out" the corporation like the C corporation at the end of the year to avoid taxes. The S corporation is not subject to the possible onerous corporate tax rate discussed earlier on every dollar of corporate profit.

Example: Using the same example cited earlier (under C corporations), if Dr. Jones has a $20,000 profit after paying her salary and business expenses, instead of paying the $7,920 of corporate tax as a C corporation shareholder, the $20,000 will "flow through" to Dr. Jones' personal tax return. Dr. Jones takes $20,000 out of the corporation in the form of what is called a *distribution*, and it is tax-free to the corporation. Dr. Jones pays personal taxes on the $20,000 distribution.

The S corporation files a Federal Form 1120S each year to report income and expenses. In order to convert to an S corporation from an existing business, the shareholder(s) must file a Federal Form 2553 within 75 days of the beginning of the tax year. When dentists incorporate at the start or purchase of a practice, the election to form an S corporation must be made within 75 days of the date the corporation is formed. For example, if you start a new practice or incorporate an existing sole proprietorship on March 15, you have 75 days from March 15, or until May 29, to make the S election. If you do not make the election within 75 days, the election will not become effective until the next year. Recently, Congress has provided generous rules if you miss the deadline and you still want to be an S corporation for the current year. For the current laws, this should be discussed with an accountant and attorney. This is a good place to mention that the tax forms mentioned in this chapter are available at www.irs.gov and/or your account.

Another loophole in the law that Congress has threatened to change for years but has not done so as of this writing applies to the Medicare tax. As a shareholder of a C corporation, Medicare tax is paid on any and all salary taken out of the corporation. There is no limit on the amount of Medicare tax, but there is a limit on Social Security tax. The Social Security tax currently applies only up to a salary maximum of $118,500 as of this writing. As mentioned above, any profit taken out of the S corporation can "flow through" to the shareholder, and this "flow through" profit is not subject to the Medicare tax (and may not be subject to Social Security tax if the shareholder's salary is under the Social Security wage base for the year).

Example: Dr. Jones's net profit before her salary is $400,000 for the current year. If Dr. Jones is operating as a C corporation, she can take out a salary of $400,000 to zero out the corporation that eliminates all profit in the corporation and any corporate taxes. However, she will pay 2.9% in Medicare tax, or $11,600 on the $400,000 of salary.

In contrast, if Dr. Jones is operating as an S corporation and she takes $180,000 in salary and then takes the remainder of the $400,000 (or $220,000) total compensation in the form of distributions, she *only* pays Medicare tax on $180,000 salary. Therefore, she saves Medicare tax on the $220,000 distribution, which results in a 2.9% or $6,380 personal Medicare tax savings for the year. For dentists who earn larger incomes, *this*

Medicare tax savings can be significant. However, the practitioner needs to be aware that some states charge state tax on S corporation profits. For example, California charges a 1.5% tax over the minimum tax on S corporation profits. This state tax can mitigate some of the Medicare tax savings discussed in the example above.

As mentioned above, the Affordable Care Act brought into the law an additional Medicare tax on wages over $250,000 and $200,000 depending upon your filing status. This tax can be avoided by an S corporation dentist/owner shareholder through proper planning. In the example discussed in the section above regarding C corporations, Dr. Jones had a salary of $400,000 and since she operated as a C corporation, she needed to take the entire $400,000 salary to zero out the C corporation.

As an S corporation shareholder, Dr. Jones could simply keep her salary at or below the $250,000 level (again, it must be a reasonable salary for a dentist) and she can take the additional $150,000 as a distribution. Dr. Jones will receive a K-1 form for $150,000 and will pay income taxes on $400,000 ($250,000 that is on a W-2 form and $150,000 that is on the K-1 form as Dr. Jones' ordinary income shown on his K-1 form). She will not be subject to the additional 0.9% Medicare tax created by the Affordable Care Act because her wages are at the $250,000 threshold and the $150,000 from the K-1 does not subject Dr. Jones to the additional Medicare tax. This Medicare tax savings is increased as the shareholder's income increases. For example, if the S corporation shareholder earns $800,000 from his or her practice and he takes a salary of $250,000, then he or she saves Medicare tax of $4,950 (income of $800,000 less $250,000 threshold = $550,000 times 0.9% = $4,950 savings).

In addition, many dentists take a salary that is at or near the maximum amount allowed to be taken into consideration for purposes of determining allowable contributions to a qualified retirement plan. The maximum salary allowed for consideration for a retirement plan for 2015 is $265,000. Therefore, if salary of $265,000 is taken in order to maximize retirement plan contributions, the shareholder dentist if married filing jointly with his spouse would only need to pay an additional Medicare tax of $135 ($265,000 salary less $250,000 threshold = $15,000 × 0.9% = $135). The salary a shareholder dentist takes requires planning and consultation with both a CPA and retirement plan administrator. In many cases, a dentist can take less than $265,000 and with modern retirement plan design can still achieve maximum retirement plan contribution allocations.

One disadvantage of using the S corporation is the requirement of complying with what are called the basis rules. Basically, in a sole proprietorship or partnership, if the owner borrows money from the bank and is personally liable on the debt, he or she is considered "at risk" and has "basis" to deduct a loss or to take a large depreciation or Section 179 item. However, the rules are different in the S corporation arena.

Let's take a simple example. Dr. Smith buys a practice and pays $400,000 for the practice. For the current year ended December 31, Dr. Smith collects in his new practice $100,000 in gross receipts and has $90,000 in overhead expenses before depreciation and loan amortization. He takes depreciation and an expense of $50,000 on the assets purchased. This creates a loss of $40,000 ($90,000 overhead expense plus $50,000 depreciation, less $100,000 gross receipts). As a sole proprietor or a partnership, there would be no question as to whether or not he could personally deduct the $40,000 loss against his personal income. But if Dr. Smith elected to be an S corporation when he bought the practice and he wants to have the loss "flow through" to create a loss on his personal taxes, he must have "basis."

For further discussion, assume that Dr. Smith worked as an associate for the first 9 months of the year and bought the practice on October 1. As an associate he earns $120,000 in the first 9 months, and he wants to use the $40,000 loss from his S corporation to offset the $120,000 of W-2 salary he earned as an associate. Without basis he cannot do this.

If Dr. Smith had the S corporation borrow the $400,000 to buy the practice, the tax code DOES NOT give Dr. Smith basis when operating as an S corporation. Basis is created in one of two ways:

- Dr. Smith creates stock basis by making a contribution of cash into the corporation.
- Dr. Smith loans the corporation money (it must be a bona fide loan with payback provisions).

Therefore, in this example, Dr. Smith can contribute $40,000 of his own money into the corporation, thereby creating stock basis. He then can take a $40,000 deduction against the $120,000 of salary. The other option is he can make a loan of $40,000 to the corporation and create loan basis that allows him to then be able to take the deduction. But the disadvantage of creating loan basis is that when Dr. Smith's corporation pays back the loan to Dr. Smith, the repayments are considered taxable income to him personally.

These provisions are very complex, and how they apply in specific circumstances requires consultation with a competent CPA or tax attorney.

Finally, there are significant tax ramifications when selling a practice and liquidating an S corporation. Congress, in 1986, put into the law for S corporations what is known as the built-in gains tax. This tax is very complex and generally doubles taxes to S corporation shareholders on any profit that existed in their corporation that was a C corporation on the date they elected S corporation status. This built-in gains tax basically provides for or results in a double tax upon the liquidation or sale of a corporation.

However, this tax can be easily avoided for S corporations. If an S corporation status is elected for on the same date you originally incorporate, the S corporation is not subject to this tax. Also, if the practice is not sold for 10 years after electing S corporation status, the tax does not apply.

Advantages of C Corporations and S Corporations

C Corporations

The advantage of the C corporation is the allowable deduction of fringe benefits such as disability insurance, medical reimbursement plans, and cafeteria plans for 2% or more shareholders. Still, as previously stated, it may not be advisable to take disability insurance premiums as tax deductions because future claims would be taxable income for the recipient.

S Corporations

The S corporation allows the shareholder to pass through profits each year without being subject to a double tax, as in the case of a C corporation. There is also an opportunity to save Medicare taxes on S corporation profits.

Disadvantages of C Corporations and S Corporations

C Corporations

The C corporation has to be "zeroed out" each year, or it is subject to double taxation on any profits taken as salary. There also is the disadvantage of double taxation upon liquidation. Finally, Medicare tax has to be paid on all salary paid to the shareholder(s).

S Corporations

The only disadvantage of the S election is the loss of deductibility of certain fringe benefits, as discussed above. The authors generally recommend that if an S corporation is going to be formed, it is best to elect on day one when forming a corporation (to avoid double taxation issues). If the owner has significant fringe benefits to pay, a C corporation may be better.

Partnerships and Limited Liability Companies: An Overview

A partnership is defined in the law as two or more persons doing business as co-owners for profit. For many years dentists and other professionals were hesitant to operate their businesses as partnerships due to the lack of liability protection. However, with the advent of the LLC, which is a combination of a partnership and a corporation (to be discussed later in this chapter), the use of the partnership form of practice entity offers the dentist advantages over the corporation whether it is treated as an S or C corporation. The advantages mostly occur in the way profits are split among partners. With more flexibility than the corporate structure, the partnership-LLC has become more popular than in years prior.

As compared with corporations, partnerships can specifically allocate profits and losses based on the agreement of the partners. This can be very appealing for the partners where different partners work different hours and days than one another. The partnership and LLC models also make it much easier to bring on additional partners and can make it easier to buy out partners who relocate or retire.

General Partnerships

Description and Ownership

A partnership is established by two or more dentists deciding to operate a practice together. All of the receipts are collected and expenses paid out of a single bank account. The partnership generally will use the name of the partners (for example, Smith & Jones Dental Partnership), as many states require the dentists to use their names as the partnership name. However, a partnership may use a d.b.a. (doing business as) title to identify itself for marketing purposes. For example, the partnership name could be Smith & Jones Dental Partnership d.b.a. Wilson Street Dental. The d.b.a., as with the sole proprietorship, needs to be published in the local newspaper so that legal notice is provided to other businesses and to the public.

A partner owns what is called a *partnership interest*. This means that the partner owns a percentage of all of the assets (and liabilities) of the partnership. Many partners, especially partners starting a new practice, will be 50/50 partners. This is the easiest form of partnership, as all income and expenses are split 50/50 or "down the middle."

One important distinction that has to be made in a partnership is the differentiation between ownership of the assets of the partnership and the splitting of profits. In most professional partnerships, profits are split based on the percentage of work done by each partner. For example, if Dr. Smith produces 65% of the revenue in the Smith & Jones Dental Partnership and Dr. Jones produces 35%, Dr. Smith receives 65% of the profits and Dr. Jones receives 35% of the profits. But regardless of the profit distribution percentages, as 50/50 partners in ownership of the partnership, if the practice were to be sold each partner would receive 50% of the sales proceeds.

Necessary Documentation

Whereas a corporation is formed by registering with the state in which it operates, a partnership has no such requirements. A partnership is formed by the creation of a partnership agreement. The agreement can be verbal, but that is generally not a good idea. Like other legal documents, the purpose of the partnership agreement is to memorialize the agreement between the partners. The agreement will generally have the following covered:

- The name and term of the partnership is in the agreement. The partners can agree that the partnership will be for, say, 50 years or until the partners retire.
- Allocation of profits and losses are also outlined in the partnership agreement. We will discuss this at length in the next section, regarding operational/management aspects.
- Ownership of the partnership assets is also covered. For example, say one dentist has an existing practice and the other dentist does not. If Dr. Smith has the existing practice and brings all of his practice assets into the new partnership, and the equipment and furnishings are worth $100,000, the partnership agreement might state that upon sale of the total practice, or if Dr. Jones buys out Dr. Smith in the future, Dr. Smith is entitled to an additional $100,000 (beyond his appraisal share) for his initial contribution of assets into the partnership. So if they are 50/50 partners and the practice sells for $700,000, the partnership agreement says Dr. Smith receives the first $100,000, and because they are 50/50 partners the remaining $600,000 would be split equally ($300,000 each).
- Buyout provisions typically are covered in the partnership agreement. This comes up in two specific instances: first, where one partner wants to leave the profession, move out of the area, or retire, and the other partner is to buy out the partner who is leaving.

  For example, say Dr. Smith and Dr. Jones are forming their partnership. They will negotiate terms as to what happens should either doctor leave the practice (other than for reasons of death or disability). While there are numerous ways to structure this, a typical scenario is for the two doctors to agree to engage the services of a qualified dental practice appraiser (many times this is a dental practice broker in the area with experience in preparing appraisals). The partnership agreement states that both doctors agree on a particular appraiser, or more typically that each doctor will get his or her own independent appraisal. If the doctors agree on a particular appraiser and he or she is still appraising practices when one of the partners leaves the practice, then they agree to accept the value of the practice as appraised by that appraiser. Under the other scenario, each doctor engages a qualified dental practice appraiser, and each appraiser establishes a value for the practice. A typical agreement might say that if the two values arrived at by the appraisers are within 10% of each other, then the two appraisals are averaged and that average is the buyout value. If the two appraisals are not within the 10% benchmark, a third appraiser is then utilized, and his or her value is used.

Once the value is established, the agreement states that the partner remaining with the practice has the right to buy out the partner who is leaving based on the agreed-upon appraisal. If the remaining partner agrees to buy out the departing partner, then partnership agreements typically also provide for terms regarding down payment, interest rate, and so on.

For example, say Dr. Jones decides to retire. Dr. Smith as his partner has the first right to buy him out at the appraised value of the practice. If this value is $700,000, the agreement might say that Dr. Smith is to make a 10% down payment ($70,000) and Dr. Jones is to carry the balance over 7 years at the current prime interest rate. Of course, as with most legal agreements, these provisions can be altered to be anything the two partners agree upon.

Second in the case of death or disability, the partnership agreement provides for buyout provisions that are usually covered through life or disability insurance benefits. This is generally the most cost-effective way for a partnership to provide the mechanism to buy out a partner who becomes disabled or who unexpectedly dies during the term of the partnership. If one or both of the dentists are not able to obtain insurance (generally for health reasons), usually a reduced total buyout value is agreed upon and is structured over a period of years. Without insurance benefits available a reduced value is used because if one of the doctors dies or becomes disabled, the value of his or her partnership practice is reduced dramatically as word of the dentist's death or disability spreads in the community.

- The partnership agreement outlines responsibilities and duties of the partners. It states that each partner is expected to devote his or her full-time professional effort to the operation of the practice. It also states whether or not one of the partners will be the managing partner (this is a responsibility that is usually rotated between partners unless the partners agree that one partner has more expertise and should be the managing partner). The managing partner will likely be paid a management fee for his or her services.

Operational and Management Aspects

When the partnership is formed, all of the gross receipts of the practice are deposited into the partnership bank account, and all of the expenses are paid out of this account. For example, Dr. Smith and Dr. Jones form a partnership. They agree to split profits equally, as they are both working the same number of days each week and expect to produce about the same amount of dentistry. Additionally, they decide to split management duties equally.

Dr. Smith and Dr. Jones expect to gross $400,000 in the first year of the partnership, and their business plan shows overhead of $250,000 for the first year, leaving an expected profit of $150,000. Each doctor needs to take a draw from the partnership to cover personal living expenses and taxes. Because they do not want to deplete all of the

Table 10.1 Drs. Smith and Jones capital account example.

	Smith	Jones	Total
Capital Account: Beginning of Year 1	0	0	0
Capital Contributed	10,000	10,000	20,000
Profit Earned During the Year	75,000	75,000	150,000
Draws Taken by Partners during the Year	−60,000	−60,000	−120,000
Capital Account: End of Year 1	25,000	25,000	50,000

partnership funds from the bank account, they each agree that they will take a monthly draw of $5,000 and leave the $30,000 balance of funds ($150,000 profit less $120,000 or $60,000 times two partners' draw) in the bank for purposes of working capital and future equipment purchases.

Dr. Smith and Dr. Jones will maintain what are called "capital accounts." *Capital accounts* are very important because a capital account is a running accounting of how much profit each partner earns and how much draw each partner takes out of the partnership. Capital accounts are used to determine how much of the remaining profit exists in the partnership attributable to each partner. These accounts are valuable in calculating a buyout of a partner deciding to leave the partnership. These accounts are also used if a partner needs to take additional personal draws. The capital account tells each of the partners if the other has "overdrawn" or "underdrawn" his or her capital account.

For example, using the above example of Drs. Smith and Jones, the partnership earns $150,000 in year 1. Each partner takes out $60,000 in draw leaving $30,000 in the bank. Let's also say that to open the partnership both doctors contributed their own cash of $10,000 each. Table 10.1 shows what the capital account would look like after year 1.

In this simplistic example, each partner has $25,000 in the capital accounts and the partnership has $50,000 in the bank at the end of year 1. If the partners decided to end their partnership at the end of year 1, each partner would receive a final draw of $25,000, which would give them back their original capital contribution of $10,000 each and distribution of undistributed profits of $15,000 each. From a practical standpoint, partners receive capital account adjustments for other items, such as liabilities of the practice, depreciation, purchase of fixed assets, and so forth. When determining the correct capital account amounts, a qualified CPA needs to be engaged.

Tax Issues

Despite the fact that the partnership section of the Internal Revenue Code is probably the most complex section of the tax code, operating as a partnership (or now as an LLC—see discussion below) has major tax advantages over the S and C corporations.

As discussed in the corporation section, in order to take tax losses in excess of basis, a dentist must be able to create basis by either loaning or contributing money to the corporation, which in many cases is not possible.

In the area of partnerships, as long as the dentist is personally liable on debt, basis is created. This can provide a huge tax advantage for a dentist who recently set up a practice and earned a large income from his or her associate position earlier in the year.

Example: Dr. Moss has worked from January through October for a private practice dentist and earns 1099 income of $150,000 (1099 is an IRS form). On November, 15 Dr. Moss and his new partner, Dr. Jeffries, open a new dental office. In the first year (a month and a half), the Moss & Jeffries Dental Partnership purchases $200,000 of dental equipment and furnishings. Additionally, they generate revenues of $40,000 and expenses, not including depreciation, of $80,000 ($40,000 operating loss).

For the new partnership, Drs. Moss and Jeffries took out a loan from the local bank for $500,000, which paid for the $200,000 in equipment and furnishings, $200,000 in leasehold improvements, and $100,000 for soft costs and working capital. Both Dr. Moss and Dr. Jeffries are personally liable on the debt to the bank.

When Drs. Moss and Jeffries send their information to their CPA, they are informed that they are entitled to the $40,000 operating loss, plus $50,000 depreciation of assets (leasehold improvements), plus $100,000 of Section 179 deduction. Therefore, the loss on their individual K-1 (tax) forms is $45,000 each ($40,000 operating loss plus $50,000 depreciation, divided by two). Each also receives one-half of Section 179 deduction ($100,000), or $50,000 apiece. In total each will receive an allowable deduction of $95,000 (the $45,000 loss on the K-1 plus $50,000 in Section 179 expense).

The entire $95,000 loss is deductible on Dr. Moss's tax return and can be used to directly offset his $150,000 in 1099 income from his associate position. This is a huge advantage for Dr. Moss, as he can limit his tax liability while building his practice.

Each doctor in a partnership receives a K-1 form, which is an attachment to Federal tax form 1065. All of the net income or expense is allocated to each partner based on his or her percentage interest in the partnership, which is found in the partnership agreement.

The partnership also allocates on the K-1 what is called separately allocated items, which have other limitations in the tax code. These items in a dental practice are generally Section 179 deductions on equipment purchases, charitable contributions, interest income, and other items in the tax code. These items are then put on the partner's individual tax returns (or corporate tax returns if the partners are corporations.

Another advantage of operating a business as a partnership is the ability to specially allocate income and deductions. For example, say Drs. Moss and Jeffries from above choose to have three locations. The partnership agreement says that the partnership owns the three locations, and that the income from location #1 is specially allocated 80% to Dr. Moss and 20% to Dr. Jeffries, location #2 allocates income equally, and location #3 is allocated 70% to Dr. Jeffries and 30% to Dr. Moss. As long as (pursuant to Internal Revenue Code Section 704[c]) the allocation has "substantial economic effect," meaning that the percentage allocations per the partnership agreement are how the profits are distributed, then the allocation will be respected by the IRS for tax purposes.

As with sole proprietorships, income allocated by a partnership to a general partner (all dental partnerships are general partnerships, which means that the general partner has unlimited liability as a partner) are subject to Social Security self-employment tax.

Liability Issues

One of the big disadvantages of operating as a partnership is that *partners in a dental partnership are personally liable for any lawsuits filed against the partnership*. This could include wrongful termination, sexual harassment, age or sex discrimination, slip and fall, and so forth. Unless the dentist has an umbrella liability insurance policy (see Chapter 25), the dentist who is a partner when a partnership is sued can lose his or her personal assets, such as the family home, savings and brokerage accounts, and so on. This is why most dentists who form partnerships first individually make professional corporations (our recommendation is an S corporation). These corporations, rather than the individuals, become partners of the partnership.

Limited Liability Company

The limited liability company is an entity that is frequently used instead of the general partnership. A limited liability company allows dentists wanting to be partners to form this new entity and have it taxed under the partnership tax rules, while also having the liability protection of a corporation.

Prior to the LLC, when partners set up a partnership, each partner would set up a corporation that became the partner of the partnership. By doing this, the dentist would not be subject to the personal liability discussed above. The LLC basically makes it unnecessary to set up a partnership of professional corporations.

The LLC with more than one member (owners of LLCs are called members) files the same federal tax form as a partnership, which is a Federal Form 1065. As noted above, the federal tax rules are exactly the same for LLCs as they are for partnerships, but dentists need to check the LLC tax rules for each particular state. California, for example, has a limited liability tax of $800 per year and a limited liability fee that is based on gross income (as of this writing it is being challenged in court as being unconstitutional).

The IRS has made it easier for tax filing for single-member LLCs. If you are the sole shareholder of a dental corporation, you have to file a corporate tax return, which requires double entry accounting (income statement and balance sheet—see Chapter 2), as well as paying a CPA to prepare that return.

With the single-member LLC, the IRS considers it a disregarded entity. In other words, if a dentist practices as a single-member LLC, the dentist does not have to file a partnership tax return and simply treats the business as a sole proprietorship for income tax purposes and reports all income and expenses on Schedule C of Form 1040, just like the sole proprietorship discussed earlier.

Advantages and Disadvantages of Partnerships and LLCs

The biggest advantage of the partnership is the ability to split profits any way the partners desire as long as the allocation has substantial economic effect. Also, the partnership offers huge flexibility in bringing in new partners, and there is no double taxation on sale of a partnership interest.

The biggest disadvantage of the partnership is the liability of the partners. As noted above, this can be easily eliminated by using the LLC.

The LLC has very few disadvantages and provides the advantage of using the favorable tax rules of partnerships, the limited liability afforded to corporate shareholders, and the use of the disregarded entities that eliminates partnership tax return and associated costs for the single-member LLCs.

What Is Right for You?

Hopefully the information in this chapter has given you some ideas as to which entity is best for you. Much depends on whether you are operating as a single dentist or with partners. The best thing to do is to put your thoughts together on paper as to what your long-term vision is for your dental practice and to meet with your CPA and attorney, who will generally give you the pros and cons of each option and will provide sound advice in order to make the decision appropriate for your situation.

As mentioned a few times earlier, several other chapters help to complement this one. Chapter 1 discusses how to choose advisors, including attorneys and accountants. The business entity of a practice obviously also has important implications in business planning (Chapter 4), buying and buying-into a practice (Chapter 7), starting a practice (Chapter 8), financing a practice (Chapter 9), and personal and business insurance needs (chapter 25), among other chapters.

As a final reminder, tax and corporate-related laws change frequently, and so it is *essential* that you and your advisory team stay current in changes at the local, county, state, and federal levels.

References and Additional Resources

American Dental Association. 1992, 1996, 2001. *Valuing a Practice: A Guide for Dentists*. Chicago: American Dental Association.

Baumann, Paul and Berning, Randall. 2013. *The ADA Practical Guide to Valuing a Practice: A Manual for Dentists*. Chicago: American Dental Association.

Collier, Sarner and Associates, Inc. Newsletter. Website: www.csa.com; e-mail: newsletter@csa news.com.

Hill, Roger K. 2006. *Transitions: Navigating Sales, Partnerships, and Associateships in Your Dental Practice*. Chicago: American Dental Association.

McGill Advisory Newsletter. E-mail: info@bmhgroup.com.

www.adcpa.org/resources.html.

www.dentaleconomics.com/. *Dental Economics* homepage

www.irs.gov/Businesses/Small-Businesses-&-Self-Employed/Business-Structures.

www.scorehelp.org/lists/types_of_business_entities.html.

Learning Exercises

1. When would you use a C corporation form of business as opposed to an S corporation form?
2. What are the advantages of the limited liability company over the corporate form of business?
3. When would it be appropriate to use a sole proprietorship, and what are its pitfalls?

Part 3
Business Systems and Related Issues: Incorporating Technology, Dental Fees and Financial Policies, Dental Benefits, Appointment Scheduling, Compliance, and Embezzlement

Chapter 11
Incorporating Technology
Thomas Terronez

Introduction

Technology is one of the most important aspects of any dental practice. Current dental practices leverage technology literally in every facet of their operations, from scheduling to patient treatment to processing claims and payments. To be without technology for any extended period of time will significantly impair a practice's ability to function. It cannot be stressed enough that as an owner of a practice or even as an associate, you should ensure that all technology decisions are taken seriously. The goal of this chapter is to provide knowledge that will help you make informed decisions about technology in practice.

Choosing a Technology Partner

Just as you choose a professional to assist with legal and accounting decisions, a *technology partner* should be chosen to help provide guidance and knowledge in important technology choices. In today's and tomorrow's environment, there are a myriad of options, choices, and situations that need to be evaluated in regard to technology, making a technological partner all the more beneficial. The complicated web of equipment and software compatibility in a dental practice alone is enough to boggle the mind. Take your time in choosing a partner to evaluate their knowledge, commitment, and reputation. Keep in mind that some options are more expensive than others, but that does not mean they are necessarily better. Chapter 1 discusses how to select other members of your advisory team, and you can use a similar process in selecting a technology partner.

Going Alone

If you consider yourself very comfortable and educated with technology, then you might also feel a technological partner wasteful. Please consider the fact that it never hurts to have at least some additional input and clarity. Just as you have spent countless years focused on learning dentistry, there are people who have done the same with

Dental Practice Transition: A Practical Guide to Management, Second Edition.
Edited by David G. Dunning and Brian M. Lange.
© 2016 John Wiley & Sons, Inc. Published 2016 by John Wiley & Sons, Inc.
Companion Website: www.wiley.com/go/dunning/transition

technology. Typically, the initial money that is saved by not hiring a partner is negated by the costs of lost production when you have interrupted to manage technology issues.

Family or Friend

It is possible that you have a friend or family member who has a strong breadth of experience with technology. If they are experienced with dental technology, then selecting that person for a technological partner is certainly an option. If they only have a general technology background, realize that person's limitations in helping with certain aspects of technology in your practice. Also, be cognizant of the fact that if they can only help after hours or on weekends, then you run the potential of having issues impact your practice for a longer than ideal period.

General IT Vendors

There are general IT vendors that have specific experience with dental practices. The more experience they glean, the more likely that they have the ability to fully partner with your practice. Dental practices have some specific needs with compliance and it is important that your vendors fully understand this. You can always choose a general IT vendor to manage just IT needs and a dental product vendor to handle the software and equipment aspects.

Dental Product Vendors

Dental product vendors provide value in the fact that they work only in dental practices. Keep in mind that most of these vendors will only support products that they sell. If you have a digital imaging solution from another vendor, then you are likely to experience finger pointing between the two vendors. The other issue to keep in mind is that the IT aspect of your technology is not their core business, so the resources available to you will likely be reflective of this fact.

Dental-Focused IT Vendors

Dental-focused IT vendors are typically a great partner as they focus only on technology in dental practices. They will support your practice no matter which software or digital imaging equipment you use. Most of the dental-focused IT vendors do not sell practice software or digital equipment, making them a more objective resource when it comes to evaluating dental equipment purchases. The downside with a dental-focused IT vendor is that their pricing may be slightly higher than general IT providers.

There is no silver bullet in choosing a technology partner. Just because a company seems ideal on the surface does not necessary mean that firm is your best option. Just as in buying or buying into a practice requires due diligence, be as thorough as possible through the process of choosing a technological partner; invest the time to interview their existing clients. Ask questions related to satisfaction, speed of issue resolution, pricing increases, and staff turnover. A good partner will go a long way in the success of your practice.

Evaluate Current Technology

As you ponder the thought of whether or not you want to purchase a practice or join an existing practice, it is critically important to evaluate the current state of technology in the practice. Updating technology often involves a major business expense. As you begin your journey, you will find practices all over the proverbial "map." Some practices will have seemingly great equipment, but it is improperly setup and used inefficiently. Some practices will have dated equipment, but setup properly and used efficiently. There are even a few remaining practices that use the bare minimum of technology based on some unfounded fear of it. Take note of the situation at each practice that you consider as it will be an important factor in your decision in finding your first home practice.

You do not need to be a technology genius to evaluate a practice's present situation, but you do need to be a bit of a detective to gather details. It is important to acknowledge that things are not always as great as they apparently seem. Start by making a list of all software as well as their versions that are being used. Be sure to collect the details on the following software: practice management, digital imaging, 3D imaging, office productivity, and operating systems. The next issue to address is the equipment. Document all of the important technology along with the age of the devices. The most important equipment to document would be server, workstations, printers, scanners, cameras, digital x-ray equipment, and pan/cone beam units. Some of the same suggestions for obtaining information about dental equipment (Chapter 6) may be utilized for technology. Finally, take the time to interview key staff members to see how major technology concerns are handled such as daily backup, HIPAA compliance, technology support, and payments. The information that you put together will give you a good overall picture to share with your technology partner, thereby facilitating a more thorough vetting about the practice's technology.

Budget for Technology

The creation of a realistic budget for the replacement, support, and maintenance of technology is a practical method to manage or transition into a dental practice. It may be surprising, but there are a surprising number of dentists who are not disciplined in managing or utilizing technology in their offices. If an adequate budget is not created, then sometimes other aspects of your practice will suffer—in the case of a technology emergency or technology investments, decisions may be made only on the basis of cost alone instead of what is best for the practice in terms of return on investment. There are multiple aspects that need to be reviewed in creating a technology budget for a dental practice.

A Proactive Approach

The best way to practice would be to mitigate as many potential surprise expenses as possible when creating a thorough budget. If you choose the right technology partner, the process should be easy as they will help you manage this. A technological partner can give you a fixed monthly fee that includes proactive monitoring of all computer equipment for issues as well as all needed support services. In addition, they will help you develop a strategy for the replacement of your equipment so that you will know when to expect those capital investments. The term for this kind of relationship is typically referred to as *managed services*. The only additional expenses are typically software support and extended warranty services on digital equipment. The downside of this method is that you have an investment every month no matter how much you need your vendor partner.

A Reactive Approach

The alternative method is to budget on the higher side to account for the worst case scenarios and engage vendors only on an as-needed basis. There are some clear downsides to this method as unexpected expenses or large issues may hit at a less than perfect time. If no one is monitoring your computer equipment, you will typically not be aware of an issue until it has already impacted you. The upside is that you can sometimes get through years with a large surplus if luck is on your side.

Business Continuity

How would your practice function if you did not have access to any of your data? It is a really scary thing to think about, but with proper planning you can protect your data and even access it within hours after a catastrophic failure. There are different levels of protection that are offered by IT vendors and you should choose the options that make the most sense for your practice. Typically, higher levels of protection and availability also involve a larger investment with hopefully better outcomes.

Local Backups

This method of backup is usually the lowest cost as there are no monthly fees with third-party vendors. You purchase the backup software and backup drives, manually completing the process on a regular basis. An additional benefit of this method is that the data can be restored almost instantly as long as there is a device with a current backup available. Some potential downsides could be device failure if only one device is used and missed or inadequate backups due to human error. If you choose this method, then (1) ensure that your backup devices are encrypted and (2) have your staff periodically test restore data to ensure the proper backup is being completed.

Off-Site Backups

This manner of backup has a monthly or annual fee with third-party vendors, but provides some additional layers of protection over a local backup. The backup is actually sent to servers in other parts of the country or world. Thus, in the event of a local disaster, your data can be restored from anywhere with internet access. The process of off-site backup is usually automated, bypassing the likelihood of most human errors. A potential disadvantage could be the restore time if there are large amounts of data that need to be sent over the internet. That concern can be mitigated by having both a local and an off-site backup concurrently. In addition, it is essential that your off-site service is HIPAA compliant. Chapter 15 explores more about HIPAA and OSHA compliance.

Disaster Recovery Systems

This process of backup is considered the ultimate layer of protection for your practice data. Generally, disaster recovery systems incorporate both local and off-site backup components, backing up not only practice data but every bit of data from the server. Some clear advantages are near instant restores of data and the ability to create a virtual version of your server should your practice be completely destroyed. This virtual server would allow your staff to use practice data and communicate with your patients while your office rebuilds or relocates. The only shortcoming of this level of protection is expense. Like the off-site backup vendors, you need to ensure that your disaster recovery vendor is HIPAA compliant.

Computer and Networking Equipment

Even if you are comparing specifications, computer and network equipment procurement can be confusing. You will find two computers that seem exactly the same but are priced hundreds of dollars apart, so what is the difference? There are distinct variances between low-grade equipment and enterprise-level equipment. Low-grade equipment is typically what you will find at retail box stores. The manufacturers of this equipment cut corners on the unmentioned components to compete on features and prices alone. The minimal included warranty is a clear indicator that the manufacturers do not back this equipment for any extended period of time. In contrast, enterprise-grade equipment is built with higher level componentry and is designed to outlast the included warranty period. If your planning does not account for enterprise-grade equipment and you are forced to utilize low-grade equipment, be sure to budget for a more frequent replacement cycle.

Servers

Servers are the one piece of equipment in which the proper and higher level of investment should be made. When your server is down, your office is typically nearly incapacitated. As you look to replace a server, start with the requirements and recommendations provided by your software vendor. The details that they provide are a great guideline for what your server should include. It is suggested that you exceed the recommended specifications so that the performance lifespan of the server is adequate for the replacement cycle. Purchasing a server that does not meet or barely meets the minimum requirements is a recipe for failure. The requirements are based on the software version available now, and it will likely not meet what is necessary for the next version or upgrade. In addition to following the specifications provided by the software vendors, it is important to ensure that your server includes hard drives in a RAID array, redundant power supplies, and a minimum of a 3-year onsite warranty with a guaranteed response time within 1 business day.

Workstations

As with servers, you should start with the requirements and recommendations provided by the software vendors. How far you exceed the recommendations is determined by how long you plan on keeping the equipment in use. If possible, opt for solid state drives in place of hard drives as they are much faster and cost marginally more. However, it is advisable not to overbuy workstations—at some point, workstations provide a diminishing rate of return due to the significant costs involved. Finally, ensure that your workstations are covered by warranty for at least 3 years.

Displays/Monitors

There are seemingly many factors to consider regarding displays/monitors in your practice, but choosing is fortunately much simpler. The quality of a display is frequently determined by the price point at which it is offered. A lower priced display may seem like a steal, but the overall quality and lifespan are going to be inferior. If the display is used for digital radiography, it is important that the typical contrast ratio be at least 1000:1 so that all gray levels are seen. Busy front desk areas can benefit from two displays, allowing staff to multitask while leaving the schedule opened on one of the displays. The size of the monitor comes down to personal preference, but with current pricing there is little reason aside from space to not use a twenty-three inch or larger monitor.

Networking

The networking equipment is probably the most unclear aspect of technology for a practice. The software vendors rarely provide any recommendations either, but most still advise NOT using a wireless network as the connectivity for a practice. When reviewing networking equipment, it is important to stay away from any home networking equipment as it typically lacks features that are required for business use. A managed gigabit switch should be used for the backbone of connectivity in your office. Should you choose to have wireless and offer access to patients and staff, make sure that the access point chosen supports network limitation and segmentation so that you can eliminate the risk of security compromises. The router or firewall chosen for your practice must be HIPAA compliant and include gateway level security features such as content filtering, antivirus, antimalware, and intrusion protection. It is essential to invest in appropriate networking equipment for your practice as concessions here can significantly jeopardize stability and security of your practice function.

Digital Dentistry

You were likely not trained to practice dentistry utilizing the nondigital methodologies. Fortunately, it is rare to find a practice that is not digital on some level. There are still a few holdouts that feel they can push until retirement without taking the full leap, but they are probably limiting themselves and delimiting their practices. Nearly all insurance companies require or at least encourage electronic claims submission, including digital supporting images. Going forward, this is the best business option for your practice. Chapter 13 reviews the process of submitting insurance claims, including electronic submission.

Digital Radiography

The use of the digital sensor has surpassed other methods of collecting x-rays for a few obvious reasons. The sensor allows instant results, which saves your staff time and increases profitability. The image quality of most sensors is as good as or better than film x-rays. As time goes on, you will continue to see improvement in image quality and a decrease in the size of the devices themselves. Phosphor plates are still in use, but are being phased out fairly rapidly. The process is much more tedious as you are basically following the same procedure as film but without chemicals. Fully digital panoramic/ cephalometric units are becoming commonplace in dental practices, but you will occasionally find a film unit that has been retrofitted to emulate digital function. As with any technological investment, complete your due diligence to choose the best product for the way that you plan to practice dentistry.

3D Imaging

The use of 3D cone beam devices has grown significantly in the last few years (Figure 11.1). 3D imaging allows a deeper and more detailed view of a patient's oral cavity and head/neck anatomy, facilitating a higher level of diagnostics not provided in 2D imaging. If you are a general dentist and do not place implants, 3D imaging is likely not going to provide a substantial benefit to your practice unless you

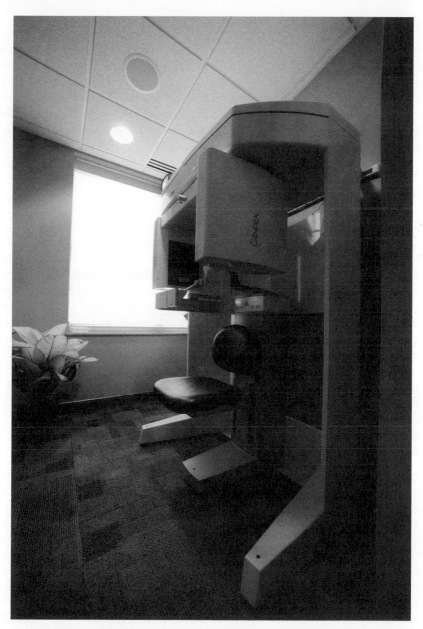

Figure 11.1. With the increasing use of dental implants, cone beam-computed tomography (CBCT) has become a vital component in the standard of care.
Source: Photograph courtesy of Unthank Design Group, www.unthank.com.

regularly diagnose and treat TMD and TMJ. Some people believe that increasing numbers of general dentists will place implants in the future, and thus 3D cone beams may become more common in general dental practices. If you are an orthodontist, endodontist, or oral surgeon, then 3D imaging can provide a significant impact on your practice. As with all purchases, be sure to analyze the return on investment potential prior to committing to 3D imaging as it is typically the single most expensive item that you can buy for a practice.

Digital Photography

There are a variety of options available to utilize digital photography in your practice. A popular combination seen in practices are webcams for adding patient photos to practice management software, intraoral cameras for case presentation, and a digital SLR camera for extraoral imaging. Some specializations such as endodontics benefit from the use of a microscope attached to a high-resolution SLR camera. The additional detail thereby provided allows for a better informed diagnosis and can be used to catalog comprehensive treatment.

Practice Management Software

Practice management software is the single most important software in your practice. Without it, you do not have access to patient information and you are unable to process insurance claims. There are quite a few options available but there are some important things to consider if you are looking for a new software system. If you are working with a small or start-up software vendor, you can likely count on bugs in software being a regular occurrence. The nature of software development is complicated, and the smaller software vendors lack the testing resources available to larger companies. Another consideration is that data from your current practice management software will not perfectly convert to the new software. There will likely be lost data or misplaced data that can cause a large inconvenience especially if you do not maintain access to your old software. Finally, there is a significant learning curve for staff to move from one software system to another. Take all of these things into consideration when deciding on whether a software change is really needed.

Cloud-based Software

There has been a large increase in cloud-based software choices available for dental practices. The concept is great and will likely be common place in the future, but there are some important concerns to be evaluated before committing to putting your practice data in the cloud. First, you must make sure that you have adequate internet connectivity performance as each workstation will be accessing the cloud individually. A best practice is to include a secondary internet connection from a separate provider to ensure consistent connectivity should your primary connection have an issue. Without an internet connection, you have no access to your practice data. Second, there will only be a small reduction in local IT investment as everything typically required for your practice to operate and maintain compliance are still required. You will still even need a server to manage security and store local practice data such as documents, book-keeping data, and in some cases digital imaging. Finally, in a sense, you basically give up ownership of your practice data to the cloud. Everything you store and update resides on your software vendor's cloud in their proprietary format. Should you wish to change vendors, the data export options are limited.

Communication Options

To ensure that your practice remains with the curve of technology, it is important that you ensure your practice is properly wired for connectivity and effectively leverages key available tools. Urban markets typically, but not always, lead rural markets in internet connectivity options. As of now, it is strongly recommended that your practice maintain a wired internet connection such as DSL, fiber optics, or cable. The performance level required will depend on your specific needs. If your practice uses a traditional phone system, local practice management software, and does not utilize audio/video streaming, then a 10 Mbps download speed and 1 Mbps upload speed is usually sufficient. If you use anything additional such as a VOIP phone system, cloud-based software or audio/video streaming, then you should consider a 20 Mbps download speed and a 2 Mbps upload speed or greater. These guidelines are provided for reference, but if your internet provider has menu of options, then it would not hurt to start out on the lower end and then upgrade as needed.

VOIP Phone Systems

There are a multitude of VOIP phone system providers that have made traditional on-premise phone systems a thing of the past. The primary caveat is similar to cloud-based software in that, if your internet connection is down, then so is the access to your phone system. However, most providers allow calls to be forwarded to a mobile phone in the case of connectivity interruptions. In spite of potential connectivity issues, a VOIP system offers several benefits in favor of adopting this technology: never needing to buy or replace a phone system, lower billing, instant call routing changes, web-based management, and integrated texting. Industry leaders, such as Fathom Voice and Weave, even include free feature additions that simply become available to customers without additional costs as they are released.

Patient Communication Tools

The key to an efficient practice is to utilize tools that automate and streamline communication with patients. Not only can these tools decrease the amount of missed appointments, but also increase the amount of income generated per patient by increasing uptake on treatment plans. RevenueWell, an integrated patient communication and practice marketing software provider, takes technology to another level by drawing in new patients as well as simplifying communication with existing patients. It is important to note that, as with all patient communication tools, you get out of them what you put into them. If you choose to adopt one of these type of options, make sure you commit adequate staff time to train and setup the system so that it will yield the results you are expecting.

Compliance and Security

No one gets excited when the topic of data security and compliance arises! Gone are the days that ignorance is bliss when it comes to compliance. There are real concerns, risks, and penalties associated with patient-data compromise. You should not think of compliance as another instance of government interference. Focus instead on being as diligent to protect and treat your patient's data as you do with their oral health. Your practice literally stores and is responsible for all the data that are needed to steal a patient's identity. You work hard to earn the trust of your patients; so, don't risk losing that trust by making avoidable mistakes.

Staff Processes

The most commonly overlooked feature of compliance focuses on staff management processes. Chapter 16 focuses on issues related to embezzlement, and Chapters 22 and 23 cover human resources and staff management. Even in a trusting work climate, your staff should all have reference and background checks prior to being hired. Individual passwords should be maintained so that team members' data access is limited to an as-needed-basis only. Further, all computer interactions should leave a per-person audit trail. A workstation should be logged off and locked down when a staff member is not using it. This will prevent the prying eyes of both patients and other people who have access to the office such as vendors, janitorial firms, and so on. These are by no means all of the management issues to consider related to technology, but the points in this section are a starting point for considering how your employees interact with practice data.

Technology Provisions

There are many necessary safeguards that should be in place at your practice to further protect data and mitigate risk of compromise. All servers and workstations should utilize current operating systems and high-priority updates and patches should be run on a regular basis. Antivirus and antimalware software should be installed and updated daily on all computers. Any drives that hold practice data should be encrypted if they are accessible to staff, especially if they are taken out of the office. A compliant firewall should be in place as well to further protect from internet intrusion and staff visiting improper websites. There are no perfect safeguards, but properly executed precautions will go a long way in protecting your patients and practice.

Patient Entertainment and Education

A more enjoyable facet of technology in your practice is patient entertainment. The ultimate goal is to make a visit to your office as enjoyable as possible which, in turn, will encourage patients to share the experience with potential patients. At the bare mini-mum level, you should have soothing background audio to taper out the sounds from other treatment areas. To take things up a notch, you can outfit the waiting areas and treatment areas with cable or satellite TV that allows patients to watch what they choose. This provides a powerful distraction for patients, diverting their focus toward something else aside from what is going on in their mouths. If TV is not a viable option, animated lighting can be added to the treatment rooms which will also distract patients but not include any intrusive sound. Some practices even go as far as providing video games or tablets for patients to play with, but this is a bit risky as patients can walk out with devices and the chemicals required for infection control can rapidly decrease the lifespan of the units. There are a variety of options that can be offered, so get creative and utilize technology to improve the patient experience.

Many educational options are available for integrating with technology today. Of particular importance are educational videos related to dental conditions, diseases, and procedures. A variety of vendors have educational videos available, including the ADA Toohiq (toothiq.com) and Caesy (www.caesycloud.com). Augmenting your chairside communication with these types of tools can potentially make your treatment time more efficient while also helping to educate and inform your patients. Chapter 19 discusses the importance of using audio-visual aids in chairside patient communication.

Marketing Your Practice

The phone book is dead in most markets and cannot be relied on to bring in new patients. Even the other alternative offerings by the phone book vendors are only mildly successful. The key to marketing your practice starts with having a good website that is reflective of your office. The website should cater to the strengths of your practice, provide a detailed listing of all services provided, introduce key staff members, highlight any differentiating factors, and be responsive so that it looks and functions well regardless of the device being used to view it. Once you have the solid web presence, you will need to increase the amount of website visitors. This can be accomplished through legacy media such as advertisements, TV commercials, and radio ads. Still, your best money is spent on investing in content marketing (formerly known as organic SEO) as well as setting up custom pay-per-click (PPC) campaigns. Legacy media still has a place in some markets, but those are rapidly disappearing. Social media and reputation management are also vital forms of marketing and should not be ignored. Facebook, Twitter, and Instagram are great ways to develop a deeper rapport with current patients but probably not as effective in recruiting new patients. Be sure to monitor your reputation by setting up a variety of Google Alerts and signing up with all review sites so that you can respond to both positive and negative feedback. There may be a point where you feel that you have all the patients that you can handle, but it is still important to invest in marketing even at a minimal level to mitigate typical patient attrition. Chapters 17 and 18 discuss external and internal marketing strategies in more detail.

Making Wise Investments

As with any investment or change in your practice, take your time and consider the benefits versus the potential issues. Utilize your network of other dental professionals of all experience levels and get as many of their opinions as possible. If you rush into an investment, the likelihood of regretting the investment is much higher. No deal is so amazing that it cannot be passed up. The most overlooked factor in incorporating different and new technology is the impact on staff. The less technologically savvy your team is, the larger the learning and adoption curve will be. In some cases, a new technology can be too much for individual team members; so keep that in mind when making major changes. Take your time and do your due diligence to ensure that your choices: (1) have an overall positive result in your practice, including ultimately ton staff; and (2) that the rate of return on investment meets your expectations.

Conclusion

This chapter reviewed a vast array of technological considerations in practice. Some of the aspects received minimal coverage. Nevertheless, the purpose is to empower you in making educated choices about your practice. Please know that technology is changing at an accelerating pace, which means what may be great now will be obsolete sooner than you might expect. As with all decisions that you must make for your practice, be sure to be strategic, making sure your decisions align with your goals and plans.

References and Additional Resources

Websites

Compliance

Waan, Olivia. 2014. *HIPAA: what do you want out of my dental practice now?* Available at http://www.dentistryiq.com/articles/2014/02/hipaa-what-do-you-want-out-of-my-dental-practice-now.html.

VOIP Providers

Weave: http://www.getweave.com/.
Fathom Voice: https://fathomvoice.com/.

Patient Communication Tools

RevenueWell: http://www.revenuewell.com/.
SolutionReach: http://www.solutionreach.com/.

Learning Exercises

A. Reach out to at least five dentists who currently own their practices and are utilizing digital dentistry. Ask them about their technology situations. Listed below are a few questions to simplify the process:
   1. How long has your practice been digital? What was the process to get there?
   2. Did you make your decisions by yourself or did you have help?
   3. If you could do it all over again, would you do things the same or differently and why?
   4. Would you pay more if your technology worked better and you had less worry?
   5. Ask them for any general tips or advice.
B. Pretend that you are building a brand new practice. Determine the approximate size, number of ops, and general layout of the hypothetical practice. Reach out to multiple vendors to determine ballpark pricing for this practice. If they want more specifics, explain that you are just trying to assemble a reasonable budget for financing. This will give you a great idea of how these vendors operate and what the realistic investment would be.

Chapter 12
Dental Fees, Fee Setting, and Financial Policies for Patients

Robert D. Madden and Eugene Heller

Introduction

A discussion of dental fees and fee setting frequently reveals insight into both the best and the worst of times of dental practice. It is the best of times for those dentists who have been paying attention to the ever-changing economic, dental benefit, and political arenas. These practitioners are keenly aware of the necessity to review their fee schedule on an annual basis. These practitioners can take comfort in seeing that their overhead stay in line with inflation and cash flow is not a problem. Change is constantly a companion for anyone who owns a business. Being prepared for that change, regardless of the nature of that change, is the sole responsibility of the owner of the business. Those who fail to exercise their due diligence to their business regarding fees look upon fees and fee setting as the worst of times for themselves and their business. These businesses frequently suffer from many disturbing financial issues. Unpaid bills, high employee turnover, and poor cash flow are but a few that could have been avoided had they paid attention and acted responsibly to what is going on in the world in which they are attempting to do business.

Dental fees are the lifeblood of a dental practice. It is the single most important instrument the dentist has to generate income and to offset the cost of doing business. The primary goals of a fee schedule are simple; generate profit and growth for the dental practice. Fees and fee increases are part of the normal process of managing a dental practice. Fees need to be high enough to permit the business to accomplish the following objectives: (1) cover the expenses of the business, (2) permit reinvestment in the business, and (3) provide a respectable rate of compensation for the owner. On the other hand, fees need not be so high as to price yourself out of the marketplace.

Dental practices have a tremendously high overhead, although arguably lower than many other types of business. Historically, overhead will range from 60 to 65% of production for a general dentist.[1] Lab fees, dental supplies, equipment, facility costs,

[1] *McGill Advisory*, May 2007, 22(5):3–4.

---

staff salaries, and taxes are just a few of the items that contribute to overhead. The doctor often has to be content with the amount that is left over after all the bills are paid for personal compensation. The amount can vary from practice to practice. It can be as little as 9% to as much as 35%+ of collections. The main point here is this: the doctor does not get anywhere near all that is collected.[2]

Practices with low fee schedules and thus low profit margins are frequently subjected to complaints from staff members about low wages. This in turn can lead to a high staff turnover rate. It can also lead to an inordinate amount of stress for the doctor having to deal with an overhead that is out of control and the financial difficulties associated with failing to realize a profit. Dental practices with healthy, well-maintained fee schedules are rarely subjected to these financial and managerial issues.

How much is a professional service worth? Ask ten different people and you are likely to get ten different answers. In dentistry, we frequently talk about professional fees being based on care, skill, judgment, overhead, and expected revenues per hour. Ideally, fees should be derived with these considerations. In reality, dental fee schedules are established in a variety of ways. Some dentists use survey data, others use tables of allowances from indemnity insurance plans, others use relative value tables, and some opt for using inherent cost of procedures in establishing fee schedules. For the most part, fees in the dental industry are determined like those in other consumer-driven entities. That is to say, prices are market driven. The range of price has been set by the marketplace. Various fee surveys reveal the range and percentile that have been established for a service in a particular geographic or zip code area. These surveys add credibility to the fact that the majority of dental fee schedules are derived in such a manner. That being the case, it makes no financial sense to charge any less than that has been established in a given geographical marketplace. Pricing established in such a fashion is referred to as *target pricing*. Target pricing is defined as being a mechanism wherein prices are set based on market penetration or price points rather than building from standard costs.[3]

The insurance industry uses this pricing model to build fee schedule profiles on its providers. It is also a means by which usual, customary, and reasonable (UCR) fee table of allowances are determined as well as preferred provider organization (PPO) fee schedules.

The reader would benefit from understanding the impact of fees and financial policies on other content in this volume. Chapter 3 discusses recommended practice performance indicators, including the percentage of gross revenue from dental benefit plans, the percentage of gross revenue in "adjustments" or discounts from dental benefit plans, and acceptable accounts/receivable. A practice's fees and financial policies on collections clearly impact those indicators. Fees and financial polices also directly impact revenue and cash flow, resulting in ramifications for business planning (Chapter 4), practice valuation (Chapter 5), and the viability of associateship opportunities (Chapters 20 and 21). Chapter 13 also provides a discussion on dental insurance, its forms, and levels of reimbursement.

---

[2] Dianne Glasscoe, RDH, BS. *Dental Economics*, March 2000, www.dentaleconomics.com/articles/print .html?id=110190&bPool=DE.pennnet.co.

[3] 12manage, The Executive Fast Track. Available at www.12mangage.com/description_target_pricing.html.

Fee Schedules and Definitions

Ethically, your practice should have only one fee schedule. The fee schedule in your office represents what you would normally charge for each procedure performed in your office and is referred to as your *usual fee schedule*. State boards and other regulatory agencies frown on practices that have multiple fee schedules. That is to say, you cannot have one fee schedule for insured patients and another for noninsured patients. The usual fee schedule in your office represents your full fee for a given procedure and has nothing to do with the amount of money contractually reimbursed by a patient's dental benefit plan.

Most dental practices accept dental insurance benefit plans. As a result, your practice may accept several different *tables of allowances*. Tables of allowances should not be confused with the usual dental fee schedule. Table of allowances are dollar amounts representing the total contractual dollar obligation on part of the dental benefit plan. They have nothing to do with your usual fee schedule!

Some dental benefit plans reimburse for specific dental services based on a *maximum allowance*. Typically these plans reimburse up to 100% of a predefined dollar amount. The dollar amount of reimbursement is based upon the financial strength of the plan as defined by the contract with the purchaser, not the insurance company per se.[4] Dentists who participate in such plans are able to collect only their contracted amount, not their full usual fee.

Frequently, dentists and patients alike are confused by the difference between the terms maximum allowance and maximum fee as they relate to a practice fee schedule. Regardless of the payment schedule, your usual fee schedule is not taken into consideration. With maximum allowances, the patient is responsible to your office for any balance due on your usual fee. With maximum fee scheduled plans (i.e., PPOs), *participating dentists* cannot collect their usual fee should a balance exist after payment. This is referred to as balance billing. On the other hand, should a patient with a maximum schedule have work done with a *nonparticipating* dentist, balance billing is permitted.

Why Do Dental Practices Need to Increase Fees?

It would truly be the best of times if you never had to raise the price for a particular good or service. Unfortunately, we live in an imperfect world. We live in world subjected to economic forces that change the outlook for everyone on a daily basis. Fees charged for dental services are subjected to the relative prices of other goods in our economy. Inflation is the primary reason you must raise fees on a periodic basis.

Inflation is defined as the increase in the price of some set of goods and services in a given economy over a period of time. It is measured as the percentage rate of change of a price index.[5]

In the long run, inflation is generally believed to be a monetary phenomenon, while in the short and medium term, it is influenced by the relative elasticity of wages, prices,

---

[4] Limoli, Jr., T. Fee survey. *Dental Economics*, September 2007. Available at www.dentaleconomics.com/articles/print.html?id=307297&bPool=DE.pennnet.co.

[5] Wikipedia, the Free Encyclopedia, en.wikipedia.org/wiki/inflation.

and interest rates.[6] Economists generally agree that a small amount of inflation carries a positive effect on our economy. There are many reasons for this justification, the principal one being it is difficult to renegotiate prices in a downward direction. One such example would be an attempt by management to lower employee wages. Modest inflationary pressure means prices for goods or services are likely to increase over time. This trend helps to keep the economy active as it encourages spending, borrowing, and long-term investment. It is for this reason dentists must keep informed about inflation and keep pace with inflation by periodically raising fees. Our economy is not stagnant and neither should be a dental professional's fee schedule!

Disturbing Trends

Not only is it important to stay abreast with inflation in raising fees, but also pay attention to what is happening to your profession. In 2004, some disturbing trends started to emerge in the dental profession. Unfortunately, most dentists in this country are not operating at or near full capacity. In a survey conducted by the *McGill Advisory* in 2006, 83% of the dentists reported not being as busy as they would like to be. Unfortunately, this lack of busyness continues to this day for many in our profession. The lack of busyness has resulted from many factors that merit discussion.

Prognosticators had previously anticipated there would be an increase in the number of retiring dentists by around the year 2000. Surveys conducted by various consulting groups, as well as the American Dental Association, have not supported the prediction. Delayed retirement by dentists has been primarily due to the lower net asset values and investment incomes of doctors. The lack of retirements has helped maintain a competitive environment in dentistry. While this is of concern, an even bigger concern is the shrinking portion of consumer disposable income.

Fueled by the Great Recession of 2007, rising gas and energy costs, inflation, the mortgage crisis, and higher short-term interest rates, consumer disposable income have lagged behind the rate of price increases in the general economy. With less disposable income available to consumers, dentists find themselves competing for the limited disposable dollars available to consumers. For the majority of dentists in our country, the results have been fewer new patients and fewer procedures being performed.

Operating costs of a dental practice have continued to mount in recent years. Dentists have traditionally relied on increasing number of units of production to sustain net income and practice growth. Survey data have shown that dental office productivity has been increasing at a rate of approximately 1.5% per year.[7] With the number of units of production in decline, dentists can no longer rely on productivity alone to sustain net income and practice growth. Fee increases are inevitable even with disturbing economic news. Unfortunately, for those dentists participating in discounted fee dental benefit programs, fee increases sufficient to offset costs have not occurred due to

---

[6] Federal Reserve Board's Semiannual Monetary Policy Report to the Congress. (http://www.federalreserve.gov/boarddocs/HH2004/july/testimony.htm)Roundtable   (http://www.federalreserve.gov/BOARDDOCS/SPEECHES/2003/20030723/Economis) Introductory statement by Jean-Claude Trichet on July 2004 (http://www.ecb.int/press/presconf/204/html/is040701.en.html).

[7] Beazouglu, T., Heffley, D., Brown, L.J., Bailit, H. The importance of productivity in estimating need for dentists. *J Am Dental Assoc* 2002, 133:1399–404.

contractual constraints by the benefit programs. Dentists participating in these programs have seen their practice profits erode and overheads skyrocket.

The ability of dentists to increase office production in the future as a means to maintain or expand their net incomes will depend on an increasing demand for dental care by people with the resources to pay for that care. The downward pressure on the utilization of services in dental benefit programs will make growth more difficult. Once viewed as an effective stimulus for the demand for dental services, dental benefit plans may be seen by some as becoming a less effective stimulus because of the downward pressure they exert on utilization and fees and the stagnation in the maximum annual benefit level over the years.[8]

Adding to the woes of the consumer is what has been happening in the insurance industry. There has been a marked decrease in dental caries. Public fluoridation and preventative oral health programs have done their job. That being the case, consumers have opted toward more cosmetic procedures, many of which are not covered by dental benefit plans. With decreasing levels of disposable incomes, even these heavily marketed cosmetic procedures have been difficult for consumers to afford.

Employers wishing to control the ever-rising cost of dental insurance premiums have switched from indemnity policies to managed care plans (see Chapter 13 for more information on these plans). Currently, over 65% of the dental benefit programs are of the discounted fee type. The result for many dentists has been, willingly or unwillingly, to become a discounted fee provider or "preferred provider." The really bad news with all of this is annual fee increases associated with discounted fee products typically only permit annual fee increases of up 1% or less.[9] If inflation is occurring at the rate of 3–4% a year, it would not take long for dentists to notice a marked decrease in profit and increase in the overhead required to run the practice. Unfortunately, many dentists fearing a lack of busyness seemingly have to opt into becoming preferred providers. Such action only adds to the problem. Practitioners, seeing their profits shrink and overheads swell, are left with only one viable solution: raise fees for patients not in discounted programs to offset the costs of those receiving the discount. Doctors who do not raise fees at least annually resign themselves to higher overhead costs and lower profits over their remaining career, since it is difficult to implement large (makeup) fee increases. Additionally, doctors participating in managed care plans must submit fees annually for approval. Most of these companies do not allow doctors to "catch up" with larger fee increases in a later year, so their fees remain lower permanently.[10] It should be noted, however, that some dental insurance companies in some markets will negotiate their fee reimbursement levels; some consultants specialize in this negotiation process.

Factors that Influence Pricing

How often should I increase my fees? How much do I raise my fees? These are frequently asked questions by young dentists. Fee schedules should be reviewed at least annually. Fee increases can vary from the percent of inflation up to whatever the marketplace will tolerate. It is a good business practice to pay attention to the consumer price index, producer price index, and the employment rate in order to ensure having a profitable, balanced, and reasonable fee schedule. Additionally, it is important to stay

[8] Guay, Albert, Dental practice prices, production and profits. *J Am Dental Assoc* March 2005, 136:357–361.
[9] *The McGill Advisory*, May 2007, 22(5):2.
[10] *The McGill Advisory*, December 2006, 21(12):3.

abreast of economic developments in your community as economic conditions can and do change. While it is important to periodically increase fees, you must pick and choose the times that are most opportunistic for the success of the business. Obviously, a dentist should think twice before increasing fees when local economic conditions fail to support this business decision. For the most part, fees and fee setting need to be reflective of economic conditions at the local, national, and international levels.

When to Raise Fees

Is there any particular time of the year when it is better to raise dental fees? The answer is yes and no. From a budgetary standpoint, it is generally agreed that fees be raised effective from the first month of the calendar year. By doing so, in the month of January, you are able to properly position your practice fees in order to ensure greater profitability in the coming year. By having a consistent time of the year for fee increases, you can better construct practice comparisons and growth indices with previous calendar years. That having been said, should economic conditions make fee adjustments necessary, you should act immediately so as to ensure profitability of the practice. One such example would be an increase in the price of gold. Drastic price changes in an upward direction of this commodity will likely lead to higher dental laboratory costs for the practice and will affect profitability.

How to Raise Fees

First, it is critical to determine where your practice's fees are positioned relative to other practices in the same geographic location. This process is easily accomplished using fee survey information. Recommended surveys include Dr. Charles Blair's comprehensive "Peace of Mind" Revenue Enhancement Program, the UCR Dental Fee Report, and the ADA Survey on Economic Research on Dentistry. One popular dental fee analyzers is Dr. Udell Webb's Current Dental Fee Analyzer. You may obtain more information about his Dental Fee Analyzer by visiting his website, www.webbdental.com. Frequently, dental practice brokers will construct fee surveys on communities in which they operate. You may locate practice brokers and fee survey information by utilizing the internet.

Doctors cannot properly set fees without first determining where their fees are positioned in the marketplace. Failing to do so can cost you thousands of dollars in the course of a career.[11] Insurance companies have access to these data from companies such as the Health Insurance Association of America and use it to establish fee reimbursement schedules. A dentist *must* access this type of information in positioning practice fees in the marketplace.

The second step in the process is determining where in the marketplace you wish to position your practice. Positioning should take into account and be reflective of the practitioner's expertise, time, skill, and judgment. Overhead associated with the practice is also an influencing factor. In short, prices should be reflective of the quality of care. It is interesting to note that many patients do not equate fees with the quality of care. Patients generally rely on the newness of the equipment, the perceived aesthetic

---

[11] *The McGill Advisory*, December 2006, 21 (12):3.

appeal of the practice, customer service, and personal interaction issues in judging the quality of care.[12]

Once deciding on which percentile is reflective of the practice, you should raise *all fees* up to that desired percentile. This is referred to as *fee balancing*. It is recommended to position your fee schedule at the 80th percentile and then adjust accordingly. Raising some but not all fees results in an unbalanced fee schedule; doing so sends an inconsistent message to the patients of the practice and to insurance carriers.[13] Ultimately, such action results in an unbalanced fee schedule.

The third step in the process is maintenance of the fee schedule. Paying attention to what is happening with inflation and the general economy is extremely important. Armed with this information, it is recommended that the doctor continue to raise fees each year thereafter to maintain market position, usually in light of fee balancing. According to practice management consultant Dr. Charles Blair, 89% of doctors raise fees annually. Eleven percent elect to raise some but not all of their fees on an irregular and inconsistent basis.

In general, doctors fear negative reactions by patients when raising fees. Change can be difficult especially for the new dentist. Having to confront conflict with patients over fees is even more trying. It has been my experience and that of many of my peers that the perception of fear in raising fees is much worse than the reality.

How Much to Raise Fees

Economists estimate that on average, our economy experiences a rate of inflation ranging from 3 to 4% annually. If you are to realize a profit at this level of inflation, you must raise fees a minimum of 5% across the board to keep pace or increase practice profitability. Once again, pay attention to the annual rate of inflation as it is reported in the economic indexes. The rate of inflation as reported by the Consumer Price Index is the primary determinant in raising fees. The *McGill Advisory* newsletter is a good resource to utilize in determining what percent you should raise fees. Annually, they make recommendations, based on our national economic environment, as to what percent to raise fees. Subscriptions to the *McGill Advisory* are available at www .mcgillhillgroup.com.

Economic Indexes that Influence Fee Setting

Consumer price index (CPI): The CPI is the most recognized measure of price inflation in retail and service goods. The CPI is composed of eight different groups, each weighted in the calculation of the CPI: housing 42.4%, food and beverage 15%, transportation 17.4%, medical care 6.2%, apparel 3.8%, recreation 5.6%, education/communication 6.0%, and other goods and services 3.5%.[14] These eight groups represent over 200 categories of goods and services whose price changes over a period of time are used to measure and calculate the CPI. The CPI uses an index number versus a dollar figure.

---

[12] *The McGill Advisory*, December 2006, 21(12):3.
[13] *The McGill Advisory*, December 2006, 21(12):3.
[14] Baumohl, B. *The Secrets of Economic Indicators*, 2nd ed. Philadelphia, PA: Wharton School Publishing, pp. 271–274.

This permits you to gain a historical perspective on how inflation has performed over various time frames. For example, assume at the end of 2016, the CPI index was 200. Measured 6 months later, the score is 202 or a 1% increase in inflation for the first 6 months. Annualized, it would represent a 2% increase in inflation.

Dr. Albert Guay, in his article, "Dental Practice Prices, Production, and Profits," states the following: "Nonetheless, dentistry functions within the general economy of the United States and its health care system, and it is influenced directly by conditions operating in those sectors. It is important for all—from health planners to individual practitioners—to understand dentistry's economic relationship to the general economy and the health care system, as well as how changes in both sectors are reflected in changes in the dental care system at all levels." His article points out the strong relationship between the CPI and dental fees charged in the United States. The trend is to run parallel to one another.[15]

Producer price index (PPI): The PPI measures the changes in prices paid by businesses during various stages of production. The index is composed of three price indexes, each representing a stage in the production cycle. Thus, the index for crude goods, immediate goods, and finished goods composes the PPI. Established in 1902, the PPI is the oldest measure of inflation for our economy.[16] From the standpoint of a practicing dentist, it is wise to pay attention to this index. A rise in this index implies the dental products we use in dentistry maybe increasing in cost, thereby signaling to dental practitioners the possible need to increase fees.

The employment rate: It represents one of the most influential economic indicators of the U.S. economy. The employment news of our economy details conditions in the job market, and household earnings. The information in the rate of employment report is important when forecasting future economic activity. The employment rate is announced the first Friday of each month and reports on the month just concluded.[17]

From the standpoint of a practicing dentist, it is nice to know what is happening both locally and nationally with employment. A rise in unemployment signals to providers of dental services that consumer spending is tending to drop off. Thus, you can expect your practice to notice a drop in production as well as collections. Armed with this information, you might put on hold any elective office improvements and watch spending on inventory more closely. Most economists agree an ideal unemployment rate would be in the range of 4.5–5%.

From the standpoint of dental fees, an increase in unemployment may cause you to think twice about instituting a fee increase. On the other hand, if the CPI is increasing at a rate of 4–5%, you would have no choice but to increase fees just to keep pace with inflation; the rationale is that you will produce less, but at a higher fee to maintain a profitable business margin. As you can see, it is a must to keep an eye on inflation as well as on what is happening to the employment rate when increasing fees. Unfortunately, most dentists when confronted with rising unemployment rates sit tight on their fees, fearing they will lose patients and thus production. The result of such action means less overall income, higher overhead, and less profitability for the practice and the dentist. If this pattern continues for 3–4 years, the dental practitioner who failed to increase fees will be playing catch-up when economic conditions improve. Playing

---

[15] *J Am Dental Assoc.* 2005, 136(3):357–361.
[16] Baumohl, B. *The Secrets of Economic Indicators*, 2nd ed. Philadelphia, PA: Wharton School Publishing, p. 283.
[17] Baumohl, B. *The Secrets of Economic Indicators*, 2nd ed. Philadelphia, PA: Wharton School Publishing, p. 25.

catch-up means fee increases beyond those of practitioners who have kept pace with inflation. This is not wise from the standpoint of maintaining patients in the practice or managing a profitable business.

It is recommended that you subscribe to economy-related periodicals such as *Business Week*, *The Economist*, or the *Wall Street Journal* to become familiar with the economy and its economic indicators. Reading economic articles will provide a perspective on what is happening in the local, national, and international economies. Understanding of what is likely to happen economically helps dentists make intelligent business decisions with regard to fee setting and general practice management.

Practice Purchase and Fee Schedule

What happens if you purchase an existing practice and are unhappy with the fee schedule? First, in an ideal situation, the former owner would have made fee adjustments before you purchased the practice. Otherwise, determine how long has it been since the fees were increased in this practice? If it has been 1–2 years, you should definitely entertain the idea of a fee increase. Generally, dentists do not like change and are reluctant to make changes to a fee schedule in a practice that is in transition in fear of losing patients. If the fee schedule is not to your liking, then change becomes a necessity and you should proceed with making the change. Long term, choosing to not do anything is a grave mistake.

Most practice brokers generally agree that fee schedules of most practices in transition tend to be too low. There are two schools of thought with regard to making changes to a practice fee schedule that is in transition. The first line of thinking would recommend an incremental increase in fees. That is to say, raise some but not all fees and do so in two to three phases during the following 12–18 months. Items that are paid by insurance carriers, exams, x-rays, and cleanings are raised to the medium-high to high percentile. Radical changes in any aspect of an existing practice made by a new owner can and may initiate problems. Once fees are at an appropriate level, fee increases should be implemented on a yearly basis. The second school of thought is to raise all fees 3–5% or more depending on where the practice fee schedule falls demographically and where you choose to position the practice in the marketplace. It should be emphasized that conditions like the one described may also have other problems associated with fees that are initially overlooked during the purchase phase of the practice. One such problem may be the lack of a written and well-communicated financial policy. Another is a high volume of PPO patients in the practice.

If the fee schedule of the practice has been raised on an annual basis and is still below the prevailing price range for the geographic area in question, what should be done? The knee-jerk reaction is to raise and balance fees to bring them into line with what is being charged in the community. Though this is the correct action to take, it merits more thought than merely increasing the fee schedule. Prior to becoming the new owner of the practice, you should take time and question the selling doctor on the philosophy of the fee schedule. It may be that the seller never felt comfortable raising fees to the prevailing level in the community. This should be a red flag to the prospective purchaser of the practice. Practices with historically low fee schedules can be difficult in which to institute fee increases without considerable conflict with patients. Additionally, practices with low fee schedules tend to have higher overhead rates, higher levels of staff turnover, and lower levels of profitability.

Discounting Practice Fees

The decision to discount fees to individual patients or in unique situations is a personal business decision for which there is really no right or wrong answer. When allowing discounts it is always nice to remember someone else is paying for that discount. With this in mind, the decision is up to the owner of the practice as to whether or not discounting of fees is permitted.

In today's marketplace people are always looking for ways in which they can get the best price. Patients of a dental practice are no different. Patients will often approach the dentist or the practice financial/accounts manager and ask for a discount of the fee. Many reasons may be cited by the patient in the hope of obtaining a discount and should come as no surprise to the dentist. In situations like this, the practice must have a clearly defined, well-communicated financial philosophy when it comes to discounting of fees. It is extremely important that the philosophy be followed, without exception, on every case in which a discount is given. It is recommended that payment for services that are discounted be made at the time of service. Payment should be made either by cash or by check. Credit cards have processing fees associated with them; so it is not recommended to be an acceptable form of payment when discounts are given. The amount of discount to be given is up to the dentist/owner of the practice. Later in the chapter, the authors discuss discounting fees when otherwise full payment is made on the same day of service.

Discounting of Fees and Dental Benefits

This complicated scenario is becoming more common:

> I have an opportunity to become a preferred provider for a particular dental benefit program. The agreement states I must use their fee schedule or discount my fees 20% and whichever fee schedule is less, is the one I will be reimbursed by. The agreement also states I cannot balance bill the patient for what the insurance company does not pay. What is the impact of participation in discounted fee programs on my fee schedule, my practice, present and future patients, and access to care?

To answer this question, you need to take an in-depth look at what is happening as a result of discounted fee dentistry. Insurance companies have developed discounted programs. The premiums paid by employers of PPO benefit programs are less expensive and thus more attractive to businesses than indemnity plans. By offering this type of program to companies, the insurance company can maintain or expand its market share and provide a product that is actuarially sound at a lower premium price to the employer. Companies electing to purchase this type of benefit program are happy because PPO premiums are less expensive and thus decrease costs and increase profit. What about the recipient of the program? What happens to them? Most commonly, they may experience higher out-of-pocket costs. Since the employer is paying less for the benefit program, the employee must pick up a portion of the costs associated with the benefit package in the form of higher co-pays or for services not covered under the discounted benefit plan. Frequently, patients may be economically forced to find a new dentist who is a preferred provider (or in the plan). A preferred provider is defined as dentist who is willing to discount fees in exchange for accepting the insurance company's fee reimbursement.

The preferred provider list of dentists is marketed to those individuals who have a specific PPO benefit plan. In essence, a "preferred provider" is agreeing to discount fees in exchange for having their practice marketed by the insurance company as a preferred provider. Dentists who become preferred providers frequently view the discounting of their fees as a marketing expense in hope of attracting more patients to the practice. If the patient refuses to change dentists, they will receive less financial benefit from their benefit program: higher out-of-pocket cost to the patient is the net result of not participating with a preferred provider. As you can see, there is a strong incentive on part of the patient to seek out dentists who are preferred providers.

The "preferred provider" dentist is also affected by agreeing to discount their fees. The cost of procedures does not go down by becoming a preferred provider. The cost of care is the same for all patients regardless of the type of benefit plan they have or may not have. Costs of providing care are very real. They do not go away. You can deny and try to negate these costs, but they do not go away. Someone always has to pay! Who is that someone? It can be the provider or the present and future patients of the practice who do not receive the benefit of a discounted fee schedule. If the provider fails to shift these costs in the form of higher fees to nondiscounted fee patients, the provider incurs a loss by being a preferred provider. Since costs remain, the overhead of the practice increases and profit margin of the practice decreases. If the provider elects to pass these costs on to the present and future patients of the practice who do not receive a discount, they will in essence be subject to increased fees beyond that needed to account for inflation and profit. The increases in fees by the provider are then passed on (assuming dental benefits are involved) to insurance companies of those patients who have dental benefits. The insurance company notes an increase in fees charged and more payout costs, and thus raises its premiums to the companies it markets its products to. The companies, who provide the benefit to the employee, then have a choice: pay a higher premium price for a benefit program or eliminate the benefit all together. As you can see, the only way one party benefits from discounted fee dentistry is at the expense of subsequent party. Michael Porter and Elizabeth Olmsted, in their book, *Redefining Healthcare*, call this *zero sum competition*. Ultimately, fee discounting and the accompanying cost shifting result in higher cost for everyone. Ultimately, less access to care is the final burden passed on to society.[18]

Impact of Fee Increases

An annual increase of fees is an economic necessity if you wish to keep pace with inflation and the ever-increasing cost of running a dental practice. Costs in the dental industry continue to climb as a result of competition for quality employees, technology, OSHA requirements, marketing, discounted fee dental benefit programs, taxation, and an increase in energy costs.

Fee structure and annual fee increases represent the quickest means available to dentists to decrease practice overhead and increase profitability. The major limitation on practice profitability is the discounting of fees through participation in discounted fee dental benefit programs. From a business standpoint, fee discounting results in less

[18] Porter, M. and Olmstead, E. *Redefining Heath Care*, Boston, MA: Harvard Business School Press, pp. 34–35.

profitability for a dental practice and ultimately higher healthcare costs for *all patients* in a given practice. It is for this sole reason, participation in discounted fee programs should be discouraged or, at minimum, monitored/limited to reasonable levels (see Chapter 3).

What Is UCR?

UCR stands for "usual, customary, and reasonable" as it pertains to fees. UCR is an acronym created by the insurance industry and appears at the bottom of explanation of benefit (EOB) forms and checks supplied to providers of dental services by insurance companies. The "reasonable" portion of this equation is on the decrease among insurance companies. The UCR is created by the following methodology. The insurance companies record the fee numbers as submitted by the practitioners on dental claims. The insurance companies sell the numbers (fees) to a company, such as the Health Insurance Association of America (HIAA). Since HIAA is not an insurance company, it can compare and analyze fees without worrying about "restriction of trade" litigation. HIAA then "sells" back the data to the insurance companies. The insurance companies then have an entire range of fees from which to compose their very own UCRs.[19]

There is no such thing as a universal "usual, customary, and reasonable fee." Rather there exists a range of fees based on percentiles created by dentists submitting fees to insurance companies. Dentists should *always* submit the fee as it appears on their *usual fee schedule* even if they are a preferred provider of dental benefits program.

What Are Percentiles?

In simple terms, percentile means, "How many out of 100 did you beat?" For example, the 80th percentile is that number or fee for which 80% of all fees fall below and 20% fall above."[20] Understanding percentiles will permit you to better position fees with those in the same geographic or zip code region.

A Benefit Provider Says My Fees Are Too High: Are They Right?

On occasion, you may receive notification from an insurance carrier stating that your fees are higher than the UCR for the geographic area. The question arises: Are my fees really out of line with the UCR for my geographic area? The answer is no. In reality, UCR varies from company to company and from policy to policy. Insurance companies generate these notices based on the *premium paid by the employer* for that particular policy. The lower the premium, the lower the table of fee allowances, thus assuring the insurance company that the policy sold is actuarially sound. *It is the responsibility of the dentist and staff to educate the patient on insurance reimbursement and coverage as it relates to policy coverage and fee-level reimbursement bought by an employer for an employee.*

---

[19] Make UCR work in your favor. *Dental Economics*, Webb, Del, July 1999. Available at http://www.dentaleconomics.com/articles/print.html?id=111096&bPool=DE.pennnet.co.

[20] Make UCR work in your favour. *Dental Economics*, Webb, Del., July 1999. Available at http://www.dentaleconomics.com/articles/print.html?id=111096&bPool=DE.pennnet.co.

Depending on the premium paid, the fee allotted as UCR may or may not be represented by your fee schedule. A good quotation to have available to patients when the above scenario presents is the following: "This action is not an attempt to establish a fee or to discuss the propriety of the provider's charge, but the expression of the obligation accruing under your plan. Please refer to your plan booklet for further information."[21]

Relative Value Unit Pricing

Just what is relative value pricing? Relative value unit pricing at this point in time is rather foreign to most dentists. This type of pricing model has been in place in medicine for over 10 years. With the Affordable Care Act (Obamacare) now law, our profession needs to become familiar with what Relative Value Unit (REV) pricing is all about.

Historically, providers of healthcare services have fee schedules based on the usual, customary, and reasonable format. The shortcoming of this form of fee schedule is the diversity in the fees charged for the same service within the same geographic area. With exploding healthcare cost in the 1970s and 1980s, serious cost-containment needs for medical and dental services prompted the investigation into alternative reimbursement methodologies. The relative value pricing model seeks to mitigate the wide variances in fees for the same service within the same geographic area. The pricing model is an attempt to standardize fees charged to patients.

The REV Model

A relative value scale (RVS) ranks services according to "value," where that value is defined with respect to a base value. All services are assigned a unit value, with more complex, more time-consuming services having higher unit values and vice versa. Values are then multiplied by a dollar conversion factor to become a fee schedule.[22]

In 1996, Resource-Based Relative Value Scale (RBRVS) was developed using the results of a Harvard University team that first identified three distinct components affecting the value of each procedure. This is a slight modification from the original REV model.

1. Provider Component
2. Overhead Component
3. Liability Component

Relative value units are assigned to each component and the sum of these composes the total value of each service.[23]

REV pricing is likely to be in the future of most dentists. You should understand that it is an attempt to standardize the cost of dental procedures within a given geographic area.

[21] Make UCR work in your favour. *Dental Economics*, Webb, Del, July 1999. Available at http://www.dentaleconomics.com/articles/print.html?id=111096&bPool=DE.pennnet.co.
[22] *Ingenix 2008 Coding Guide for Dental Services*, 5th ed., p. 16.
[23] *Ingenix 2008 Coding Guide for Dental Services*, 5th ed., p 16.

Definitions

The following is a list of definitions that may be of help in understanding fees and various forms of fee schedules and allowances. Chapter 13 includes a more extensive glossary of terms related to dental benefits/insurance.

Customary fee: The fee level determined by the administrator of a dental benefit plan from actual submitted fees for a specific dental service to establish the maximum benefit payable under a given plan for that procedure.

Fee schedule: A listing of charges for services rendered and agreed upon by the dentist of a particular practice.

Maximum allowance: The maximum dollar amount a dental program will pay toward the cost of a dental service, as specified in the program's list of provisions.

Maximum fee schedule: A compensation arrangement in which a participating dentist agrees to accept a prescribed amount as the total fee for one or more covered services.

Reasonable fee: The fee charged by a dentist for a specific dental procedure that has been modified due to the nature and severity of the condition being treated. This fee may be different from the dentist's usual fee or the insurance company's customary fee.

Table of allowances: A list of covered services with an assigned dollar amount that represents the total obligation of the benefit plan with respect to payment for such services. The table of allowances does not necessarily represent the dentist's full fee for that service.

Usual fee: The fee that the dentist most frequently charges for a given service within the practice.

Why Financial Arrangements Are Necessary

To own and operate a dental practice, you must be a skilled clinician and business-person. The goal of any business is not to break-even but to earn a reasonable profit. It is rather simple: without a profit, there is no practice. It is important to have not only a balanced fee schedule but also a system to collect the money owed to the business. Collections of fees for provided care are the lifeblood of the practice and a necessity if the practice is to remain a going concern. Overhead commonly runs ~60 to 65%+ in dentistry, and bills must be paid on time. Additionally, you deserve to be compensated for professional services. Unfortunately, dentists have traditionally been overly sensitive to the financial needs of their patients. By placing the financial needs of the patient first, far too many dentists have found that financial problems have become the norm and practice failure a reality. To avoid this set of unfortunate circumstances, it is important to have a written, well-communicated financial and collection plan. A payment policy needs to be in place prior to starting the practice of dentistry.

The dentist is not a banker. However, most patients feel as though all dentists, from the day they graduate from dental school and get their degree, are independently wealthy. Therefore, unless prior financial arrangements are made, these patients' idea of adequate financial arrangements is $10 per month for the rest of the doctor's natural life (and they believe they are doing the doctor a favor by being so generous). These patients are unaware that the average new dentist today graduates with ~$225,000+/− in educational debt, have not had a decent job for 8 years while in college, and then borrow another $300,000–750,000 in debt to purchase and equip a dental practice.

Raising your fees, instituting a state-of-the-art "Marketing Program," and selling all the dental services possible will not help if the patient does not pay you. A well-designed "Financial Policy" that states your position on the various financial matters between you and your patient is critical to maintaining an acceptable level of accounts receivable (defined as ~1 to 1.5 times the average monthly collectible production) while also depositing sufficient money to pay operational expenses with enough leftover to pay for your personal groceries, rent, and so on. Office collections should average 98.5% of collectible fees (discounts for cash, senior citizens, medical assistance, and so on are not collectible and must be deducted prior to calculation of the collection percent). To maintain these levels, financial arrangements must be made for all patients.

From the patient's perspective, it is your responsibility to help make financial arrangements that will allow them to accept and receive the care they need. Most patients want to know what is expected of them. Furthermore, patients with outstanding balances and no financial arrangements are no longer friends of the practice, are more critical of the care received, more likely to sue the doctor, and do not refer other patients to the practice. As humans, we tend to resent people to whom we owe money, especially if they seem to be in a better financial position than we are. The practice simply must make financial arrangements for the benefit of everybody involved.

The Best Financial Arrangement: Cash at the Time of Service

There is no doubt that a "Cash Only" practice has very few "collection" problems and a low accounts receivable. However, after working with and reviewing information from hundreds of practices over the past 20 years, an interesting set of data and trend has emerged. The "Cash Only" practice has on average a case acceptance rate of approximately 50% of total services offered/rendered versus the practice that offers "minimum" financial arrangements and/or assistance in securing necessary third-party financing for dental care (i.e., other than the dentist providing the financing). This means two things: (1) the average annual expenditures per patient is only 50%, that is, while the average patient spends $600 per year for dental services, the average "cash only" practice patient spends only $300 per year, and (2) "cash only" practices grow at a considerably slower rate as a result of fewer referrals for existing patients who are embarrassed to refer their friends to a dentist whose only concern is "cash."

Prefinancial Arrangement Considerations

Financial arrangements begin with the patient's first visit when they are asked to sign a *Payment Policy Acknowledgment* (PPA) form. This form is handled as part of the first appointment, either in combination with other preliminary forms or at check-out when it is time to pay for today's services. This form sets the stage for future financial arrangements and office policies. From both an informational and a financial perspective, this form states what is expected of the patient *unless other prior financial arrangements are made*. Most patients will readily and voluntarily comply with what is expected of them, if they are told what that is. The purpose of the Payment Policy Acknowledgment form is to simply inform the patient what is expected relative to payments due to your office for services rendered.

One special note is required regarding this form. The patient is not agreeing to anything when they sign the PPA form other than an acknowledgement that they have received and read the form. What is important is that they have received and *read the form*. They are not agreeing to anything, and the staff person should not push the occasional patient who refuses to sign the form. When that happens, the staff person who presented the form adds a note that says "Patient Refused to Sign," dates it, and the staff person signs their name to the form, which is scanned into the patients record/chart. A copy of this Payment Policy Acknowledgment form appears as Appendix A at the end of this chapter and a modifiable version is available on the website accompanying this book.

Financial Policy Worksheet

For other prior "financial arrangements" to be made, the staff must know what the doctor expects and wants. This is the reason a doctor needs to complete a *Financial Policy Worksheet*, thereby giving the staff guidelines as to what the dentist expects relative to the financial aspects of a dental practice. The Financial and Appointment Coordinators should have this internal financial policy memorized. A sample copy of this Financial Policy Worksheet appears as Appendix B and an editable version is available on the website accompanying this book.

Financial agreements should be done privately, that is, in a private setting by the Financial Coordinator or another qualified person. If a private area is not available, the discussion can be held in a treatment room but should never take place where other patients can hear or see. Financial arrangements should never be done by the doctor: this should be delegated so that the doctor can move on to other more productive activities. While the doctor should quote the fee being presented, explanation of the available financial options should be left to the trained staff person. This also avoids the opportunity for the patient to negotiate the terms of the financial arrangements directly with the doctor. The staff member will advise the patient, in the event they are unable to reach arrangements as specified in the Financial Policy, that they will discuss what would be an acceptable alternative to the policy with the doctor. When faced with this, 50% of the patients will subsequently agree to a more acceptable arrangement without involving the dentist.

Financial Arrangements for Insurance Patients

When making financial arrangements for patients with insurance, you are only making arrangements for their deductible and co-insurance. Therefore, only refer to these numbers when discussing these arrangements with the patient rather than referring to the entire fee (usually a much larger number). The psychological benefits of dealing with the smaller number makes acceptance of the treatment and financial arrangements much easier for the patient. This is a sales lesson learned years ago by the auto industry: at the time of sale, the focus is not on the total cost of the vehicle under consideration, but rather the "low monthly payment."

Formula for Successful Financial Consultations

The first step in making financial arrangements is to be certain that the patients have accepted and are ready to proceed with the proposed treatment plan. Patients generally desire the treatment until the fee is announced. Once the fee is announced, however, they may not want the treatment unless they perceive that the service suggested is a better value than the money that they are asked to exchange for the service. Throughout your conversation, it is necessary for you to continue confirming in the patients minds how they will enjoy and benefit from the proposed treatment. This will make your task of making the necessary financial arrangements much easier.

Once the treatment plan has been presented, the doctor should "casually" mention the fee. "Mrs. Smith, the fee for your treatment will be $XXX and I will now ask Suzy to cover what insurance will cover, and make the necessary financial arrangements for your treatment. Before I turn you over to Suzy, what further questions do you have regarding the proposed treatment?" It is very important that you do not just end the conversation with the fee, but rather incorporate the fee into a continuous sentence indicating that it is no big deal. On the one hand, you are telling the patient you are not afraid to tell them how much the proposed treatment will cost, but that another staff person will work out how the patient will pay for the proposed treatment.

The next step is to hand the patient off to the financial coordinator who will review the office financial policy with the patient. "Mrs. Smith, as you are aware (providing she has signed a Payment Policy Acknowledgment), we expect treatment to be paid for on the day services are rendered, 'unless other prior financial arrangements are made'. Your *estimated* portion will be $XXX. Will you be able to take care of that on the day of your appointment?"

Remember, even if you are not a "Cash Only" practice, your first goal is still to get all of the money up front and ideally in advance. It is very important that the Financial Coordinator present options only one at a time, starting with the offices preferred method, and waits for the patient to respond to each alternative before offering the next. It does not take a rocket scientist to figure out that if all alternatives are presented at once, the patient will select the alternative that is most desirable for the patient and least desirable for the practice.

Discounted Treatment Rules

To encourage payment prior to or on the day of treatment, many doctors have adapted what is commonly referred to as a "pretreatment courtesy bookkeeping adjustment." Before instituting such a policy, you should confirm with your local attorney that this is acceptable in your state.

Historically, if the patient also has dental insurance, insurance companies have claimed that you are charging less for a cash patient and you are charging the insurance company the full fee to maximize benefits. The insurance company then calls this "insurance fraud." However, again historically, because the insurance carrier is offered the same arrangements, that is, a discount for payment prior to the rendering of treatment, that argument has been largely lost. The insurance company of course will never pay up front.

That said, prepayment discounts are still covered by local and State Dental Examining Board rules and regulations, so legal input is mandatory prior to offering a "pretreatment discount." If allowed by your state, even payments made on the day of treatment can be qualified as "pretreatment" if, so that the patient does not need to deal with payment after the appointment, the staff offers to handle the "bookkeeping," including the agreed to payment due, prior to seating the patient.

If your attorney approves the use of a pretreatment discount and your office allows for a "pretreatment courtesy bookkeeping adjustment," then the following can be added to the initial "payment at time of services" opening statement: "If you can pay for this prior to your appointment, I can offer you a pretreatment bookkeeping adjustment of $YY that will make your balance due $ZZZ." Most senior citizens have the money and will take advantage of this. They are the easiest group with which to make financial arrangements.

The second insurance-related rule that applies is the fact that while you can charge a patient who does not have insurance a higher fee than you charge insurance-covered patients, you cannot charge a patient who has insurance a higher fee than you charge fee-for-service cash paying only patients. Other than the "pretreatment discount," if you give the insurance-covered patient any type of discount (friends and family, professional courtesy, etc.), whatever the discounted fee is, that is the same fee you must file on the insurance claim.

Again, watch the body language of the patient and their initial response to the suggested payment option, and do not proceed to the next option until the patient indicates that this option is unacceptable.

Alternative Financial Arrangements

If the patient is unable to pay the entire fee in advance or on the day services are rendered, the next choice is half of the fee due on the day of service and the balance within 30 days. The third choice is one third at time of treatment, with the second third due at 30 days and the final third due at 60 days. Your final choice would be one fourth on the day of service and three monthly payments. You can also offer to take a postdated check if the patient only needs a short postponement.

If these alternatives are not acceptable, it is now necessary for you to *get additional financial data*. "Mrs. Smith, it really sounds like your financial situation is a little tight right now. What do you think you can afford to do?" If what she offers is unacceptable, you will need to attempt to *create a money source* that she may not have thought of.

"It really sounds like you want to have the treatment done that the doctor recommended if we can work out the financial arrangements. What I'd like to do is to share with you some ideas that other patients who have had a similar problem have done. All of our patients have had to give up something to receive the dentistry they needed and wanted. For our wealthy patients, it is usually more the time and inconvenience that they must give up. For our not-so-wealthy patients, it is other things. And it is these patients who don't have a lot of money who can least afford to have the work they need done cheaply and have to be re-done at a later date. Or worse, not do anything and have conditions present that, if neglected, may further compromise patient health and be significantly more expensive to treat in the future."

"Some of our patients have had other assets they could use like savings accounts, stocks, bonds, or things like that. Would any of those be a possibility for you? A lot of our patients just put the balance on their credit card." Wait for a response. If the patient tells you that he/she is at their credit card credit limits, suggest that they check into getting the limit raised. If he/she pays promptly and has had no problems, this is usually done with a simple phone request to the bank issuing the card. "Some of our patients have had to take a bank loan, or get a loan from a finance company, or better yet if you are a member of a credit union, which is the least expensive loan source. Some patients just ask the bank to add to an existing loan. Would that be a possibility for you? . . . Is there a relative who could help you out?" Especially for young adults, this is frequently a source of available assistance.

Two other possible sources of funding include special "dental" credit card programs currently available (such as CareCredit) and some offices have actually made arrangements with a local bank for special financing for some of their patients. The bank arrangements can take several forms. In one program, the office merely agrees, unknown to the patient, to co-sign the loan. It is important that the bank understands that the patient should not know that the note has been guaranteed or co-signed. The advantage to the office is that the money is received upfront and the patient is much more likely to pay the bank than the doctor. The advantage to the patient is that he or she can spread the payments out, they usually get a lower interest rate than credit cards, and they establish an ongoing credit history.

Another bank program used by some offices involves the office receiving a discount on the fee paid from the lender. This allows the patient to receive, in effect, an interest-free loan. The office receives 85–92% of the face value of the amount financed and the patient pays the face value back to the bank. If the fee was $1000, the office receives $850–$920 and the patient pays the bank $1000. While these notes are sometimes nonrecourse, the majority are recourse (if the patient fails to pay the bank, the dentist must repay the balance due). If the doctor feels that the patient is a good risk, recourse notes are a good option.

The banks like this arrangement because if the patient pays the note off in 1 year as scheduled, they collect a net interest rate of about 18%. If the patient prepays the note, the net rate is considerably higher (and so is the bank's profit when calculated as a return on their investment, that is, the interest "rate" actually received by the bank on the money they have loaned). The term is usually 1 year but can be longer.

The entire loan application is handled by the doctor's office that forward the information to the bank. Approval is usually obtained less than a day. There is usually a $300–500 minimum transaction because of the banks cost to process the loan. The discount rate must be negotiated with the bank by the doctor.

Most "bank dental loans" will be recourse, which means you are guaranteeing the loan. Again, the justification for the dentist to assume this risk in exchange for getting their cash upfront is the fact that most patients will readily make their bank note payments versus dental fee payments to the dentist. Therefore, if the only alternative is for the dentist to finance the work needed, getting the money upfront from the bank minimizes the risk that the dentist would not be paid if they were carrying the financing themselves.

If all attempts at finding financing sources are unsuccessful, then the only other alternative is to break the treatment down into manageable financial increments (phase treatment). This allows the patient to receive ideal care they can afford to pay as they receive treatment. For many patients, they may really want the care but may be facing a short-term cash flow problem. This is frequently seen with young families and families with children in college.

It is important that the person making the financial arrangements be empathetic with the patient and not lose the patient altogether while attempting to make arrangements. Remember, most dentistry is discretionary in nature. It is okay for you to compete against the patient using their money for a new car or golf clubs instead of dentistry. However, you must also be sensitive to the patient who may legitimately not be able to afford anything and is struggling to just put food on the table. By maintaining this sensitive attitude now, you may get to do the work in the future and you will keep the patient in the practice as an ongoing referral source.

Additional Considerations

For those cases requiring laboratory procedures, at least the laboratory fee must be collected prior to or on the day of preparation. If the patient does not pay the fee on the preparation date, then the laboratory work should be held and not sent to the laboratory until payment is received.

If the case is of a complete or removable partial denture, unless the doctor's policy is clearly stated to the contrary, the treatment must be paid in full prior to final insertion and delivery of the appliance/prosthesis. It is common knowledge that the prosthesis will fit better if it is paid for.

If a patient's financial arrangements for fixed prosthetics is to be paid in full prior to insertion, the verbal skills are as follows. The patient should be approached as soon as they arrive at the office. "Mrs. Smith, we have a couple of minutes before they will be ready for you in back. Why don't we take care of the necessary paperwork now so that as soon as you are completed, you can just leave. Let's see. My note here says you were to make a payment of $XXX today. Will that be cash, check, or credit card?"

If the patient does not make the payment as agreed or none at all, the doctor should be alerted. The doctor can do the final seating and try-in, but it is amazing how there is always something a little wrong that will require one more trip back to the laboratory for correction. On the second appointment, the same approach should be used. If the patient fails to make the required payment a second time, the patient should be informed that you are sorry but you cannot deliver the final prosthesis until it is paid for and you will be happy to reschedule the appointment as soon as it is. It may be necessary for you to remake financial arrangements at this time.

One final note: For patients with either a poor credit history prior to becoming a patient in your office or who have demonstrated poor payment habits while a patient, the only financial arrangement possible is *cash*.

Account Registration Form

In addition to a medical/dental history form, an informed consent form, and the payment policy previously discussed (see Appendix A), patients should be given an account registration form to complete. The account registration form should include the following for patients with or without dental insurance benefits:

Account Registration Form Components

1. Person responsible for the account
2. Driver's license number
3. Address information
4. Phone number
5. Insurance information
6. Preferred payment option (cash, check, or credit card)

The information in the Account Registration Form then becomes a part of the patient record. The hardest part of any payment policy is the follow-up and continuity with all patients of the practice. If not strictly adhered to and audited every month, the policy becomes worthless.

Disclaimer

Any discussions related to "Financial Arrangements" have a legal component, from a Federal, State, and local Dental Examining Board perspective. In addition to Federal rules that include the need to follow "Truth in Lending" guidelines for any financing done by the dentist with terms exceeding three payments, there are also State regulations that vary from state to state. The authors of this information are not providing "legal advice," and any "Financial Policies" should be reviewed by the dentist's legal advisors prior to implementation.

Importance of Cash Flow

According to a survey conducted by American Express of healthcare professionals, 32% of dentists identified cash flow as the most important management priority for the next 6 months.[24] In order to improve cash flow, payment policies need to be enforced. Payment involves more than just stating to the patient that payment will be made by cash, check, or credit card. It starts by having a written and well-communicated treatment plan.

The components of the treatment plan should include the items to be addressed, cost, priority, treatment options, estimate of dental benefits, and the number of appointments required. The patient should be consulted about the treatment plan and asked if they have any questions. The patient is given a copy of the treatment plan and financial arrangements are made with the office accounts manager. A comprehensive treatment plan enables the accounts manager to become more familiar with the treatment, sequencing of treatment, and associated fees prior to making financial arrangement with the patient. By handling treatment in this fashion, you can avoid performing treatment the patient did not expect or for which they were unaware of the cost. In private practice, the best surprise to the patient is no surprise when it comes to fees and comprehensive cost of care.

How Much Can You Afford to Finance?

While financial arrangements are important, you must ask who is in control of the process. Patients want arrangements that are affordable and advantageous for their personal budgets. On the other hand, patient financing is a liability to the dental practice. With this in mind, you should make financial arrangements accordingly.

Acceptable financial arrangements are those in which risk to the practice is minimized. The first step in the process to minimize risk is to know the overhead of the practice. The overhead percentage is the key if you are to have an in-office financing program. As an example, if the overhead of the practice is 60%, the practice can only afford to finance 40% of the patient's expected bill. By not financing the variable cost of the treatment, your cash flow remains intact and risk is minimized. Bills associated with treatment are covered by not financing more than the profit margin of the business. The idea of a financing is to be flexible enough to oblige patient but strict enough not to put the practice at any undue risk.

[24] Langwith, Elizabeth. Adopt a strict payment policy without losing patients. *Dental Economics*, April 2005.

Once the financial policy has been established, it is extremely important that follow-up on the arrangements are carried forth by the accounts manager. This step is frequently left to lapse in many practices. If you expect to collect what you have produced, it is an absolute necessity that this step not be ignored.

The authors recommend to set reasonable limits on how much you are involved in the business of extending credit to patients. CareCredit is a better alternative to offer patients whom to pay for services over time. CareCredit offers the patient flexibility and convenience when managing the cost of healthcare. Applying for approval is easy and quick. Numerous payment alternatives are available to patients. Some options offer no interest if paid in full within 6 or 12 months. If you wish to incorporate CareCredit into your financial policy, contact CareCredit at www.carecredit.com. CareCredit is not new to the dental industry. Over 165,000 providers currently provide this alternative service to their patients.

Credit Cards

Part of a good financial policy is accepting credit cards for services provided. The use of credit cards allows for a strict payment policy while simultaneously keeping the widest range of patients. Recent estimates show that 144 million Americans carry at least one general-purpose credit card.[25] Surprisingly, many dental offices today still do not accept payment by credit card. The primary objection to credit card payment is the associated costs of establishing and maintaining a credit card system. When you consider the benefits—payment, out of the office financing, ease at which business can be transacted—it seems wise to have this service available to patients.

Utilizing Collection Agents

In spite of efforts to have and administrate a good financial policy in your practice, bad accounts still occur. There are two schools of thought with regard to utilizing a collection agency when this situation arises. One line of thought centers around the fear of getting sued by the patient if the account is turned over to a third-party collection service. It is interesting that people cannot find the money to pay dental bills but always have enough money to pay to an attorney to file a law suit against the one trying to collect for professional services. Nonetheless, fear results in no action and a financial loss to the practice. The downside of such an approach is that your practice gets a reputation in the community of being "soft" on financial issues. The saying "birds of a feather tend to flock together" really holds true to having a soft hand with regard to those people who are delinquent on their accounts.

The second school of thought is to use a collection agent when all in-office attempts have failed to result in payment of a delinquent account. It is important to be aware of state and federal standards governing the use of collection agents. You should take the time to interview and discuss with the third-party collector its policies and adherence to state and federal law. Hiring a collection agency with a good reputation and adherence

[25] Langworth, Elizabeth. Adopt a strict payment policy without losing patients. *Dental Economics*, April 2005. Available at http://www.dentaleconoimics.com/articles/print.html?id=228171&bPool=DE.pennnet .com%.

to state and federal law is of utmost importance if you are to avoid litigation. Whether you attempt to collect accounts in-house or via a third-party agent, the Fair Debt Collection Practices Act (FDCPA) governs issues as to how to communicate with debtors and how payments must be processed. The FDCPA became law in 1978 and prohibits any harassment, abusive conduct, and the use of false or misleading statements in the collection of patient debt by third-party debt collectors. The provisions of this act do not apply to businesses that collect their own debt. However, it does apply to collection agencies, lawyers, and other third-party agents, who in the regular course of their regular business collect debt for others.[26] A word of caution when you choose to collect accounts in-house: state law can be stricter than federal law when it comes to collection of delinquent accounts. Adherence only to the FDCPA guidelines may not protect you from litigation. You should consult an attorney prior to the collection process to ensure you are in compliance with laws of your state.

When turning an account over to a third-party collector, it is your responsibility to ensure information about the person and the account is correct. Additionally, the collection agent cannot use any prohibited acts as stated in the FDCPA to collect a delinquent account. Violations by the collection agent can result in federal litigation should the patient file a complaint and a violation of the FDCPA is noted. As result, dental practices using third-party collection agencies face the very real risk of countersuits.

Summary

Creating and maintaining a balanced fee schedule purposefully positioned in the marketplace is a primary tool available to a dentist to generate income to help offset the cost of doing business. Our economy is influenced by a number of factors that cause it to be in a constant state of flux and impacts a dentist's fees. Economic indicators help us measure these changes and help us understand our rate of inflation. Inflation is the primary reason why fees need to be increased on a periodic basis. Discounting of fees must be carefully monitored and has a tremendous impact on the cost of doing business and the level of profitability recognized by the business. A well-communicated treatment plan and clearly defined and communicated financial policies for patients will help ensure that a practice collects money owed by patients.

Book Companion Website

The book companion website at www.wiley.com/go/dunning/transition includes editable versions of Appendices A and B for you to download and use. Please see 'About the Companion Website' at the start of the book for details on how to access the website.

References and Additional Resources

Abdullah, L.R. 1996. The credit and collections game. *Dent Econ*, October. Available at http://www.dentaleconomics.com/articles/print.html?id=123112&bPool=DE.pennnet.com%.

Baumohl, B. 2005. *The Secrets of Economic Indicators*, 2nd ed. Philadelphia: Wharton School Publishing.

[26] Abdullah, Larry R. The credit and collections game. *Dental Economics*, October 1996. Available at http://www.dentaleconomics.com/articles/print.html?id=123112&bPool=DE.pennnet.com%.

Beazouglu, T., Heffley, D., Brown, L.J., and Bailit, H. 2002. The importance of productivity in estimating need for dentists. *J Am Dent Assoc* 133: 1399–1404.

Federal Reserve Board. 2003. Introductory statement by Jean-Claude Trichet on July 2004. http://www.federalreserve.gov. http://www.ecb.int/press/presconf/2004/html/is040701.en.html.

Federal Reserve Board. 2004. Federal Reserve Board's Semiannual Monetary Policy Report to the Congress. http://www.federalreserve.gov.

Glasscoe, Diane. 2000. Our fees are too high! *Dent Econ*, March. Available at www.dentaleconomics.com/articles/print.html?id=110190&bPool=DE.pennnet.co.

Guay, Albert. 2005. Dental practice prices, production and profits. *J Am Dent Assoc* 136(3): 357–361.

Ingenix. 2008. *Coding Guide for Dental Services*, 5th ed. Salt Lake City: Ingenix, p. 16.

Langwith, Elizabeth. 2005. Adopt a strict payment policy without losing patients. *Dent Econ*, April. Available at http://www.dentaleconoimics.com/articles/print.html?id=228171&bPool=DE.pennnet.com%.

Limoli, Jr., T. 2007. Fee survey. *Dent Econ*, September. Available at www.dentaleconomics.com/articles/print.html?id=307297&bPool=DE.pennnet.com.

McGill Advisory, 2006. 21(12): 3.

McGill Advisory, 2007a. 22(5): 2.

McGill Advisory, 2007b. 22(5): 3–4.

Porter M., and Olmstead, E. 2006. *Redefining Health Care*. Boston: Harvard Business School Press.

12manage, The Executive Fast Track. Available at www.12manage.com/description_target_pricing.html.

Webb, Del. 1999. Make UCR work in your favor. *Dent Econ*, July. Available at http://www.dentaleconomics.com/articles/print.html?id=111096&bPool=DE.pennnet.co.

Wikipedia: The Free Encyclopedia. en.wikipedia.org/wiki/inflation.

Learning Exercises

1. You have recently purchased a dental practice in which the fee schedule appears to be competitive within the geographic area. The practice broker reaffirms the fact that the fee schedule has been well maintained and is competitive. You notice the collection/production ratio of the practice is in the low 90% range and the overhead of the practice is higher than the national average at 73%. What are the possible reasons for what is going on in this practice? What can you do to resolve this problem? What areas of practice management would you investigate?

2. A disgruntled patient tells you that your fees are too high? What do you tell this patient? What can you do to possibly prevent this situation from happening again? Should the actions of this patient concern you? Why or why not?

3. How does managed care impact fee setting? Do you think it is unethical to participate in cost shifting? Why or why not? Do you think the ADA should have an ethical statement concerning cost shifting?

4. Why does increasing fees offer more benefit to those practices with higher overheads?

Appendix A: Payment Policy Acknowledgement Sample

Dr. I am a New Dentist
1234 Any Street
Somewhere, Montana 76543
987-654-3210

Payment Policy Acknowledgment
SAMPLE

Dear Patient:

In an effort to control fees, we recognize that one of the best methods is to *control costs*. We have therefore instituted the following policies as an aid in controlling bookkeeping overhead expenses.

For those Patients who do not have dental insurance, payment in full is expected for services rendered on the day of service, unless prior financial arrangements have been made.

If the Patient or Responsible Party has an insurance program, the Office will produce and send claims to the insurance carrier (usually within 24 hours of the appointment), provided evidence of benefits (insurance card, employment verification) is presented to the Office.

Any portion of services not covered by insurance is due on the day services are rendered unless prior financial arrangements are made.

The Office will not be responsible for follow-up of delayed insurance payments or for negotiation of any settlements on any disputed insurance claims regarding any services rendered by the Office. When there is a delay in receiving payments from the insurance carrier, it is the responsibility of the Patient or Responsible Party to investigate the delay. The Responsible Party will be requested to make payment in full when an insurance claim is delayed beyond 45 days of the date of service.

If it is necessary to change your reserved appointment time, we request notification of at least 24 hours in advance of the appointment. Notification of an appointment change must be made during regular business hours. Failure to keep a scheduled appointment or provide appropriate notification may result in a charge for the appointed time.

Any questions regarding payments should be directed to the Financial Coordinator.

By my signature, I acknowledge receipt of a copy of the office payment policy.

_____   _____
Patient or Responsible Party   Date

Appendix B: Financial Policy Worksheet (with recommended policies)

(from Dr. Eugene Heller)[*]

Each office must have a policy for each of the following categories for the financial coordinator to be successful at making financial arrangements. Please complete each category for your office policy.

1. **Quoting Fees/Shoppers:**
   The Goal is to get the patient in for a quick, no charge exam by Dr. who will then quote fee.
2. **New Patient Routine Visit**: Cash not required for initial visit.
3. **Emergency:**
   New Patient Emergency Visit: Requires patient to bring $100 cash or credit card.
   Active Patient Emergency Visit: Cash not required.
4. **Accident Emergency:**
   School Related: Handle under normal policy. Do not agree to wait for insurance settlement.
   Auto Related: Same as above.
   Industrial Related: Same as above.
   Worker's Compensation: Same as above.
5. **Hygiene**: Payment per visit for non-insurance patients.
6. **Insurance:**
   1. Will you accept assignment? Suggested response -Yes.
   2. Co-pays/deductibles less than $100, paid at time of service.
   3. Co-pays/deductibles over $100, make financial arrangements.
7. **Restorative:**
   Non-Insurance-Routine (Amalgam, Resin, Endo, etc.)
   Under $100: Cash at time of visit.
   Over $100: Make financial arrangements.
   Insurance-Routine (Amalgam, Resin, Endo, etc.)
   Under $100: Paid at time of service.
   Over $100: Make financial arrangements.
8. **Restorative-Accident Related (Insurance)**
   School Related: Handle under normal policy. Do not agree to wait for insurance settlement.
   Auto Related: Same as above.
   Industrial Related: Same as above.
   Worker's Compensation: Same as above.
9. **Prosthetics:**
   Fixed: Normally 33-50% Paid at time of service to cover lab fee, otherwise same as 7 above.
   Removable: Make financial arrangements/offer alternative finance services.

Remember, editable versions of both Appendix A and B are available on this book's companion website: http://www .wiley.com/go/dunning/transition

    Implants: Make financial arrangements/offer alternative finance services

    Cosmetic: Make financial arrangements/offer alternative finance services

10. **Benevolence (providing discounted or no fee dentistry for people in financial need):**
    1. Will you accept and treat patients in this situation in life, and, if so, what criteria will be utilized?
    2. Will you/can you legally limit the number of these patients you accept or the treatment provided?
11. **Medicaid**: Same as Benevolence
12. **Payment Per Appointment:**
    Remember, Cash Practices tend to produce 50% less per patient than practices providing minimal financial arrangements and grow at 50% the rate of practices with minimal financial arrangements.
13. **Monthly Payment Plan:**
    Not recommended beyond 3 months.
    More than 3 payments requires adherence to Truth in Lending and Regulation Z.
14. **Credit Cards:**
    If a 5% discount for payment before or on the day of service is allowed, will you allow this discount for credit card payments considering the credit card company will charge 2-4% of the amount paid this way?
    Recommendation: No.
15. **Children:**
    1. Parents responsible.
    2. If divorced parents, parent presenting child responsible unless prior financial arrangements made with a different party.
16. **Out-of-Town Students**: Cash or credit card.
17. **Adjustments/Discounts:**
    5% discount for payments before or on the day of service as a bookkeeping courtesy adjustment.
18. **Broken Appointments:**
    Only charge a fee for those patients you desire to dismiss from the practice.
    If charging a fee, it is typical to give patients a pass on the first one or two missed appointments.
19. **Credit Checks:**
    Check with your state to determine whether legal to conduct. If legal, an excellent idea.
20. **Other:** _____
21. **Other:** _____

ORDER OF PAYMENT PREFERENCES

1. **Cash or Credit Card on or before the day of appointment**
2. **One-half on the 1st day of appointment, one-half on last appointment**
3. **One-half on the day of appointment, balance in 30 days**
4. **One-third day of 1st appointment, one-third day of last appointment, one-third in 30 days**

Chapter 13
Dental Benefits

Kristen Strasheim, RDH, BSDH

Dental Benefits Overview

A dental benefit plan or dental insurance policy is a contract in which the dental benefit organization agrees to pay for some or all of your covered dental care costs. Nearly 192 million Americans have dental benefits, which represents 60% of the population in the United States (2015 NADP/DDPA Joint Dental Benefits Report).

There are two types of dental benefits: publicly funded and commercial. Of the Americans that have dental benefits, 19% were covered by public funding and 82% were covered by commercial dental benefit plans. The government agency or organization processing and paying may be called "third-party payers."

Dentists working in private practice reported that 65% of their patients were covered by commercial dental insurance, 7% were covered by public assistance, and 28% had no dental insurance (American Dental Association Health Policy Institute). This is a total of 72% of patients seen in private practice having some type of dental benefits. These statistics indicate that your future dental practice will likely have some involvement with dental benefits.

Additionally, research shows that having dental insurance drives utilization or patient demand for dental services. Among those who hadn't seen a dentist in the last year, 33% stated that the lack of a dental plan was their main reason for not visiting a dentist (Consumer Survey Dental Health and Health Care Reform May 2012).

As with any specific area of study, understanding terminology is vitally important. As you read through this chapter, refer to the glossary near the end of the chapter if you need to learn the meaning of an insurance-related term with which you are unfamiliar.

In addition, several chapters in this volume relate to dental benefits/insurance. Chapter 3 discusses recommended practice performance indicators, including the percentage of gross revenue from dental benefit plans and the percentage of gross revenue in "adjustments" or discounts from dental benefit plans. A practice's involvement in dental insurance will likely also impact practice valuation (Chapter 5) and the viability of associateship opportunities (Chapters 20 and 21). Chapter 12 also provides a discussion on dental fees, dental insurance, and financial policies for patients.

Dental Practice Transition: A Practical Guide to Management, Second Edition.
Edited by David G. Dunning and Brian M. Lange.
© 2016 John Wiley & Sons, Inc. Published 2016 by John Wiley & Sons, Inc.
Companion Website: www.wiley.com/go/dunning/transition

Publicly Funded Dental Benefits

Publicly funded dental benefits refer to dental care paid through the federal and state government. These programs are *Medicaid, State Children's Health Insurance Program* (SCHIP), and *Medicare Supplemental Plans.*

Medicaid is a government program for low-income and special-needs (disabled) people whose resources are insufficient to pay for health care. It is a collaborative program by both the federal and state government. The federal agency Centers for Medicare and Medicaid Services (CMS) monitors the programs in each state and sets standards for how the programs are managed and financed. Each state establishes and administers its own Medicaid program, and determines the type, amount, duration, and scope of services. And these programs vary greatly in the services covered and the patient population eligible for services. For example, in some states adults may not have dental Medicaid benefits.

SCHIP is the program that extends coverage to uninsured children and pregnant women with incomes too high to qualify for Medicaid. Another name for this program is the Children's Health Insurance Program (CHIP).

Medicare is a federal program for people aged 65 and older. Medicare doesn't cover dental procedures except in very rare cases integrally related to another covered procedure (for example, reconstruction of the jaw following an accident). However, dental coverage may be offered under Medicare supplemental plans.

Commercial Dental Benefits

Some dental plans sold are individual plans (7%) or are dental plans integrated with medical plans (less than 1%). The vast majority of dental plans are group dental plans (92%). This is when the employer chooses the dental plan and contracts with a dental benefit organization or third-party payer to provide dental benefits to an enrolled population. Several variables determine the type of plan the employer chooses for their employees: the company benefit budget, company contribution amount, employee affordability, what benefits will be valued by the majority of their employees, whether employees need more than one plan, location of employees, and dependents. There is a very wide variety of plans available to accommodate what the employer wants to purchase, literally hundreds of thousands of potential plan configurations. Although the employer chooses and purchases the plan, most of the time employees pay some of the premium (70%).

Commercial Dental Plan Models

Employers have many options when choosing a dental plan for their employees. One of the first decisions is to provide a fully insured or self-funded dental plan.

A *fully insured plan* is when the employer purchases a dental plan from a dental benefit organization. This is the more traditional way to structure an employer-sponsored plan. The dental benefit organization assumes the risk that the expenses of the dental claims may exceed the premiums paid. The dental benefit organization sets the premium based on demographics and location of the group. The employer pays the premium monthly. The premium rates are fixed for a year and are based on the number of employees enrolled in the plan each month. The monthly premium changes during the year only if the number of enrolled employees in the plan changes. The dental benefit organization processes and pays the dental claims according to the dental plan the employer selected. Fully insured plans are subject to state insurance regulations. The covered persons, employees, and dependents are responsible to pay any deductible amounts or co-payments required for covered services under the policy. Employees often share in paying some of the insurance premium as part of a payroll deduction.

A *self-funded plan* can also be referred to as a self-insured plan. This is when the employer provides the funds necessary to pay the dental claims for its employees and assumes the financial risk. The employer is responsible for paying the dental claims that its employees incur instead of paying a fixed premium to an insurance company. The employer must have the financial resources to meet its obligations, which can vary each month. The employer must have enough money to cover the cost of the claims. If not, the payment of the claims may be delayed or suspended. Some plans may be partially self-funded. The partially self-funded plan sponsor may use stop-loss insurance (a maximum benefit amount) to protect against the risk of unanticipated higher utilization.

Larger employers are more likely to offer a self-funded plan than small businesses. This type of plan may be identified by looking for phrases such as "administered by" or "administrative services only (ASO)" on the covered person's insurance card. Self-funded plans are regulated by federal law under the Employee Retirement Income Security Act (ERISA).

A self-funded plan may be administered by a third-party administrator (TPA) or a commercial third-party payer. They process the claims and may provide other administrative services such as customer service, preparing claim reports, and provider network access. The TPA may charge a fee per claim or a fixed monthly administration fee based on the services provided.

Fully insured or self-insured plans can have the following plan elements: managed care, indemnity, and direct reimbursement.

Commercial Dental Benefit Plan Types

The plan types are managed care plans, indemnity or fee-for-service, direct reimbursement, and discount dental plans.

- *Managed Care* refers to a cost containment system that directs the utilization of dental benefits by restricting the type, level, and frequency of treatment. It also limits access to care with provider networks and controlling the level of reimbursement for services. There are three types of managed care plans:
  - *Dental Participating Provider Organization* (DPPO or PPO): There is a contract with dentists for a discount from their usual and customary fees. Dentists are paid on a discounted fee-for-service basis after each dental care service has been completed. Dentists are paid at the agreed discount if they are in the DPPO network or at a rate set by the plan if they are not in the network. When using a dentist in the network, patients are not billed for the difference between the negotiated or discounted fee and the usual and customary fee that the dentist charges. Enrollees usually pay less when dental services are done by a dentist in

the DPPO network. They may have dental services completed outside the DPPO network, but will usually pay more for those services. Enrollees can see a specialist without a referral. Payments from the dental benefit organization typically are made directly to the dentist.

- *Dental Exclusive Provider Organization* (DEPO): Enrollees *must* use an in-network dentist to receive benefits. Payments from the dental benefit organization typically are made to the dentist. Care from out-of-network dentists is *not* covered except for emergencies. Like a DPPO, members can see a specialist without a referral. These specialist visits are covered as long as the dentists are in the network.
- *Dental Health Maintenance Organization* (DHMO) or also known as *Capitation*: Provides comprehensive dental benefits at fixed dollar co-payments. Enrollees must go to a dentist in the DHMO network for dental services. Dentists in the DHMO network are paid a monthly fee for each person that signs up and selects that dentist. Claims are not filed for each service provided by a DHMO network dentist. Nonemergency services received outside the network without prior approval are not covered by the plan.

- *Dental Indemnity Plan or Fee-for-Service Plan*: This is a nonnetwork dental plan so there are no restrictions on which dentist the enrollee can visit. There are no discounted provider contract arrangements whereby the provider agrees to accept a fee below their usual and customary fee. It often has a deductible. After the deductible, it pays a certain percentage of charges for services completed. Payments from the dental benefit organization can go to either the enrollee or to the dentist.
- *Direct Reimbursement*: This is a self-funded program in which the enrollee is reimbursed based on a percentage of dollars spent for the dental care provided, and allows enrollees to seek treatment from the dentist of their choice. Dentists receive payment directly by the enrollee/patient.
- *Discount Dental Plan or Dental Saving Plan*: A type of dental plan that is not "insurance" per se. A group of dentists agrees to perform services at specified discounted fee or discount their customary fee. The enrollee pays the dentist the discounted fee for the services received.

Structure of Commercial Dental Benefit Plans

Dental benefit plans may have cost-sharing components such as deductibles, co-payments, or co-insurance. A *deductible* is the amount enrollees pay for covered dental services before the plan pays. On most plans, the enrollee must pay the deductible amount each calendar or plan year. The average annual deductible is $50–99. A dental plan covering several family members may have both an individual and a family deductible. The family deductible is the overall limit on what a family will pay before the dental plan pays—namely, deductible satisfied by combined expenses of all the covered family members. For example, a dental plan with a $25 deductible may limit its application to a maximum of three deductibles, or $75 for your family, regardless of the number of family members.

A *co-payment* requires the enrollee to pay a fixed dollar amount for each visit to a provider or for a specific procedure. Co-insurance is when the enrollee shares the cost of the dental procedure. It is calculated as a percentage of the covered procedures expense.

If a person is covered under more than one dental plan, then the benefits must be coordinated between the dental benefit organizations so that payments do not exceed the allowed charges. This is called *coordination of benefits*. It will need to be determined which plan is considered the primary dental plan (determined by state law) and is based on the National Association of Insurance Commissioners (NAIC). The primary dental plan pays first, and then the second plan pays. The second plan's payment covers the balance due for dental services; however, the second plan will never pay more than they would have paid had they been the primary plan.

Dental benefit plans typically cover preventative care, restorations, endodontics, oral surgery, orthodontics, periodontic, and prosthodontics. These types of procedures are then broken into three categories: diagnostic/preventive services, basic services, and major services.

The diagnostic/preventive services are often paid by the dental plan without deductibles or co-payments. Typically included here are exams, cleanings, radiographs, fluoride treatments, sealants, and space maintainers. These may also be called Class I, Group I, or Type A services.

Basic Services generally include restorations/fillings, extractions, root canals, and scaling and root planning. These typically include patient co-payments or co-insurance. These could also be referred to as Class II, Group II, or Type B services.

Major services generally include crowns, dentures, implants, and oral surgery. Patient co-payments or co-insurance are the highest for these services, usually at 50%. These may also be referred to as Class III, Group III, or Type C services.

Dental plans often contain a detailed list of covered procedures. A covered procedure is a procedure for which benefits are provided in the dental plan. There could be frequencies applied to the covered procedure that may affect the benefit being covered. The plan may have limitations that restrict conditions such as age, length of time covered, and waiting periods. It may also limit the extent or conditions under which certain services are provided. The plan may also exclude preexisting conditions—a dental condition that exists prior to enrollment in a dental plan. A common preexisting condition is a missing tooth.

A dental plan may have an alternative benefit clause or a plan provision called the *least expensive alternative treatment* (LEAT). This provision is not intended to dictate a course of treatment. Instead, this provision is designed to determine the allowable amount for a submitted treatment when an adequate and appropriate alternative procedure is available. The enrollee may choose to apply the alternative benefit amount determined under this provision toward the payment of the submitted treatment. An example of a LEAT would be a posterior resin composite restoration completed, but the plan gives an alternative benefit of a posterior amalgam.

The majority of plans have an annual maximum (94%). This is the most the dental plan will pay toward the cost of the enrollees' dental services. After the plan pays this amount, the enrollee must pay the total expense of the dental services, but at the discounted fee if the dentist is in a PPO network. The common annual maximum amounts are $1000–1499 (48%) and $1500–1999 (43%). On average only 3–5% of people with dental benefits reach the annual maximum each year (NADP Dental Benefits Report: Premium and Benefit Utilization Trends 2015).

Participating Provider Organization (PPO) Obligations

Managed care plans dominate the market because this is the type of dental plan employers are purchasing. So, market share and associated patient demand for services definitely influence dentists choosing to join a PPO Network. According to the NADP Consumer Survey, nine out of ten consumers use a dentist in their plan's network.

When a dentist joins a PPO network, there is a credentialing process. A completed application and contract are required along with copies of the following items: a dental license, specialty license or diploma, Federal Drug Enforcement Administration Certificate, and Professional Malpractice Liability Certificate of Insurance.

Some dental benefit organizations lease their provider network to other companies, meaning the dentist may also become by contractual agreement a PPO provider for other third-party payers. Becoming a PPO provider means the dental benefit organization will advertise your practice on their website and in a directory that may be given to employer groups and their employees. This arrangement allows your practice to be advertised to a wider range of potential patients.

The PPO contract may require that payment from the third-party payer be made to the provider and require the provider to file the dental claim for the enrolled member.

The contract requires the provider to be reimbursed at a fee that is established by the dental benefit organization, which is called a PPO fee schedule. If either the dentist or the dental benefit organization wants to terminate the contract, it must be done in writing.

Submitting Claims

All dental claims should be submitted using the current ADA dental claim form. Claims may be submitted electronically or on paper. Approximately 61% of claims are submitted electronically, and this percentage will probably increase in the future. Submitting claims electronically is more efficient and cost-effective for both the dental office and the dental benefit organization. Some dental benefit organizations offer incentives to the provider for submitting claims electronically. Chapter 11 discusses the technological infrastructure necessary for submitting claims electronically.

Most dental benefit organizations offer claims performance guarantees. The most common guarantees are: claim financial accuracy, and turnaround time for claim payment. A median range for processing dental claims is 96% within 6–10 days (NADP/LIMRA 2014 U.S. Group Dental Claims Processing Metric). This means that half of all dental claims are processed/paid in less than 6–10 days, and half in more than 10 days. Part of the reason for the quick turnaround time is that approximately two out of three claims are auto-adjudicated, meaning an the electronic processing of a claim without human intervention.

Current Dental Terminology © American Dental Association (CDT) is the code set to be used in all dental transactions and is used for dental claims processing. CDT codes are used to describe the clinical procedures performed. CDT is updated annually; so, make sure you use the current version of the codes. Claims should be submitted in a timely manner. Many plans have a timely filing clause such that claims submitted after that time period will not be reimbursed.

Some claims may undergo a professional review by dental professionals either employed or contracted with the dental benefit organization. This is called *utilization review* or *utilization management*. This is when criteria are designed to monitor the use of or evaluate the appropriateness or the medical necessity of the dental procedures performed. When this is done, supporting documentation may need to be submitted with the dental claim. The supporting documentation required may be radiographs, periodontal charting, or narratives. Generally, there is a time limitation in which to submit the supporting documentation. If it is submitted after that time period, the claim will receive an administrative denial due to lack of information to make a benefit determination.

A *pretreatment estimate* (PTE) (also sometimes referred to as a predetermination) is a process where a treatment plan is submitted to the dental benefit organization prior to starting treatment. This is done to determine potential benefits, but is not a guarantee of benefits. PTEs are typically submitted on complex and costly procedures.

After the claim is submitted, an *explanation of benefits* (EOB) will be sent either electronically or by mail to the enrollee and an *explanation of payment* (EOP) will be sent to the provider. This is a detailed summary from the dental plan explaining if the dental procedures submitted were a covered benefit or not, and the allocation of related deductibles, co-payments from patients, and insurance benefit amounts. The EOB or EOP could include payment. If the dental procedures submitted were not a covered benefit, then information will be included on how to appeal the decision. An appeal is a formal request for the dental plan to review denied or unpaid claims. Either the enrollee or the dentist can file an appeal. As a reminder, Chapter 12 addresses the importance of having financial policies for patients, including recommendations related to collecting co-pays.

An Overview of Dental Benefits

Table 13.1 provides a high-level overview of dental benefits that lists each type of dental plan, enrollment information, an overview of the dental benefit plan, if there is a contract for the provider, typical claim submission and payment, and the average reduction in the fees for providing dental services.

A Glossary of Dental Benefit Terms

Accepted Fee: The fee accepted as full payment under the dentists' contract.

Allowable Amount: Highest amount payable for covered services. This may also be called maximum allowable amount.

Allowed Charge: The maximum amount the dental plan will pay for a dental service. For in-network providers, the allowed charge is based on the provider's contract. For out-of-network providers, the allowed charges may be the same as for in-network providers or the Usual and Customary (U & C) charges.

Alternative Benefit: A dental plan provision basing payment for a particular dental service on the least expensive treatment that is effective. The plan provision does not limit treatment options. Sometimes referred to as the least expensive alternative treatment (LEAT).

Annual Maximum: The most a dental plan will pay toward the cost of the enrollees dental services. After the plan pays this amount, the enrollee must pay the total cost of the dental services, but at the discounted cost if the dentist is an in-network provider.

Table 13.1 A Summary Overview of Dental Benefits.

Type of Dental Plan	Plan Enrollment	Overview of Plan	Provider Contract	Claim Submission and Payment	Fee/Reimbursement
Medicaid, State Children's Health Insurance Program (SCHIP) and Medicare These programs focus on providing care for low-income and disabled people.	Precise enrollment not known but an estimated 30%–40% of dentists nationally participate at some level in Medicaid/SCHIP. Further, more dentists provide preventative services than regular dental care.	Medicaid and SCHIP is a publicly funded federal and state government program. Each state establishes and administers the program. Medicare is a federal program for people age 65 and older. Dental coverage may be offered under Medicare supplemental plans.	Yes	Provider submits claims and each state determines the process. Some states only accept claims electronically. Receive payment directly for services provided from dental benefit organization.	The fee varies greatly from state to state. It could be a deep or negligible discount. Doesn't necessarily have the lowest fees. Provider agrees to discount their usual and customary fee. The reduction in fees could depend on the dental procedure and if patient is a child or an adult. The reimbursement range is 10–100% of their usual and customary fee.[a]
Dental Participating Provider Organization (DPPO)	The percentage of dentists that participate in a provider network for DPPO is 60.6%. The mean (average) number of networks a dentist participates in is 5.7. 82% of all commercial dental plans sold.	A managed care plan in which the enrollees pay less when dental services are done by a provider in the PPO Network. Enrollees may use a provider not on the network, but will pay more for those services.	Yes	Provider submits claims and receives payment for services provided from dental benefit organization and patient.	Provider agrees to discount their usual and customary fee. The average reimbursement is 72% of their usual and customary fee.
Dental Exclusive Provider Organization (DEPO)	<1% of all commercial dental plans sold.	Enrollees must use an in-network dentist. Care from out-of-network dentists isn't covered except for emergencies. This is a managed care plan.	Yes	Provider submits claims and receives payment for services provided from dental benefit organization and patient.	Provider agrees to discount their usual and customary fee. The average reimbursement is 60% of their usual and customary fee.

Plan	Description			
Dental Health Maintenance Organization (DHMO)	The percentage of dentists that participate in a provider network for DHMO is 12.8%. The mean (average) number of networks a dentist participates in is 1.9. 8% of all commercial dental plans sold.	Enrollees must go to a dentist in the DHMO network. Dentists in the DHMO network are paid a monthly fee for each person that signs up and selects that dentist. This is a managed care plan.	No	Claims are not filed for each service provided and receives payment directly for services provided from dental benefit organization.	Provider is paid a monthly fee for each person that signs up and selects that dentist. Payment received is typically lower than their usual and customary fee.
Dental Indemnity Plan or Fee-for Service Plan	6% of all commercial dental plans sold.	This is a non-network plan so there are no restrictions on which dentist you can visit.	No	Provider submits claims and receives payment for services provided from dental benefit organization and patient.	Provider is paid their usual and customary fees.
Discount Dental Plan or Dental Saving Plan	The percentage of dentists that participate in this type of plan is 37.7%. The mean (average) number of networks a dentist participates in is 2.2. 4% of all commercial plans sold.	A type of plan not considered insurance. A network dentist agrees to perform services at a specified discounted fee or discount their customary fee.	Yes	Provider may or may not submit claims and receives payment for services provided from the patient.	Provider agrees to a specified discounted fee or to discount their fees.
Direct Reimbursement	<1% of all commercial dental plans sold.	Enrollee is reimbursed based on a percentage of dollars spent for dental care provided and can receive treatment from the dentist of their choice.	No	Provider submits claims and receives payment for services provided from the patient.	Provider is paid their usual and customary fees.

[a] A ten-year national study by Nisseh, Vujicic and Tarbough (2014) found average reimbursement rates for Medicaid services to be at these respective levels compare to commercial dental plans: 49% for pediatric services and 41% for adult services.

Appeal: An appeal is a formal request for the dental plan to review denied or unpaid claims. Either the enrollee or the dentist can file an appeal.

Assignment of Benefits: The benefit payments may go to the dentist or to the enrollee.

Balance Billing: When providers bill for the difference between their fee and the allowed amount.

Basic Services: A category of dental services. Usually includes fillings, extractions, root canals, and root planning. Also called Class II, Group II, or Type B services.

Beneficiary: A person covered on the dental benefits contract. Beneficiaries are eligible for benefits.

Benefit: The amount the dental plan pays on a covered service.

Benefit Summary: An outline of your dental plan. It may include co-insurance percentages, deductibles, maximums, and noncovered services. Also referred to as benefit highlights.

Benefit Year: The 12-month period used for deductibles, maximums, and other plan provisions. Also called a plan year.

Billed Charge: The amount billed by the provider for services.

Claim: A request for payment under a dental benefit plan. It is a statement listing services rendered, the dates of services, and itemization of costs. The completed request serves as the basis for payment of benefits.

Co-insurance: The enrollee shares of the cost of dental services. It is calculated as a percentage of the covered procedures expense.

Coordination of Benefits: The enrollee has more than one dental plan, and so payments do not exceed allowed charges. The primary dental plan pays first. The second plan pays after the first plan pays.

Co-payment or Co-pay: The enrollee pays a fixed dollar amount for each visit to a provider or for a specific service.

Cost-sharing: The portion of the dental costs the enrollee pays. This can be a deductible, co-payments, or co-insurance.

Covered Procedures or Services: The dental procedures or services the dental plan covers.

Current Dental Terminology (CDT): CDT code is the code set to be used in all dental transactions and is used for dental claims processing. CDT is copyrighted by the American Dental Association (ADA).

Deductible: The amount enrollees pay for covered dental services before the plan pays.

Dental Exclusive Provider Organization (DEPO): A type of managed care dental plan. Enrollees must use an in-network provider. Care from out-of-network provider is not covered except for emergencies.

Dental Health Maintenance Organization (DHMO) (also known as Capitation): A type of dental plan. It provides comprehensive dental benefits at fixed dollar co-payments. Enrollees must go to a dentist in the DHMO network for dental services. Dentists in the DHMO network are paid a monthly fee for each person that signs up and selects that dentist. Nonemergency services received outside the network without prior approval are not covered by the plan.

Dental Indemnity Plan: A type of dental plan. A nonnetwork dental plan, and so there are no restrictions on which dentist you can visit. There are no discounted provider contract arrangements whereby the provider agrees to accept a fee below their customary fee. Also called a fee-for-service plan.

Dental Participating Provider Organization (DPPO): A type of managed care dental plan. There is a contract with dentists to discount their usual and customary fees. Dentists are paid at the agreed discount if they are in the DPPO network or at a rate set by the plan if they are not in the network. When using a dentist in the network, individuals are not billed for the difference between the negotiated or discounted fee and the customary fee that the dentist charges. Enrollees usually pay less when dental services are done by a dentist in the DPPO network. Enrollees may go outside the DPPO network but will usually pay more for those services.

Dental Plan or Dental Insurance Policy: A contract in which the dental plan agrees to pay for some or all of the enrollees' covered dental care expenses. The employer and/or the enrollee pay premiums for the plan. The enrollee may also have to pay deductibles, co-pays, or co-insurance as part of the contract.

Dependents: Enrollees' spouse and/or children covered on the plan. This is generally defined by terms of the dental benefit contract.

Diagnostic or Preventive Services: A category of dental services that are often paid by the dental plan without deductibles or co-payments. Usually includes exams, cleanings, x-rays, fluoride treatment, sealants, and space maintainers. Also called Class I, Group I, or Type A services.

Direct Reimbursement: A type of self-funded dental plan in which the enrollee is reimbursed based on a percentage of dollars spent for dental care provided and allows enrollees to seek treatment from the dentist of their choice.

Discount Dental Plan or Dental Saving Plan: A type of dental plan that is not insurance. It is a network of dentists that agrees to perform services at specified discounted fee or discount their usual and customary fee. The enrollee pays the dentists the discounted fee for the services received.

Eligibility Date: The date the enrollee and dependents are eligible for benefits under the plan. Often referred to as the effective date.

Enrollee: Individual covered by a benefit plan. See beneficiary.

Expiration Date: The date the dental plan expires and the enrollee is no longer eligible for benefits. May also be called a termination date.

Explanation of Benefits (EOB): A detailed summary from the dental plan to the enrollee explaining if the dental procedures submitted were a covered benefit or not. If the dental procedures submitted were not a covered benefit, then information will be included on how to appeal the decision. It could include payment.

Explanation of Payment (EOP): A detailed summary from the dental plan to the provider explaining if the dental procedures submitted were a covered benefit or not. If the dental procedures submitted were not a covered benefit, then information will be included on how to appeal the decision. It could include payment.

Family Deductible: The combined amount enrollees pay for covered dental services for all covered family members before the plan pays.

Fee Schedule: Reimbursed at a fee that is established by the dental benefit organization for in-network providers.

In-Network: Dentists and other licensed dental care providers that contract to provide dental services on the dental plan.

Insured: Individual covered by a benefit plan.

Insurer: The party promising to pay a benefit if a specified loss occurs in an insurance contract.

Limitations: Restrictive conditions stated in a dental benefit plan such as age, length of time covered, and waiting periods. The plan may also exclude certain benefits or services. It may limit the extent or conditions under which certain services are provided.

Major Services: A category of dental services. Typically includes crowns, dentures, implants, and oral surgery. Co-payments or co-insurance is the highest for these services, usually 50%. Also called Class III, Group III, or Type C services.

Managed Care: Refers to a cost containment system that directs the utilization of dental benefits by restricting the type, level, and frequency of treatment. It also limits access to care with provider networks and controlling the level of reimbursement for services.

Maximum Allowable Amount: See Allowable Amount.

Medicaid: A government program for low-income and disabled people whose resources are insufficient to pay for health care. It is a collaborative program by both the federal and state government. Each state establishes and administers its own Medicaid program, and determines the type, amount, duration, and scope of services.

Medically Necessary Care: Health care services or supplies needed to diagnose or treat an illness, injury, condition, disease, or its symptoms and that meet accepted standards of medicine.

Medicare: A federal insurance program for people age 65 and older. Medicare does not cover dental procedures. Some insurance plans offer dental coverage under Medicare supplemental plans.

Member: An individual enrolled in a dental benefit program.

Noncovered Charges: Expenses for dental services that the dental plan does not cover. In some cases, the service is a covered service, but the insurer is not responsible for the entire charge. In these cases, the enrollee will be responsible for any charge not covered by the dental plan.

Noncovered Services: Dental services or procedures not listed as a benefit. Noncovered services or procedures will not be paid by the dental plan. The enrollee will be responsible for the full fee.

Open Enrollment or Open Enrollment Period: Time of year when an eligible person may add, change, or terminate a dental plan for the next contract year.

Out-of-Network: Care from providers not contracted with the dental plan. Generally, the enrollee will pay more out of pocket when receiving dental care by an out-of-network provider.

Out-of-Network Benefits: Coverage for services from providers who are not under a contract with the dental plan.

Out-of-Pocket Expense: The amount enrollees must pay for dental care. Includes the difference between the amount charged by a provider and what the dental plan pays for the service.

Overbilling: Stating fees as higher than actual charges. An example is when the enrollee is charged one fee and the dental plan is billed a higher fee.

Participating Provider: Dentists that have a contract with a dental plan. The contract includes set service fees.

Payer: Party responsible for paying the dental claims. It can be a self-insured employer, insurance company, or governmental agency.

Preauthorization: A process that the dental plan uses to make a decision that a particular dental service is covered. The dental plan may require preauthorization for certain services, such as crowns, before being completed. Preauthorization requirements are generally waived if you need emergency care.

Precertification: Confirmation by the dental plan of eligibility for coverage.

Preexisting Condition: A dental condition that exists for a time period prior to enrollment in a dental plan. The common preexisting condition for dental plans is a missing tooth.

Premium: The amount an employer or enrollee pays to a dental insurance company for dental coverage. The dental insurance company generally recalculates the premium each policy year.

Pretreatment Estimate (PTE) or *Predetermination:* A process where a dentist submits a treatment plan to the payer before treatment begins. The payer reviews the treatment plan. Then the payer notifies the enrolled and the provider about one or more of the following: eligibility, covered services, amounts payable, co-payment, and deductibles and plan maximums.

Primary Payer: The dental plan with first responsibility in a benefit determination.

Provider: A dentist or other dental care professional, or clinic that is accredited, licensed, or certified to provide dental services in their state and is providing services within the scope of that accreditation, license, or certification.

Provider Network: Dentists and other dental care professionals who agree to provide dental care to enrollees of a dental plan under the terms of a contract.

Purchaser: Often employer that contracts with the dental benefit organization to provide dental benefits to an enrolled population.

Schedule of Benefits: A list of dental services and the maximum benefit amounts an insurer will pay for each.

Self-Funded Plan: A benefit plan in which the plan sponsor bears the entire risk. Some plans may be partially self-funded. Third-party administrators may process claims and provide other administrative services. They do not bear any of the risk of utilization of the plan.

Self-Insured Plan: The employer pays the dental claims and establishes the plan design. The benefits may be administered from a third-party administrator (TPA) or a dental benefit organization.

Third-Party Administrator: Claims payer who assumes responsibility for administering dental benefit plans without assuming any financial risk. Some commercial insurance companies also have TPA operations to accommodate self-funded employers seeking administrative services only (ASO) contracts.

Usual and Customary (U & C): The base amount that is treated as the standard or most common charge for the dental service.

References and Additional Resources

American Dental Association Health Policy Institute, July 2015.

Consumer Survey Dental Health and Health Care Reform, May 2012.

Centers for Medicare and Medicaid Services www.cms.gov.

NADP Dental Benefits Report: Premium and Benefit Utilization Trends, January 2015.

NADP/LIMRA 2014 U.S. Group Dental Claims Processing Metrics, September 2015.

Nasseh K., Vujicic M., and Yarbough C. *A ten-year, state-by-state, analysis of Medicaid fee-for-service reimbursement rates for dental care services*. Health Policy Institute Research Brief. American Dental Association, October 2014. Available at http://www.ada.org/~/media/ADA/Science%20and%20Research/HPI/Files/HPIBrief_1014_3.ashx.

2015 NADP/DDPA Joint Dental Benefits Report: Enrollment, September 2015.

2015 NADP/DDPA Joint Dental Benefits Report: Network Statistic, October 2015.

Learning Exercises

1. What is defined as "A form of dental cost sharing in a dental plan that requires the enrollee to pay a fixed dollar amount for each visit to a dentist or for a specific service"?

2. What percentage of enrollees typically reach their annual plan maximums?
   a. 3–5%
   b. 6–8%
   c. 9–11%
   d. 12–14?
   e. 15–17%

3. According to the American Dental Association Health Policy Institute, what percentage of patients in private practice have private dental insurance?
   a. 45%
   b. 50%
   c. 55%
   d. 60%
   e. 65%

4. What is also referred to as fee-for-service plan?

   Key: 1. Co-payment or co-pay; 2. a; 3. e. 4. Dental indemnity plan.

Chapter 14
Appointment Scheduling Strategies
Dunn H. Cumby

Appointment Scheduling Policy and Philosophy

A commitment to oral health as a component of the patient's general health should be a core value reflected in the culture of the business created to serve as a particular market of potential patients. The *value* of an appointment should be established and demonstrated by both the staff and the doctors. The reality that this commitment can only be achieved by active participation of both the dental team and the patients should be conveyed to the patients and to the dental team as well. An "appointment/scheduling policy" based on this core value must be developed and maintained if this commitment is to be realized. The key to honoring this commitment in a dental practice can be achieved by planning, implementing, and continually evaluating a disciplined but flexible scheduling system. In order to be effective, this system must be centered on the patients in the market that the practice is designed to serve.

Honoring and being on time for appointments is one of the first messages that must be shared with new patients at the time of their admission into the practice. The business must constantly strive to attract patients who are willing to participate in the culture of the practice. The entire dental team must continually reinforce the importance of this value. This culture is promoted in many positive ways and, if necessary, in ways that may be interpreted by the patients as being negative. The appointment/scheduling policy should be given to every new patient, and stressed with existing patients on an ongoing basis. "If you don't control your schedule, your schedule will control you!"

If an office can control the numbers of No Shows and Last Minute Cancellations, the patients can benefit by the office being able to better control the costs of delivering dental treatment. Controlling the cost of dental treatment is an ongoing challenge in the dental business. Salaries, supplies, lab fees, and equipment are constantly increasing in the dental market. One thing that drives up costs is the need to raise prices to offset the lost income that is caused by No Shows and Last Minute Reschedules. A well-orchestrated schedule reduces the stress of achieving preset production goals, which are challenged by missed appointments. When patients keep their appointments and the dental offices are on time, a very efficient low-stress environment is created. When patients have to wait, it increases their stress. When patients are late or don't show up for appointments, it increases the stress for the dental office providers. Having an

Dental Practice Transition: A Practical Guide to Management, Second Edition.
Edited by David G. Dunning and Brian M. Lange.
© 2016 John Wiley & Sons, Inc. Published 2016 by John Wiley & Sons, Inc.
Companion Website: www.wiley.com/go/dunning/transition

efficient appointment/scheduling policy is foundational to establishing and maintaining a productive and efficient dental business model.

All production and revenue generated by the practice is the result of collected patient fees generated by the provision of dental services. These fees result from the effective and efficient use of time. Dentistry can be described as a service business that sells time. This time is broken up into units that are used to assign patient appointments into daily scheduling. How this time is allocated and managed first depends on the number of hours available to the dental office.

The typical dental office is not open for business every day of the calendar week. Most dental offices use a 4-day workweek. In addition, by providing 7 holidays and 2 weeks of vacation each year, the average dental office may be open for production a total of 196 days per year. Most offices can count on the dental providers losing other production days due to personal or family illness or other emergencies. Time away from the office must also be allowed for professional continuing education. In large practices, time units are also lost to staff meetings and strategic planning and/or facilities maintenance. All of this means that out of a typical year (365 days), the dental office may be open for business about 50% of those days.

Since time is the most valuable product for sale in the dental practice, the best use of this resource is accomplished by establishing a scheduling policy and philosophy that allows for the effective use of this resource. The policy, along with its philosophical principles, should be written, implemented, maintained, and periodically reexamined to verify that it remains relevant within the desired context and will provide the desired results. The document should be kept in the office in a place where all the staff have access to it and can refer to it on a daily basis, as necessary. Some offices refer to this as a "recipe or system strategy" for scheduling. But whatever name is given to it, it should be a documented systematic approach to appointment scheduling that works for a particular office as long as the logic and steps are followed.

Many scheduling strategies exist among dental offices. Generally, these strategies are rooted in philosophical principles. Unless an office has scheduling principles from which an appointing strategy can be implemented, the true potential of the dental office will not be achieved. In addition, the office will not come close to receiving its highest return on investment while simultaneously providing scheduled patients with excellent care. Whoever schedules the appointments in a dental office is like the conductor of a symphony. If an appointment is not scheduled, production cannot be realized, and if appointments are not scheduled properly, office production will never reach the fullest potential. No scheduling strategy will work if there is a lack of commitment by the doctor(s) and staff. In other words, for the scheduling system to work, it must *be* worked. A scheduling system is worked by the consistent application of the principles involved in its management. Any decision to change the system should be decided collectively. Two of these philosophies are briefly discussed.

The first of these principles results from a relatively simple philosophy: *Just keep the doctor busy and everything will work out in the end. Keep all the chairs full during office hours.* Offices using this philosophy generally schedule several appointments within the same time slot just in case one or more of the patients scheduled do not show up or cancel the appointment at the last moment. The doctor, then, may also be scheduled in two or more treatment rooms at the same time. The type of treatment procedures planned for the time slot is not taken into consideration when these appointments are made. The philosophy is to just keep the doctor busy. These are the kind of scheduling philosophies found in clinics where the patients expect to wait for extended periods of time, and usually only very basic types of dental treatment are provided. Another way to understand this philosophy is to view it as similar to an emergency room at a local hospital, where patients are treated on a first-come-first-served basis. This principle is to do *something* for each patient and to do *more* only if time allows.

On the other hand, some offices "orchestrate" time slot utilization. This orchestration is based on production goals, finely tuned and timed procedures (systems), disinfection and preparation time needed before and after each treatment procedure, the doctor's time to perform each procedure, and the preferences of doctors and patients. The principles in this type of scheduling can be relatively simple or extremely complex. Some doctors prefer to schedule more complex treatment early in the day, while others prefer to schedule this treatment in the middle of the afternoon or at the end of the day. Some doctors prefer to appoint children early in the morning rather than late in the afternoon. These schedules require the complete coordination of clinical and clerical staff as well as provider staff to maintain smooth office workflow.

Either of the philosophical approaches to scheduling will work in a variety of dental settings. There are, however, many other types of scheduling that fall somewhere between these two. For the purposes of this chapter, we focus on the merits and challenges involved in the principles of orchestrating an appointment scheduling system.

Types of Appointments

In order to orchestrate appointments, thought, purpose, and intent must be used to schedule all appointments before they are written in the appointment book. Appointment time increments in dental computer software are usually broken down into units of either 10 or 15 minutes. The daily appointment objective is to maintain a productive flow of patients throughout the practice day. Scheduling and production efficiency are critical to patient wait times. Appropriate scheduling with low no-show rates results in a most effective and efficient patient-satisfying practice. Additionally, appropriate scheduling is more likely to meet daily provider production goals. As scheduling is discussed in this chapter, consider an ideal small clinic or practice to have three chairs (operatories) and two assistants per dentist. Also consider the ideal larger practice as a six-chair (operatory) dental clinic with two dentists, four assistants, and one hygienist.

There are many strategies to developing and using scheduling blocks. Many offices have successfully used quadrant dentistry by scheduling one or two patients per hour per dentist, classifying an appointment as either exam or operative (child or adult) or emergencies (or walk-ins). Many others have used the physical operatory as the scheduling block. Some use the open access method of appointment scheduling by appointing daily call-ins and seeing call-ins the same day of the call. Some leave blank time intervals in the schedule for potential emergencies that are filled as emergencies or when new patients call in for appointment times either the same day or the next day. Providers or assistants may elect to schedule next appointments from the chair based on treatment evaluation, and suggested follow-up time intervals requiring a later reconciliation with the front desk scheduler. There are advantages and disadvantages to any strategy chosen. Provider preferences and the target market served generally dictate the best strategy for managing scheduling blocks.

Appropriate scheduling blocks and sequencing of procedures are important to the efficiency of the practice as well as to establishing patient goodwill. Time demands, scope of the treatment plan, patient requests, and treatment sequencing are aspects of scheduling that are impacted by the type of procedure provided to the patient. In other words, all aspects complement one another, and none are stand-alone considerations. Other aspects to consider along with the procedure itself include office staffing availability, provider absences, other office facilities and equipment availability, style and philosophy of the provider, and the proficiency of the dentist or provider complementing the individual need of the patient to tolerate particular treatment demands. In this section, we do not incorporate or address these aspects specifically, although we do acknowledge their existence. Instead, we refer the reader to other sections of the chapter.

Units of Time

There are many ways to utilize time to get the best production from providers and to most efficiently utilize operatories. Time units can be scheduled in 10-or 15-minute intervals. An example of a 10-minute interval appointment book is shown in Table 14.1. A 1-hour time block can comprise as many as six appointments for each of the doctors, as shown on the appointment book in Table 14.1.

An example of a 15-minute interval appointment book is shown in Table 14.2. A 1-hour time block can only comprise as many as four appointments for each of the doctors as shown.

Consideration must be given to doctor preferences and the most frequently delivered treatment procedures prior to selecting time intervals for a practice.

Operatory Availability

An example of a 10-minute appointment interval using operatory scheduling is shown in Table 14.3.

Operatory appointment booking allows for doctor, space, assistants, and facility use to be included in planning for the appointment. Each operatory is assigned an assistant,

Table 14.1   Ten-minute appointment book interval.

Time Units	Dr. Zip	Dr. Dip
8:00 a.m.	Ms. Happy (child exam)	Mr. Loner (emergency)
8:10 a.m.		
8:20 a.m.		
8:30 a.m.	Open slot	
8:40 a.m.	Open slot	
8:50 a.m.	Open slot	

Table 14.2   Fifteen-minute appointment book interval.

Time Units	Dr. Zip	Dr. Dip
8:00 a.m.	Ms. Happy (child exam)	Mr. Loner (emergency)
8:15 a.m.		
8:30 a.m.	Open slot	
8:45 a.m.	Open slot	

Table 14.3 Operatory appointment booking.

Interval	Operatory No. 1/ Assistant W	Operatory No. 2/ Assistant Y	Appointment Name/Op No.	Dr. Zip
8:00 a.m.	Prep and seating	Open	Crown—Ms. Sad/OP No.1	Open
8:10 a.m.		Open		Open
8:20 a.m.	Dr. Zip	Open		OP No.1—Asst. W
8:30 a.m.	Dr. Zip	Prep and seating	Crown—Ms. Glad/OP No. 2	OP No.1—Asst. W
8:40 a.m.	Dismiss			Open
8:50 a.m.	Decontaminate	Dr. Zip		OP No. 2—Asst. Y
9:00 a.m.	Open	Dr. Zip	Open time	OP No. 2—Asst. Y
9:10 a.m.	Open	Dismiss		Open
9:20 a.m.	Open	Decontaminate		Open

Operatory No. 1 (OP No.1)
Operatory No. 2 (OP No. 2)
Assistant W (Asst. W)
Assistant Y (Asst. Y)

in this case Assistant W and Assistant Y. Some time slots shown on Table 14.3 indicate assistant functions where the doctor is *not* involved and present in the operatory. These may or may not be included in an actual appointment book. These slots are prep and seating, dismissal of the patient, and disinfection of the operatory. The dental assistant is primarily responsible for these required functions.

Preparation (prep) of the operatory may include the assistant reviewing a checklist of items that are needed for the appointed procedure and subsequently ensuring that those items or supplies are available prior to the doctor's entry into the operatory. In addition, "seating of the patient" ensures that the patient and his or her chart are brought to the appropriate operatory and the patient is greeted, made to feel comfortable, and draped for the procedure. The assistant may also preliminarily converse with the patient and generally address today's treatment event. Also of interest in this demonstration is that the time slot is unavailable when the operatory is being disinfected, in spite of the fact that the patient is not physically present in the operatory.

The patient appointed to the time slot and the procedure planned is included under the fourth column in Table 14.3. Ms. Sad's treatment is planned as a crown preparation and final impression. She has been scheduled in operatory No. 1 with Assistant W. A 1-hour total operatory time slot has been allotted to this procedure. Dr. Zip has been given only 20 total minutes to complete the procedure. The amount of time required for this treatment procedure (by this doctor) can only be known by the scheduler and/or doctor through trial and error over a period of several months. As an example, an additional 10 minutes could be made available to him by decreasing the amount of prep and seating time required for this patient and/or procedure. Ms. Sad, however, may be elderly with co-morbid conditions requiring several blood pressure readings or more time to prepare her for the procedure. In this case, time must be made up in the dismissal and/or disinfection time slots or through the doctor's increased efficiency. A doctor could also alternatively make up time through efficient use of the second operatory.

The opportunity to make up time through use of another operatory makes operatory scheduling more desirable, given a flexible and efficient staff. Notice the staggered scheduling required in order to effectively utilize the provider's time between two operatories. Whenever both an operatory and a dentist are shown to be *open in the same time slot*, there is an opportunity for another appointment to be inserted. However, the amount of *open time* available dictates the procedure that can be performed within that time frame.

Disinfection and Preparation Time

The procedure determines the amount of preparation time and disinfection time that it takes to prepare a treatment room between patients. Hygiene procedures are the simplest and fastest types of dental treatments to prepare for in setting up an operatory and in disinfecting a treatment room. Hygienists use the same instruments on most all procedures. They have two basic trays: one for prophylaxis and one for deep scaling and curettage. Dentists, on the other hand, have many different types of treatment procedures requiring different instrumentation and equipment, as well as different time frames to complete these functions.

Root canal treatments have become very sophisticated when rotary instrument systems are used instead of hand instrumentation. Many of the rotary files can only be used once, and those that can be recycled must be monitored with each usage and inspected for damage before being used for the next procedure. Some practices that offer implants and other surgical procedures have specially designed rooms to be used specifically for those types of procedures. It may take up to 20 minutes to properly set up a room for an implant procedure. If they have the space, for efficiency, some practices use other rooms for patient sedation before moving the patient into the surgical treatment room. Documentation of the specific manufacturer and brand name of implants used in the procedure must be recorded. Sometimes it takes longer than was allotted in an appointment time slot to provide proper sedation for the patient. When this happens the doctor or hygienist has to wait and try again. All of this takes time that may or may not have been planned.

For every procedure performed in a dental office, the proper time needed to set up and disinfect before and after the treatment should be factored into the time that the treatment room is not available for any other procedure. These functions also occupy the assistant's time both before and after the treatment procedure. Care should be taken when using operatory scheduling to consider procedure type, especially when scheduling a patient for treatment that requires the presence of both the assistant and the doctor. Some appointments, like denture adjustments and healing checks, do not require an assistant.

There are hundreds of different dental procedures that can be provided to patients. The doctor or assistant uses a basic exam instrumentation setup (mirror, explorer, and cotton pliers) for many of these procedures. Some offices use a tray and tub system in which all the materials and instruments are placed on a tray and all the supplies and equipment are placed in a tub that is either color coded or labeled for use with a particular procedure. Other offices stock each operatory with the basic supplies and only bring the necessary instruments from the sterilization room into the operatory. The tray and tub systems are broken down and disinfected away from the operatory. Those offices that stock supplies in the operatory treatment room must take the time to restock each room periodically, in addition to disinfecting after each use of the operatory.

Time Units by Procedure

The time it takes to set up and disinfect an operatory is easier to gauge than the time a particular doctor needs to perform a specific procedure. This is especially true of new doctors or even an experienced doctor who has incorporated a new procedure into the practice. Just remember that with every new thing there is a learning curve. Repetition leads to efficiency, and efficiency leads to decreasing the time needed to perform different dental procedures. An excellent idea is to periodically record the time doctors and hygienists need to perform different procedures.

The more information the scheduler has concerning a particular appointment prior to the appointment time, the more likely the appointment will be scheduled within the appropriate time slot. The specific tooth number, the surfaces to be treated on each tooth, and the total number of teeth to be treated at the next visit are "minimal information." No scheduler will ever complain about being given too much information about the dental visit being scheduled. Typically doctors err on the side of giving too little information to the scheduler about the next appointment. This is not a desirable behavior.

Ten-minute time units allow for more flexibility in scheduling an appointment. When 10-minute time units are used in scheduling, it is much easier to salvage time over the course of a normal workday. "Ten-minute cultures" must be established over time in the dental office. Much of appropriate appointment scheduling is orchestrating a practice/patient rhythm. Procedures can be measured in terms of 10-minute time units. Hygiene appointments can be used as a basic example. Some offices schedule one hygiene appointment per hour. Not all prophylaxis takes the entire hour to accomplish, but even if finished before the hour is over, the hygienist must wait until the next patient arrives for the next appointment. If, however, the hygiene appointments are scheduled every 50 minutes or five "10-minute" units of time for each appointment scheduled, 10 minutes are saved with each appointment. If appointments are scheduled on the hour, using the 50-minute time for cleanings, the next appointment will be scheduled for 10 minutes before the hour, the following appointment will be scheduled for 20 minutes before the next hour, and so on. For every eight appointments, eight units of time are saved (1 hour and 20 minutes in potential production time by the end of a typical 8-hour day). This will allow the hygienist to see nine patients instead of eight and have two units of time to "spare" at the end of the day.

Let us take this hygiene example and put some numbers with it. If the average hygiene appointment is a $100 production, the hygienist can treat five more patients over the period of 1 week. That increased production accumulates over a 1-year period to 300 more patients treated. Using these very conservative figures, an additional $30,000 in production could be scheduled for the year. These "spare units" can be thought of as "spare change," which adds up to increased production, as well as efficiency in utilizing the resources of the practice.

Scheduling by Provider

This section includes a discussion of the four basic dental aspects that impact scheduling (type of procedure, order and sequence of procedures, variability of provider work habits, and patient preferences).

Patients form opinions about the dental office at all these levels, starting with their first contact with the office, whether it is on the phone, in person, or on the internet.

Attention to details in all these levels of sequencing is critical. The recurring question that must be constantly asked at all levels is: how can we do this better? We must always look to the patients for the answers because all that we do is under their continual scrutiny.

Creating an efficient and productive schedule is similar to accomplishing successful dental treatment. There are certain principles that need to be honored, and there are systems that need to be followed. Schedulers must first be taught how long it typically takes each provider to do the different procedures that will be scheduled. They must be educated as to the setup and disinfection time it takes for particular procedures. It helps if this person has a working knowledge of the different procedures, but if not, the level of understanding of the procedures from a time standpoint can be taught. Not to have this working knowledge of the dental procedures limits the scheduler's potential to achieve excellence in this area.

Type of Procedure

Procedures can be classified in many ways. Separate consideration of appointment time units can be given based on classes of dentistry. These class divisions could be made based on the following: examination and consultation, prophylaxis (with dentist review), diagnostic (referral to specialists), episodic treatment (hurting), simple restorative, cosmetic, evaluation of previous treatment effectiveness, treatment follow-up, and implementation of comprehensive long-term treatment plans. There are other ways to classify dentistry with regard to appointments, and remember, our concern is with our commodity—time.

Classes of dental appointments can be viewed strictly from the time requirements. There are long, intermediate, and short procedures. The long procedures would be those that require at least 1 hour of the doctor's time. Intermediate appointments would require 30 minutes of the doctor's time, while short appointments only require 10 minutes of the doctor's time. An example of a long procedure could be a root canal, crown and bridge (preparation and final impression), or an implant procedure. An intermediate procedure could be fillings, extractions, or impressions for dentures or partial dentures. Short appointments are healing checks, denture adjustments, or hygiene and treatment planning exams.

Dentistry can also be classified according to the dollar amount of production for the different procedures. Using the cost of a crown as the basis for production, we divide these classes into primary, secondary, or tertiary. Primary procedures are procedures that use the cost of a crown or above. Secondary procedures are those that are about half the cost of a crown. Tertiary appointments are procedures that have no out-of-pocket cost to the patient at that appointment. In other words, the exam may simply be a follow-up exam or check-up to assess healing from a previous treatment.

Examples of primary procedures are partial dentures, veneers, implants, root canals, or completing several fillings during one appointment. Examples of secondary procedures are fillings, some surgical procedures, extractions, and teeth bleaching. An example of a tertiary appointment is a healing check exam. It is very important that when appointments are scheduled, these appointments are translated into production dollars by the scheduler. If the scheduler is not very conscious about these differences, a very busy schedule will be created, but if slots are filled with mostly tertiary appointments, there is no dollar value to the day's production.

Dental consultant Cathy Jameson of Jameson and Associates refers to primary, secondary, and tertiary appointments as rocks, pebbles, and sand, using complementary definitions of each, as provided previously. She recommends preblocking the schedule for the placement of primary appointments in the schedule, with the daily goal to have at least half of the production scheduled in primary appointments and then building secondary and tertiary appointments around the primary appointments. This is an excellent system that makes primary appointments a priority for the scheduler and helps prevent being busy but not being productive. This sometimes requires negotiation skills on the part of the scheduler to gain patient acceptance in scheduling a primary appointment on a day and in a time slot that may be less desirable from the patient's viewpoint.

Sequence of Procedures

Before an efficient and productive schedule can be sequenced properly based on the treatment required, the person scheduling the appointments must have a working knowledge of dental treatment procedures. Sequencing is the understanding of the steps necessary for treatment completion and how these steps integrate with appointment scheduling. For example, scheduling appointments involved in developing a patient denture includes an understanding of when the treatment sequence requires an appointment and what steps must be completed by the laboratory before the next appointment can be scheduled relative to this treatment procedure. Consider the following sequences in the development of a patient's denture:

1. An appointment is required to take oral cavity impressions (models are created).
2. No appointment is needed to send models to the laboratory, but wax rims must be returned prior to the next appointment.
3. An appointment is required to establish vertical relationships and dimensions and to take measurements for teeth.
4. No appointment is needed to send these articulated models to the lab so that teeth can be set in wax.
5. An appointment is, however, required for try-ins.
6. No appointment is required to send the try-ins back to the lab for processing and finishing.
7. An appointment is required for delivery when laboratory finishing is complete.

Many dental offices do not have schedulers with dental backgrounds. Schedulers must be educated in this area. There are certain principles that need to be honored, and there are systems that need to be followed in order to accomplish successful scheduling. Let's deconstruct components of a crown procedure resulting from a previous *diagnostic* patient visit. For the current visit (treatment follow-up), the patient will be greeted by the assistant and prepped while seating. The dentist will apply a topical anesthesia and develop the operative model. The dentist spends time on tooth preparation to include taking the final impression. The assistant, depending on state rules, can complete the temporization of the prepared tooth. After the temporary is prepared the dentist returns and examines the temporary that has been fabricated for the tooth, makes any needed adjustments, and cements it. For this procedure, an hour has been allotted on the appointment book to accommodate the way Dr. X and

Assistant Y work together. This procedure may require 30–40 minutes of doctor-devoted time. However, Dr. Z and Assistant W may require less or more time depending on their speed and efficiency.

Notice on Table 14.3 (operatory availability) that the dentist is not involved in all of the time that was allotted for the patient on the appointment book. This means that if the doctor works two operatories (side by side), another patient can also be seen during this time period. If the second patient is also a primary procedure (like the crown procedure), then staggering the appointment time by starting the first patient on the hour and the second patient on the half hour would allow the dentist to walk away from the first patient to the second patient and complete them both in about an hour's time. However, without two assistants, this would not be possible.

Let's deconstruct components of an examination for a 6-year-old child. The first dental visit should be allotted a full 30 minutes. This allows time for the assistant to make both the child and the parent comfortable and then seat the child, describe prophylaxis techniques, expose a panoramic radiograph of the child's teeth, and determine how the child will respond to the examination. The panoramic radiography should be completed and available for the dentist to review prior to his or her entering the operatory. The dentist primarily spends time explaining the panoramic results and developing a plan of action, if necessary, for the child's next visit. Within this 30-minute appointment interval, this examination procedure may require only 5–10 minutes of doctor-devoted time. However, over time each provider establishes his or her ease in interacting with child patients. Some dentists may require more than 10 minutes to establish the relationship and conduct the examination. Others require less time.

Comprehensive treatment plans can be difficult to schedule and sequence. The patient should be informed during the consultation of the total number of appointments that will be required, as well as the total estimated length of time it will take to complete the whole treatment. If this is a treatment plan that involves perio, oral surgery, fillings, implants, and crown and bridge, the sequence of the appointments is critical to the timely completion of these appointments. This is where the philosophy of the doctor is critical. The traditional way to treat these types of cases is to start out by getting the foundation healthy. This approach requires that the gums and tissue be treated first. Whenever possible the teeth that need to be extracted need to come out very early in the treatment so that as these sites are healing while other treatment is being accomplished. After the foundation is healthy, the remaining teeth are restored and then the missing teeth are replaced. What you do not want to happen is that the treatment is interrupted over periods of time while you are waiting on something to heal. Sometimes this cannot be avoided, but every attempt should be made to keep the treatment moving forward toward its completion as soon as possible. Every attempt should be made to get as much treatment accomplished as possible at each appointment. One of the major challenges in dealing with comprehensive long-term treatment plans is keeping the patient informed and motivated to complete the treatment.

Variability of Provider's Work Habits

How examinations and consultations are coordinated can vary tremendously by provider. The variation is dependent on how inclusive the doctor wants the patient's information to be prior to initiating treatment, as a reflection of the philosophy of the doctor. Comprehensive exams usually refer to exams conducted for patients new to the practice. Comprehensive appointments consist of hard and soft tissue examinations with x-rays taken of all the teeth and surrounding structures. A complete medical history and evaluation, which can also include intra-oral and extra-oral photographs, is usually taken at this time. Diagnostic impressions can also be taken during this time, as indicated. Another philosophy would be to conduct limited examinations. These exams are usually conducted on established patients or on patients having specific problems to resolve at the time of the visit. These exams are limited to a particular part of the oral cavity and can be as specific as a particular tooth. Emergency examinations can be simple and straightforward, or they can be rather complex and time-consuming if the cause of the emergency is obscure. An example of this is a patient presenting with referred pain. The cause of the pain is perceived by the patient as coming from a particular tooth when in fact on thorough examination, it is discovered that the cause is from another part of the mouth, the jaw, or the sinus cavity.

Some doctors want fully orchestrated consultations for their patients, requiring separate appointments, while others want the patients to have simple time-conservative consultations done immediately after all the necessary information is obtained from the patient either at chair-side or in a separate consultation room. These orchestrated consultations may be scripted for the staff, as are scripts used by the doctor. All the bells and whistles are used at this time because part of this process is "selling the treatment plan and closing the deal." Some consultation rooms in the high-tech offices are the most elaborate rooms in the dental office, and they take on the appearance of a multimedia room. No matter what the philosophy is regarding consultations, after consultations are conducted, the patient or responsible party must agree to the financial arrangements before treatment begins.

The work habits of each provider are different. Some prefer a fast-paced, high-volume practice day, while others prefer to concentrate on a few patients. Some prefer a variety of treatment procedures, while others would be perfectly happy to have similar schedules day in and day out. Some providers are perfectionists, while others are production driven and try to save time whenever possible. Both hygienists and doctors vary in this area. Some providers are time conscious, while others do not even wear a watch. This provider's only concern is doing the very best for each patient no matter how long it takes. This may drive the entire staff crazy, and there has to be a conscious effort on the part of the staff to keep the provider aware that a schedule even exists, especially if the staff wants to go to lunch or get home at a reasonable time. This difference in work habits can be very problematic in group practices. The scheduler is required to take into consideration the work habits of each provider in the practice as the patients are scheduled.

Some providers are morning people and are at their best early in the morning, while others do not get fully focused until midmorning, after the third cup of coffee. Some providers are very personable people and must be given time to visit with their patients, while others would prefer to limit this type of interaction.

Dentistry is a profession with a plethora of new toys and gadgets. If the dentist is not careful, he or she may end up buying every new gadget that comes out, and supply sales people will love to call on that office. The disruption to the office caused by sales people calling on the provider may contribute to inefficiency and ineffective workflow in the practice workday. Any interruption that is not a part of the planned appointment workday can create a backlog in the day that is never resolved. The dental provider must protect the time commodity by insisting that sales people call at the completion of the day or by appointment only.

Patient Preferences by Provider

Every dental student has an ideal practice that he or she envisions while in dental school. After the student has been out of school for a few years, this ideal is integrated and blended with reality and shaped into a new or similar vision. One of the reasons that many people are attracted to dentistry is that the profession offers such a variety of practice models. There are cosmetic practices which are very popular with many dentists today. In order to have this type of practice, dentists must be able to attract enough of the right kind of patients who can afford what they have to offer.

Other providers may be more community-oriented and simply want to offer a variety of services to a diverse population. This is known as a "blue collar" model that is usually insurance dependent. This model treats a large volume of patients, but a much smaller dollar per patient is generated when you compare this model to the cosmetic model.

Whatever practice model the doctor chooses, relationships are built with the patients. The more loyal the patients are to the doctor, the more they do not want to be treated by anyone other than that particular doctor. This makes it difficult for the schedulers. The busier the practice gets, the less appointment availability there is. Patients want to continue to be seen by the doctor in the customary way as when the practice was not as busy. The more a doctor successfully delegates to the staff, the more the patients can have the same level of satisfaction at the appointment and not occupy as much of the doctor's time.

This works especially well if the staff have been with the office for long periods of time. The patients get to know them and form relationships with them. This allows a practice to "get large and remain small at the same time." The patients do not feel neglected because as the practice has grown, the staff has filled in some of the time that was spent with the doctor. This allows the office to provide the same type of "one-on-one" treatment as it grows. The patients still feel like kings and queens when coming to the office.

This preference for a particular provider creates some challenges when the office brings in a new associate. Many of the patients do not want to see the *new* doctor. Patients want to see "their" doctor. This requires a well-thought-out, scripted transfer of value from the *old* doctor to the *new* doctor by the staff, as well as by the old doctor. Both have to literally sell the new doctor to the old doctor's patients in order to make this work. It helps when both the old and new doctor share treatment responsibilities for these patients during this initial period. As hard as the doctor and staff try to make this happen, some patients will leave the practice and go somewhere else if they are not allowed to see "their" doctor. Those patients who simply refuse to see the new doctor are labeled as such and their wishes are respected, although some may have to wait longer for appointments. It is prudent for the staff to always offer the availability of the new doctor in an attempt to decrease appointment wait time.

Integrating Appointment Scheduling with Other Business Systems

Appointment scheduling is only one of the systems needed for a dental business to function like a well-oiled machine. There is a dependent relationship that exists among all the systems that make up the business. The dental business is a system of systems applied within a constantly changing context. Because of these constant changes, the systems used to run the business must be dynamic and adaptable to keep the office current.

The first task in systematizing the dental office is to identify all the generic business and clinical systems that must be either created or improved, and then create a systems development plan for the office that will serve as a road map for this process.

The system starts with the patient calling on the phone for an appointment or physically walking into the office and being greeted by the staff. Scripting of telephone conversations is used to get the new patient to schedule an appointment. Asking the right questions to determine what type of appointment to schedule is important. At this point, a working knowledge of the various dental procedures that are available in the clinical area is a must. The sequencing of processes to create a patient chart and corresponding documents that collect all pertinent information will save time, and will later be invaluable to both the clinical and the business staff. Determining how the perceived dental services will be paid for and by whom must be handled in a very sensitive way so as not to alienate the patient and make a bad first impression before the patient ever meets the doctor. The ability to give the patient as much information as requested, without attempting to diagnose the condition for which the patient may have originally sought an appointment, is also dependent on a working knowledge of treatment procedures among the staff. Most of the time, a checklist is a valuable tool for the business office staff to ensure that all the necessary processes are complete before the patient is allowed to enter the clinical area.

The appointment sequencing occurs once the patient is brought from the clinical area to the business area. There must be a checklist of processes to follow before the patient is allowed to leave the office. The procedures that were delineated during the clinical part of the visit should be repeated, along with the corresponding charges for the procedures. Again, a working knowledge of dental procedures is a must to communicate this to the patient. Insurance benefits for today's appointment should be explained again, if necessary. Any payment due for today's procedures should be collected at this time. All these procedures need to be scripted and evaluated for their effectiveness. Finally, the patient should be reappointed for his or her next appointment and dismissed.

Well-Balanced Patient Load

A well-balanced patient load consists of a good mix of first-time appointments, children, cash and emergencies, and filler appointments. These are all categories of patients that are welcomed into the dental office and should be tracked for evaluation purposes. Well-balanced patient loads do not just happen. Systems must be set up with these groups of patients in mind. User-friendly, patient-centered systems will facilitate the attraction and maintenance of the desired mix of patients.

How does one determine a well-balanced patient load in terms of scheduling? The practice should determine by policy the maximum number of new patients that can be seen on a particular day given the number of total patients scheduled. If children pose a problem for the practice, then children should be limited to certain times of the day and/or limited to a certain percentage of the total patient load on a given day.

Emergency patients should not make up more than 10% of the number of patients scheduled for appointments in a practice. Some solo practitioners may want to keep that number even lower. For example, if 5% of the thirty patients encountered in 1 day in a solo practice were emergency patients, this would mean that one or two patients the doctor plans to treat would require at least an hour of his or her time, whereas the average time planned per patient might be 30 minutes. Even if only one emergency patient was encountered, total time added to the workday schedule could be 30 minutes, but if two emergency patients were encountered, total time added to the workday schedule would be closer to an hour.

First-Time/New Patient Appointments

One very important piece of information that should be noted in patient charts is the way that contact was made with the dental office for the first time. This will give the office valuable information on trends in the market about which modes of communication are growing or decreasing. Patients should also be asked how they wish to be contacted by the office in the future. An office cannot have too much information in a patient's chart about how to get in contact with them.

First-time patients and patients of record who have not had an appointment for a period of time are primary sources for scheduling patient appointments. When these patients call in for appointments, the first thing that the scheduler must do is to categorize the appointment as an emergency or nonemergency. If it is a nonemergency appointment, then it needs to be classified as a problem-specific appointment or a general evaluation appointment. If it is a problem-specific appointment, as much information as possible should be gathered about the problem and passed on to the clinical staff. This information will help the clinical assistants and the doctor as they prepare for the appointment.

The scheduler should not attempt to diagnose the patient's problem before the doctor examines him or her. As an example, a patient calls and states that he or she needs a tooth pulled. The scheduler should pass this "chief complaint" information on to the clinical staff, but should not schedule the patient for an extraction based on the request of the patient. It may turn out that the tooth, after examination, can be saved with a simple filling, or it might require a root canal and crown.

If this first-time patient wants a general evaluation, then he or she is appointed for what many offices call the "new patient experience." New patients are the future of the dental practice. Because you only have one chance to make a good first impression, the manner in which new patients are serviced is of utmost importance to the dental practice. When the new patient arrives in the office, the receptionist should greet them by acknowledging the fact that this is the patient's first time in the office, and that the entire dental team has been looking forward to meeting him or her. The patient can be given a limited tour of the office on the way to the treatment room and be introduced to as many members of the dental team as possible. The entire team needs to make sure that this is not viewed as just being a routine procedure. The new patient is treated like a guest who enters your home for the first time and who you had been looking forward to meeting. Business systems are put in place to properly service new patients and convert them into loyal returning patients and sources of other new patients.

One barrier to an excellent new patient experience can be the wait time. What happens if the new patient calls in for an appointment just to have an oral prophylaxis? The office will have to establish a policy on how to integrate the "new patient experience" with the prophylaxis appointment. Decisions will have to be made as to who sees the patient first, the doctor or the hygienist. This is where the systems used by the hygienist and the doctor will have to be integrated.

Children

Children bring diversity to the office. They also provide rewarding and healthy challenges to the dental office. Their presence paints a different color on the flow of the day in a most positive way. It is rewarding to have the privilege to work with children and to watch them grow and develop. Dentistry can place the dentist in a very influential position in the life of a child, to serve as a mentor or role model.

There can, however, be a downside to treating children and adults together. Sometimes children are difficult to manage, and this can really challenge the doctor or hygienist to stay on schedule. For example, if a practice decides that the maximum number of children to be treated in a normal day is six, and two of those six children take an extra 30 minutes to treat due to management problems, an extra hour of the doctor's time is required to treat those children. This means that other patients will have to wait, and the staff may either have to work through part of their lunch time, or work late. An ill-behaved, uncooperative child can stress the entire staff as well as other patients in the office.

To minimize disruptions that can be encountered when treating children, blocks of time during certain parts of the day can be used. Screening techniques for predicting behavioral problems during the initial visit can be used to decide how to properly schedule the child for clinical visits. This approach can also be used to decide if it is best to refer this child to a pedodontist. One of the worst things that can happen in the office is to have one of these challenging children ill-behaving while new patients are in the office. Even with these downsides to treating children, the benefits outweigh the liabilities.

Cash and Emergencies

Cash and emergency patients can have a devastating effect on the daily schedule, especially if provisions for them are not made. However, they also provide an excellent opportunity to provide care for patients who are in pain. Care must be taken when deciding how much treatment to provide these patients. The objective of treating emergency patients is to get them comfortable, and then reappoint them when the schedule permits if there is not enough time in the current day's schedule to adequately treat them. This is easier said than done, because doctors are trained to help people, especially when they are hurting.

This is where the schedule of many offices gets in trouble—while they are treating cash and emergency patients. Here is an example of what can happen. A cash and emergency patient comes in with a toothache. The doctor diagnoses the problem and recommends that the tooth be extracted. Then the business manager makes financial arrangements with the patient, and the doctor proceeds to extract the tooth. At first it appears to be a simple extraction, but the tooth breaks off and the doctor ends up having to do a surgical extraction. It takes an hour to complete the extraction. By the time everything is finished and the room is disinfected, the operatory has been tied up for 2 hours. To make matters worse, when the patient is informed that the doctor had to do a surgical extraction, the patient informs the business manager that he or she is not able to pay for the treatment just rendered. In the meantime, two of the scheduled patients reappoint and the doctor and the clinical assistant end up not having lunch. A better way to handle this would be to make the emergency patient comfortable, have the patient pay cash for the visit, and reschedule for the next available appointment to receive additional treatment.

Filler Appointments

Filler appointments are patients who have indicated that they can possibly come into the office for treatment on very short notice. This kind of appointment is available to some people who have flexible work schedules or live short distances from the dental office. These appointments are worth their weight in gold if the patient can actually come in on short notice. When a patient is 5 minutes late for an appointment there should be someone on the phone calling that patient to see if they are going to keep the scheduled appointment. This means that someone in the office must be time conscious and aware of patient arrivals and delays. In some offices this may be the doctor's clinical assistant or some other designated person at the front desk.

Filler appointments are schedule savers when offices have no-shows, last-minute cancellations, and rescheduled appointments. Every patient who is scheduled for a restorative or hygiene appointment should be asked if they could be called on short notice to fill open slots in the schedule. If patients can be available for filler appointments, they should be placed on a call list with their contact information and planned treatment procedures. Care should also be taken to ensure that the patients on the filler or short call list do not have outstanding account balances. The object is to replace lost production with good production, and not to increase the accounts receivable.

Over-the-Counter Follow-Up Appointments

When a patient is dismissed from the clinical area and is at the checkout counter, there should be a list of the treatment planned for the next few visits. The goal of all the activities that occur with patients standing at the counter is to get them rescheduled for their next appointment. This is an opportune time, when the patient is physically present in the facility at the same time the doctor and the hygienist are in, just in case their input is needed for scheduling the next appointment.

Getting It on the Books

It is an excellent idea to begin the rescheduling process with an explanation to the patient as to what procedures were accomplished during the current visit and what treatment remains to be completed. The scheduler will then discuss with the patient what treatment the doctor has recommended to be scheduled next and how long the procedure will take. At this time, the cost of the planned procedure should be discussed with the patient. If the patient has dental insurance and the planned procedure is covered, the patient's co-pay can be discussed. The patient should know what will be done at the next appointment, how long it will take, and the amount that will need to be paid. If a treatment plan has been presented and financial arrangements have already been made with the patient before the treatment was started, this discussion serves only as a reminder to the patient and should be a very quick process.

Scheduling this appointment can interface with several aspects of the appointment system. For example, the next appointment listed in the patient's treatment plan calls for a crown preparation and final impression. The patient wants to schedule the appointment for the following Tuesday. On observation the scheduler notes that the doctor has four major procedures already scheduled for that day. It is the policy of the office to not schedule more than four major procedures in a typical appointment day in order to maintain a well-balanced patient load. The scheduler now has to negotiate with the patient for an alternative day where another major procedure can be accommodated and one that fits the patient's schedule. It is always a good idea to present the patient with at least two alternative dates, giving him or her a sense of some control over the appointment. The scheduler may have to sell this appointment day and time to the patient. The doctor and the hygienist could also help assist the scheduler in negotiating the appointment time that bests fits into the office scheduling system.

Understanding Patient Behaviors

While all these activities are going on it is the task of the check-out person to observe the patient's behavior. This can be done by watching and listening. Systems should already be in place to gather information about the scheduling preferences of a patient. Does the patient prefer morning or afternoon appointments? Does the patient prefer to pay by cash or credit card? Does this patient get agitated when he or she has to wait at the counter for a short period of time? Does the patient prefer a certain provider? This is especially important in a group practice where there are multiple providers. Matching the appointment with the provider time needs to be negotiated with the patient. A patient's preferences must be factored in as part of the process.

The scheduler must motivate the patient to reschedule for further treatment. This is especially true when a lengthy treatment plan is being followed. This is the juncture where scripted conversations are useful. The scheduler as part of the initial training process must practice scripts, and periodic retraining must be completed. The scheduler must serve as both a motivator and a concierge to help get the patients to do what is needed in order to complete the recommended treatment. The next appointment is scheduled with an explanation of what will be done and how much it will cost. The patient is then given a reminder card with the date and time of the next appointment, is thanked, and is then dismissed from the office.

Telephone, E-mail, and Internet Appointment Scheduling

The telephone is still the main artery supplying life to the dental practice. E-mail and internet scheduling are rapidly expanding and should be used to supplement and leverage the effectiveness of the telephone. Many people use cell phones as their primary—and in many cases their only—phone service. This is a part of the information that should be noted in every patient's chart. E-mail addresses are very helpful in contacting patients because many people check their e-mails during normal business hours.

One of the advantages of having a well-developed website is the information you can allow the patient to access. Directions to the office can be obtained from the website. Many websites are able to take the viewer on a virtual tour of the office as well as introduce the staff. Potential patients and current patients can ask questions through the website.

Confirmations

Confirmations are an ongoing challenge to the dental staff. First the office must establish a policy about just what is considered a confirmation. Is it just leaving a message on an answering machine? Is the confirmation done at the time that the appointment is made? Does the staff actually speak with the patient, or is talking to the patient's spouse enough? Do the same rules apply to hygiene recall appointments that apply to appointments to see the doctor? These are just some of the considerations that have to be sorted through when patients are confirmed.

E-mail and the internet can serve as tools to leverage the communication capabilities between the office and the patient/households. One of the most dynamic usages of the internet is remote access to the computer by the doctor or staff. One of the most effective ways to confirm a patient's appointment is to call the patient after regular business hours during the evening. This can be accomplished by simply subscribing to a remote access company. GoToMyPC is one of the larger companies, but there are several. These companies will establish a link to your computer that will allow total access to a designated computer that is left on at all times. Doctors can thus review patients' charts and x-rays (if they have digital x-rays) while away from the office.

Recalls

In an office without a hygienist on staff, the doctor must perform recall appointments. If recall blocks are not limited, the scheduler can fill up the doctor's time with recall appointments and leave no room for restorative appointments. This type of scheduling will not allow the practice to meet its daily production goals. To complicate things even more, the insurance eligibility dates for recall on prophylaxis must be factored into these negotiations.

In well-established practices that have hygienists, time for the doctor to examine the hygiene patients must be factored into the schedule. Offices will have to establish systems and procedures for the doctor to examine the patient in an efficient and timely manner. Time can be lost in hygiene production when the hygienist is waiting on an exam by the doctor before he or she can dismiss the patient and turn the room around before seating the next patient. The placement of the proximity of the doctor's treatment rooms with the hygiene rooms should be taken into consideration in designating operatories for hygiene treatment. The closer the doctor's chairs are to the hygienist's chairs, the more the time will be saved in both the doctor's and the hygienist's schedule.

Patient Account Balances

The office financial policy spells out in detail how the office will collect money from the patients for the services rendered. It is strongly recommended that dental offices do not finance dental treatment. There are companies that specialize in financing dental procedures. There must be a written financial policy in the office. Financial policies need to be objective and clear. Any decisions to make exceptions to the financial policy must be cleared with the doctor. This is not a decision that should be made by the staff if it deviates from the policy. There should be a written sequence of activities (systems) to collect these unpaid balances incorporated in a progressive time that tells the staff exactly what to do about an account balance as it ages. Patients with outstanding balances cannot continue to be rescheduled for more treatment until the balances are cleared up.

Laboratory and Preparatory Results

Most dental offices may use more than one dental lab. Each lab has a different time line to finish a case and return it to the office for delivery to the patient. The clinical staff must work closely with the scheduler to coordinate the patient's return appointment to have a crown or a partial denture delivered. The patient should not be scheduled for an appointment to have a crown delivered before the lab finishes the crown. This is a waste of production time, not to mention the impression that it leaves with the patient when treatment cannot be completed on the day agreed upon.

Some dental offices have the technology to make crowns and deliver them on the same day that the teeth are prepared for the crowns and the impression is taken. Patients should not be asked to wait more than 2 weeks for crowns. As a general rule, no dental treatment that involves lab work should take more than 2 weeks to deliver. This includes dentures and partial dentures.

Who Is Responsible for Scheduling?

In most offices scheduling is centralized in the business area. The key to effective scheduling is to have a scheduling system. Those who are not familiar with the system should *not* be allowed to schedule because they will create more problems than they will solve by scheduling improperly. There should be one person in the office ultimately responsible for all scheduling. Even though that person does not actually make every appointment, he or she has the responsibility of coordinating the schedule and making sure that the system is being followed. This person is constantly monitoring the schedule, making sure that production goals are being met and coordinating with the clinical staff on the status of all laboratory cases ready for delivery on an appointed date. Any decentralized scheduling must be limited and strictly coordinated or it will cause problems.

Computerized and Paper Appointment Schedules

Dental offices are moving away from paper appointment schedules and incorporating computerized appointment schedules. In addition to simple web-based appointment scheduling systems, there are many dental software developers that have included appointment schedule modules in their practice management software packages. Converting from a paper appointment system to a computerized one is simply a matter of selecting start and stop dates and beginning the demographic data conversion process. Once the computerized software has been installed and personnel trained, staff can begin to appoint into the computerized software. As time permits, appointments from the paper appointment book are simply moved to the computerized system until all appointments have been converted. Simultaneously, new appointments are not put in the paper system and are entered directly into the computerized scheduling software application.

Computer Interactive Scheduling/Web-Based

Web-based appointment systems are new innovative ways of empowering the patients to make their own appointments. While the use of web-based systems has not become commonplace in the dental practice business, the technology creating the possibilities for a web-based appointment scheduling system are well defined. Like web-based accounting systems, all of the appointment scheduling data is maintained at the host server site unless the dental practice has the expertise to be responsible for maintaining the web-based system (data) for both software and hardware. Some of the risks associated with privacy issues for medical and dental providers have not been resolved to the satisfaction of many providers. This may be one of the main reasons web-based scheduling has not been adopted more quickly.

Most of these systems are organized in much the same way as paper appointment systems from the user's perspective. Most are designed to take the user through a series of questions that, when answered, lead to an appointment being placed on the system. Patients using the system are generally established patients of the practice as opposed to new patients, since medico-legal releases and consents, as well as web-site access permission, must be obtained prior to utilizing the web-based system. Demographic documents used by the dental practice office staff can also be placed on the web-based system so that patients can complete much of this information prior to coming into the dental office for the appointment.

In addition to a web-based appointment scheduling systems, many dental offices elect to use practice management appointment scheduling software. The advantage of using practice management software is the ease of integration with other business system applications, which are usually developed by the same company. Each company has its own set of modules comprising the practice management software. In contrast to practice management systems, web-based appointment scheduling systems are generally stand-alone but can be connected to other office software so that the data collected through web access can be downloaded and used with other office applications.

Components of the scheduling application generally include a comprehensive system of interactive modules that share patient, household, treatment, and financial information. The computerized schedule can enable staff to list all patients due into the office that day by operatory room along with the name of the chosen providers and notes or medical alerts pertinent to the appointment. Information about the treatment procedure such as tooth number and surfaces may also be included. Unlike what is available using a paper appointment schedule, a large amount of data can be collected, manipulated, and stored for various uses in the dental practice. The collection of this amount of data for a particular appointment enables staff to quickly review and understand patient needs for the day's appointments.

A computerized appointment system is also critical for the dental recall system. Using the computer, office staffs are able to classify patients by the number or type of recall notice and print personal or generic messages on each or all of the notices. Address or responsible party labels can be printed at the touch of a few buttons, as opposed to paper systems that must be manipulated and re-manipulated to get the necessary information for sending correspondence to patients or households. The complexities and intricate workings of the recall system are not as burdensome when computerized since basic inquiry parameters are set and can be reset as needed and the computer quickly executes those parameters. Staff can run missed appointment reports and conduct patient tracking as necessary. Tickler files can be used and confirmation and/or end-of-day callback lists can be printed quickly and easily. The use of the computerized short call list can substantively increase achievement of practice production goals, maximize practice revenue, and contribute to increased patient satisfaction by getting patients in to see the doctor sooner. Effective use of this list and the quick and easy generation of it through the computer may justify the expense involved in purchasing and using practice management appointment scheduling software.

Completing an Appointment Unit

Appointment scheduling is involved at patient check-out, over the telephone, and at walk-in. Completing an appointment unit varies by whether a patient is new, established, or an established or new patient emergency. For brevity, we use the perspective of an established patient physically present at check-out as the prototype for explaining the process involved in completing an appointment unit in an appointment scheduling application software. This prototype is likely to represent the most inclusive procedure and the most frequently encountered patient type.

At checkout, the patient has completed a treatment procedure by the doctor or hygienist in the back office and likely has a router or other document with instructions for follow-up. The scheduler or front office staff review the physical router/document (some offices may utilize a computer screen router that never becomes paper). The patient's account history and medical alerts are also reviewed. Front office staff must balance the patient's financial responsibilities to the practice with the need to get the treatment completed while at the same time negotiating a future appointment.

Front office staff explains the time interval suggested by the doctor for the return appointment. The patient is asked whether a certain day of the week is better and whether a certain time of the day is better than another. After obtaining the patient's response, the front office staff reviews available appointment days and times with the appropriate doctor in the scheduling system to determine a match with any of the days and times preferred by the patient. The appointment system can quickly display the schedule for the requested time interval and the days and times available for that particular doctor. If there is no match, the patient is provided a day and/or time that is closest to the preferred time.

The appointment is physically entered into the system, blocking off the estimated amount of time needed to deliver the planned treatment, assigning the operatory and doctor, and ensuring that a current phone number is available for the patient so that the confirmation call can be made. The patient may be asked if it is acceptable to receive a confirmation call at the number provided. Other financial information is given and received from the patient at this time. Minimum information needed for most offices to complete an appointment time unit within a computerized system could be patient name, contact phone number, ID or account number or date of birth, date and time of the appointment, estimated treatment time block, planned treatment procedure with information about tooth/surfaces and so forth, operatory or doctor, premedication instruction/alerts, and how the treatment cost will be paid.

One of the most vexing decisions for front office staff in the checkout process is the patient's need to complete treatment in consideration of the fact that the patient may have an outstanding balance from previous treatments and may not have made appropriate financial arrangements for full payment. Placing the appointment on the schedule becomes a difficult process when the practice has difficult patients with regard to bill payment history. When this is the case, office policy must be referenced by the staff to ensure that patients are treated alike with regard to this process. Many times, the front office staff must get special permission from the manager or doctor to forego making a future appointment until financial arrangements for full payment of previous charges are made. In this case, notes are made in the computer system as to the disposition of the patient with regard to the future appointment. It is important to add a tickler so that when the payments have been made, the computer can alert the scheduler to call the patient so that the treatment appointment can be made.

Chair-Side Scheduling

Chair-side scheduling is another innovative dental practice showing promise for increased production goals. It requires that the dental office be equipped with computers in the patient operatories and consultation rooms. Through these connections, integration of other technologies such as digital radiography, intra-oral cameras, digital photography, and patient education videos or tutorials can be established. It also requires that back office staff (doctors, hygienists, and assistants) be trained to use the scheduling application software. The extent of the training for doctors and other back office staff, however, can and should be limited to very rudimentary aspects of inquiring, viewing, and entering an appointment.

Computerized appointment scheduling allows for back office interaction with the activities of the scheduler and checkout staff. Back office staff can view any and all appointments previously scheduled for the patient to include no-show and cancellation activities. Staff can also quickly view any future appointments already scheduled with family members or the patients themselves to increase coordination of household activities. With appropriate training back office staff is able to enter follow-up appointments.

Many times, not enough information has been supplied from the back office staff on the encounter form or router for the scheduler or front office checkout personnel to determine the time interval for the next appointment based on the procedures completed today. Back office staff generally has more knowledge about the length of time that may be required for a particular patient to heal and/or information about how the patient will respond to treatment. Back office staff is in the best position to set a follow-up appointment time interval for evaluation of treatment progress while the patient is available and able to contribute to the follow-up appointment time interval negotiation process. When the patient observes the doctor setting the next appointment, emphasis is placed on the importance of the follow-up examination to treatment progress from the patient's perspective. One disadvantage of chair-side scheduling is that most offices do not and should not get back office staff involved in patient financial matters that may be connected to future appointments. Most of this can be accommodated through policy and computerized security levels.

Accessing and Monitoring Schedules

Appointment schedules are monitored throughout the day by most all of the dental office staff, which includes the doctor, the assistant, and the hygienist as well as the scheduler and front office staff. The schedule is the backbone of the dental practice and on forms the foundation for operation of the business. Since the front office staff create the schedule (even in a paper scheduling office), the back office can usually only receive the information secondarily. Accessing and monitoring appointment schedules by the back office staff is dependent on timing and on front office staff completing the necessary paper documents to make the schedule available either physically or through the computer. In many cases, a day's schedule is dynamic; that is, write-ins for added appointments and deletions for no-shows and cancellations could make the paper schedule convoluted and hard to read. In addition, back office staff must constantly coordinate with front office staff to ensure that up-to-date information has been placed on the paper schedule. Computerized appointment scheduling with back office staff access to the operatory scheduling module of the software enhances this process. There is increased capability to utilize a dynamic schedule without much of the inefficiency of constant coordination between front and back office staff with regard to the living document—the operatory schedule.

Back office staff can use the computer screen to constantly view the operatory schedule and any changes made to it by the front office staff or the scheduler. Added appointments could be color coded for the back office staff as an alert; cancelled appointments could be similarly coded. Some applications also allow for alerts for patient arrivals and treatment completion so that most coordination between the front and back office staff can be simply viewed on the computer screen, as opposed to the walking and verbal coordination necessary with paper systems.

For dental offices that want to monitor patient arrival-to-treatment wait times and other intraoffice time management components, appointment scheduling software applications are the ideal solution. Software applications enable the practice to monitor other evaluation measures as well. These may include no-show rates, cancellation rates, number and dollar amount of treatment plans initiated or completed, operatory and provider production forecast by treatment codes, number of recall notices sent, and so forth.

Appointment Scheduling Maintenance

All recall systems begin with the doctor. The doctor's philosophy for having a recall system is the driving force that determines what resources of the practice are allocated and how those resources will be managed. Some doctors set up recall systems and hire hygienists as profit centers in the practices. Some doctors set them up so that they will be able to dedicate more of their time to other procedures that bring more income into the practice. Some doctors view them strictly as referral sources for restorative treatment. Some doctors view them as the only way to offer patients comprehensive care, while others see them as the means to never having to clean teeth again in this lifetime.

Recall System

The traditional approach to scheduling patients for recall (prophylaxis) appointments will be discussed in this section along with two nontraditional options. The traditional recall system and the two nontraditional options are all based on a 6-month recall plan. The traditional plan begins with scheduling a patient for his or her next appointment as the patient checks out of the office after having a prophylaxis. The appointment is set up for a specific date at a specific time 6 months from the current date. The paper process to this recall plan is described. At this appointment a recall card is made with the patient's name and address on the front of the card. The card is filed 6 months from the date of the current appointment. For example, if a patient has a prophylaxis in January, the card is put in the July section of this recall system file. Six months later all the cards in that current month are pulled from the file and the cards are mailed to the patient as a reminder of the appointment.

Since these cards are already addressed it makes mailing a matter of simply placing a postage stamp on each card and dropping them in the mail. Some offices have the patients address their recall cards to themselves as an attention-getting device. When they unexpectedly receive mail addressed to them in their own handwriting, they are pleasantly reminded. These cards are typically followed up with a phone call to confirm the appointment with the patient. This 6-month recall system can also be accomplished by using a computer. In some of the more technically advanced offices these notices are sent in either text messages or e-mails to the patients.

Another approach toward scheduling is the "next 2 weeks" system. There are no cards sent out. There are no self-addressed cards employed. All patients who are eligible for recall (prophylaxis) appointments are tracked and utilized to fill up not only today's schedule, but also for the next 2 weeks. Today's schedule always takes precedence over all recall efforts, but when all is exhausted on making a schedule happen today, then the focus is moved to the next 2 weeks. This approach allows the staff to focus on the near future as well as setting and maintaining short- and long-range production goals. The hygiene scheduler is the primary focus of the "next 2 weeks" method. And these next 2 weeks are filled by any means necessary. The danger of this system is allowing patients to fall through the cracks. It must be closely monitored and maintained to prevent this from happening.

A third approach, which can be utilized, is a combination of the traditional recall approach and the "next 2 weeks" approach. This is a hybrid of the two. Recall cards are addressed and reminders are made in the traditional manner. Appointments are confirmed in the traditional manner. Confirmations are made in the traditional manner. However, the traditional system is merely a starting point for this hybrid "next 2 weeks" approach to scheduling. Even though patients are scheduled for the next 6 months in advance, the dental office sets very specific criteria for confirmation of those patients. Once patients scheduled 6 months ago are confirmed, their appointments remain on the schedule. Those patients who are scheduled appointments 6 months ago but did not confirm are removed from the schedule, and those times are filled with other patients requesting hygiene appointments. This method not only cleans up the appointments that could not be confirmed, but it also creates capacity in the upcoming daily schedule for the next 2 weeks. This capacity can be used for appointing new patients and for old patients who are reactivated. This alternative can be very difficult to implement if the traditional approach to recall has historically been utilized in a practice, and patients have been allowed to just show up for an appointment without confirming. If a dental office decides to transition from a traditional system to this recall system, it must be prepared when two patients arrive at the dental office at the same time—each with a scheduled appointment. This transition can be accomplished in 6–8 months.

Each office must track the effectiveness of the recall system being used to determine if it is giving them the results expected. No matter which system is employed, any system is better than none. The systems, if properly developed and maintained, will allow the office to leverage ordinary people and reap extraordinary benefits. The more successful an office is in keeping patients, the more successful the business. The rate of return of recall patients is a good measure of sustainable growth and the maturity of a practice. It is also a good way to measure customer satisfaction among the patients.

A recall patient list can also serve as a mailing list for newsletters, as well as Christmas cards or any other mailings that the office decides to make a part of its overall marketing plan. Some offices offer special incentives to patients who have a prophylaxis every 6 months. An example of such an incentive would be to guarantee a crown or a partial for 5 years if a patient never misses a 6-month recall appointment during that period.

No-Shows, Last-Minute Cancellations, and Reschedules

No-shows, last-minute cancellations, and reschedules are schedule breakers and a scheduler's nightmare. No-shows and last-minute reschedules must be tracked, and a policy should be established as to what happens on the first, second, or third time. Some offices automatically send a letter to the patients who no-show telling them that no-shows are grounds for dismissal from the practice. The patient is reminded of how committed the office is to providing excellent dental care for them. The letter also states that continued competent care cannot be provided if appointments are not kept. This is a very positive approach that initially has no consequences to the patient, but if no-show rates are high, then office policy should outline a strong plan of action for staff.

Some offices try to control the patient's behavior using negative enforcement. Patients are charged and sent a bill for not showing up for the appointment. The rationale is that the office had reserved that specific time for them and as a result could not schedule anyone else in that time. Because the patient did not show up, the office lost production time and the patient was sent a bill. Another approach is to have the patient put a down payment on the next appointment before he or she is rescheduled. Some offices simply do not reschedule the patient in the near future. Patients are made to wait for a period of time before rescheduling.

Treat the first scheduled patients of the day with special care, and educate them so that they understand the importance of showing up for their appointments. When possible, appoint these time slots with patients who routinely keep their appointments. These can be time slots that the scheduler intentionally offers to patients who keep their appointments routinely. The fact that the patients will not have to wait at all if they are the first patients of the day is a good selling feature. Never schedule patients who have a history of missed appointments for any reason in the first time slots of the morning or afternoon sessions. Time lost is potential production lost, and once it is lost it cannot be recovered.

Replacing Rocks with Pebbles

A well-orchestrated schedule is a thing of beauty. There is an easy workflow and spacing between patients. Even though the schedule does not look busy, the production numbers are excellent. The daily schedule results in production goals reached or even exceeded. The downside of having only a few patients scheduled is that it only takes one of the major production appointments to reschedule, or not to show for the appointment, to turn the day into a disaster, which leaves everyone in the office hustling, just trying to salvage the day. Any production is better than none is the attitude that prevails at this point.

Offices that try to schedule a percentage of their production in primary appointments (rocks) must decide when they will let these appointments go if they are not filled within a certain time interval. If this plan is used, these time slots must be closely monitored by the scheduler. This gets even harder to monitor if more than one person schedules appointments. The scheduler needs to have a very clear understanding about the profitability of the different procedures in the dental office. Several small but very profitable procedures (pebbles) in a time block may produce more net income in the office than one major procedure that carries with it a small profit margin.

Late Providers and Late Patients

Most patients usually are very understanding when the doctor is running a little late. There is that unspoken understanding that if the doctor was with me and it takes longer to complete my treatment, I expect the doctor to stay as long as it takes to finish the job and do it right. The motto for the appointment is "it's over when it's over." However, if this is the norm rather than the exception, patients will grow tired of this and go somewhere else for their dental treatment.

Offices need to create a culture that time is valuable. The patients should be kept informed if the doctor is running behind. This sends a message to the patient that the office is concerned about honoring the appointment time. We have discussed adding filler appointments to salvage production. There is also a need to condense an appointment time slot in order to get back on schedule. If the doctor gets behind in the morning or evening, the work flows into the lunch hour or late work hours. This produces stress and tension in the staff. Some patients may prefer to reschedule if the wait time is excessive.

In a group practice, the doctors can help keep each other on schedule by helping out with each other's patient load until the partner gets back on track. The same is true for multiple hygiene practices. The added number of producers adds flexibility. It also allows for expanding an appointment if the partner is not busy and can see some of the doctor's patients while the patient's appointment is being expanded to do more treatment. Even if the patient prefers to wait on the doctor with whom they are scheduled, the ability to offer such a choice is a valuable resource.

On the other hand, how does an office handle late patients? This is extremely critical in hygiene. The appointments are set on the half hour or hour. Time has been allocated to accomplish a precise number of procedures during that time. If a patient is late, the hygienist has to decide whether or not to treat him or her. If the patient is treated and given all of the scheduled procedures, there is a guarantee that the next patient will also finish late even if he or she shows up on time.

It is a very difficult thing to refuse to do any treatment on patients who come in late because of all the effort that it takes just to physically keep an appointment. The issue then becomes, how late are they? If the patient is 45 minutes late for a 1-hour appointment, the hygienist does not have much time to get anything done. However, if the patient is only 10 minutes late, most of the scheduled treatment probably can be accomplished.

If an office refuses to treat a late patient, what happens the next time the doctor or hygienist is late? What options are the patients given? A practice that refuses to treat late patients creates negative goodwill with its patients. Staff and doctors are also late from time to time, and the schedule seldom proceeds without some adjustments. The scheduler must be an excellent negotiator. If the doctor is late coming back from lunch or arriving in the morning, the scheduler must quickly inform the patient and inquire of the patient how the appointment should proceed. The scheduler is working to accomplish two outcomes simultaneously. The first outcome is to produce the major treatment production goals for the day. The second outcome is to be able to treat the patient who was late or who was made late by the doctor without a major disruption to other patients on the schedule.

The principles involved in appointment scheduling for late patients and late providers vary based on whether the schedule becomes 10, 20, or 30 minutes late. If the schedule is delayed 10 minutes, major time units may not be affected. However, if the schedule becomes 30 minutes late, then major treatments planned will affect the production goals for the day. The principle is to deliver the major treatment planned to preserve the achievement of the day's production goals. The scheduler must observe time units and treatment types planned for the remainder of the day's schedule, make some preliminary decisions about preferred outcomes, and then talk to one or more patients about the doctor's lateness or need to reschedule. If the scheduler is able to accomplish the scheduled day within a reasonable time frame by continuing the planned treatment for all patients, including the late patient, then that is the preferable outcome for which the scheduler negotiates.

The practice should recognize, however, that patients must be given options as to how their time is to be used. If the lateness delays the majority of patients on the day's schedule, each of them must be notified immediately and given the option to reschedule or continue with the planned time units. Sometimes patients are willing to deal with a longer wait to get the planned treatment completed, preventing the need to return on another day. Also, there are some treatment procedures that the doctor may provide as easily during the next appointment, saving valuable time in the day's schedule. These time unit savers are sometimes invaluable to a scheduler's ability to negotiate.

Keys to Productive Scheduling

The key to productive scheduling is to create and maintain a production-based schedule, and to change only when it no longer accomplishes the desired results. Always keep the patients at the center of this endeavor, but remember to create a win-win enterprise for both the patient and the dentist and his/her staff. Design a scheduling policy that gives the patients what they want and the dentist what he/she expects from the practice. Income must be generated for the success of this activity, but keep in mind that success can be measured in various ways. To some it may be profitability, while to others it may be in working a schedule that fits their lifestyle. To others, it may be providing very cost-effective dental treatment in access-to-care challenged areas. In Stephen Covey's book, *Seven Habits of Highly Successful People*, one of the seven habits is to "begin with the end in mind." First, envision what the successful business will look like when it is fully developed, and then implement scheduling policies that help you create the business and achieve success however you define it. These same principles can be followed to create all the other systems required in a successful dental practice.

When establishing production goals for providers, fixed and variable expenses must be considered. Examples of fixed expenses are rent and utilities, while examples of variable expenses are providers' salaries, laboratory expenses, and supply costs. According to Paul Woody, CPA and dental practice consultant, on average one-third of the collected income is paid to the producer, one-third is used to pay expenses, and one-third is retained by the business. The traditional providers in the dental business are the dentist and the hygienist. With the implementation of new mid-level providers, this model is changing. Salaries should be multiplied by 3× to establish the production goals for each provider. This information is very useful in scheduling, because "if it's not scheduled, you can't produce it!" Daily production templates for each provider should be established. The goal of a daily provider template is to schedule 1/2 of the daily production goal with major procedures.

Flexibility is a very important asset in the art of scheduling. Contrary to popular opinion, dental patients do not come in a single line, orderly formation at the times that are convenient for the practice. Instead, they come in waves, and sometimes they all seem to show up at the same time, needing similar procedures. According to E-Myth, people make decisions from an emotional side, and then their rational side attempts to justify the dental treatment that they have agreed to have done. As much as 70% of diagnosed treatment that leaves the office is never treated according to Shelly Short, a practice management consultant. All patients who are diagnosed with dental needs should be asked; "Would you like that done today?" Accomplishing this calls for an adjustment in the dentist's schedule, or else you run the risk of patients changing their minds or going elsewhere for their treatment. Part of the challenge in meeting the patients' needs is being flexible enough to treat patients when they want to be treated, especially if it involves significant treatment that warrants changing your schedule to accommodate them. Dr. Dick Barnes suggests that there must always be room in your schedule to "clear the deck" to accommodate these exceptional patients. These patients may make the difference in meeting your daily or sometimes weekly production goals. This must be a delicately performed task that is accomplished by a skilled scheduler, which creates some room in your schedule either immediately or within the next 24 hours. Clearing the deck is easier to accomplish in a group practice than it is in a solo, one doctor, practice, but it is a valuable tool that can have a significant impact on the success of any dental office.

An efficient, structured, apparently seamless, orchestrated schedule is a true art form. It addresses one of the core values, which is a commitment to oral health as a component of the general health of the patient. Scheduling is one of the foundational systems that is very well integrated with other systems and make up the matrix of the practice. An efficient scheduling policy allows patient's needs to be met in an organized and timely manner, producing success for the dental provider, although success is defined.

References and Additional Resources

Bridges, G. 2007. *Dental Reception and Practice Management*. Hoboken, NJ: Wiley-Blackwell Publishing.

Covey, S. 2004. *Seven Habits of Highly Successful People*. Simon & Schuster.

Gerber, M. 2001. *The E Myth Revisited*. HarperCollins Publishers.

Homoly, P. 2005. *Isn't It Wonderful When Patients Say "Yes."* Bloomington, IN: AuthorHouse.

Jameson, C. 2002. *Great Communication = Great Production.* Tulsa, OK: Pennwell Books.

Levoy, B. 2004. *201 Secrets of a High-Performance Dental Practice.* St. Louis: Mosby. www
.schedulinginstitute.com.

Learning Exercises

1. Dr. Powell's office has a yearly production goal of $350,000 per year. There is only one doctor and one hygienist in the practice and 25% of the production is hygiene. The gross collection rate for this practice is 95%. Using a 4-day and a 5-day workweek, 5 holidays, and 2 weeks of vacation time for each producer, what must the daily production be by provider in order to produce the yearly production goal?

2. Create a template for daily production so that half of the production goal is in primary appointments, "Rocks." This is an 8-hour day and the doctor has two treatment chairs.

3. Go online and choose three remote access computer companies like GoTo-MyPC and compare what services each offers and the cost of the service.

4. Obtain demo disks from three dental software programs and compare the dental appointment scheduling pros and cons of each.

Chapter 15
Compliance with Government Regulations

Ronda Anderson

There are several government regulations in the dental office that you will deal with on a regular basis and that will affect your practice on a daily basis. The Occupational Safety and Health Administration (OSHA), the Health Insurance Portability and Accountability Act of 1996 (HIPAA), and the Centers for Disease Control and Prevention (CDC) are the specific areas of regulation addressed in this chapter. Obviously, these areas are not exhaustive within the scope of government regulation. For example, employment law is covered in Chapter 22 in this book, and amalgam waste management is not addressed here (refer to the American Dental Association website listed in the references section). Government regulations in the areas of OSHA, HIPAA, and the CDC have changed how dentists practice and will continue to do so in the future.

What Is OSHA?

The basic answer: OSHA was created to oversee compliance with the Occupational Safety and Health Act passed by Congress in 1970. This is a worker safety law. Before this law, as an employee you were left to the goodwill of your employer as to whether your workplace was safe or not. For example, when building San Francisco's Golden Gate Bridge, the engineer insisted that it be a safe workplace. He insisted on tethers for all workers working on the high wires and even built a net under the entire bridge to catch anyone who fell. Even with these precautions, eleven men died during the construction. These workers were lucky. Brooklyn Bridge workers were not so fortunate. Twenty to thirty men died during its construction—the number being uncertain because records were not kept with any consistency. Because of this law, many lives are saved on a daily basis across many industries.

Many people in health care sometimes lose sight that OSHA is a worker safety program and not a patient safety program. In fact, most of the subparts of the OSHA law have nothing to do with health care-specific items, and even those sections can apply to any industry. However, becoming compliant with OSHA regulations does

Dental Practice Transition: A Practical Guide to Management, Second Edition.
Edited by David G. Dunning and Brian M. Lange.
© 2016 John Wiley & Sons, Inc. Published 2016 by John Wiley & Sons, Inc.
Companion Website: www.wiley.com/go/dunning/transition

make our patients safer as well. This law has to be broad because it applies to *all* employers who have employees.

We discuss the subparts of this law and the specific applications to the dental office. It is your responsibility to provide a safe workplace for any employee. This is not only the right thing to do, but it is also the law.

Subparts

Walking and Working Surfaces

This, like many of the subparts, is common sense–oriented. It has to do with safety requirements for aisles and passageways, guardrails, and the use of ladders. Basically it requires you to keep all passageways clear of debris or any obstacle that would prevent safe travel in that area. This could include a wet floor, a rug that causes tripping, or storage of inappropriate items in these areas. The ladder portion refers to the act of ensuring that the ladder is in good condition and that another person holds the ladder for the person climbing it. This subpart should be easy to comply with.

Means of Egress

This section states that you must provide an unobstructed means of exit from any place in the office. All exits should be indicated with either a lighted or glow in the dark sign. OSHA requires you to place a map of the office with the exits, fire extinguishers, smoke detectors, fire alarm, and sprinkler systems located on the map. These should be placed in areas where the employee can easily view them in case evacuation of the facility is necessary. This subpart also requires you to create an emergency action plan for your office. This should include a fire prevention plan that lists any fire hazards in your office and provides training for employees on the fire hazard of materials located in the office. The emergency action plan also includes a list of any employee who has medical or first aid training, and the location of the first aid kit. Emergency evacuation directions should also be included. The scenarios should include in case of fire, chemical spill, and weather-related emergencies such as hurricanes, tornadoes, blizzards, and floods. One of the most important features that should be included is a meeting location outside the facility in case you must evacuate so all employees can be accounted for. This subpart sometimes is neglected because people don't think it will ever happen. However, when it does, you will be happy you have rules in place.

Noise Exposure

The requirement for the employer to provide hearing protection is based on the exposure time equal or in excess of an 8-hour time-weighted average of 85 decibels. This is a very rare situation in a dental office. The sound of a sander is measured at 85 decibels. Since we are rarely exposed to something that loud and should never be so exposed for an 8-hour period, this is not applicable to the dental office. Nevertheless, you should be aware of the requirements.

Ventilation

Fortunately, there are not many items that we use in a dental office that require ventilation, but there are some. In the lab, work with monomers can be very overwhelming. Also, if you grind many models, dust particles can be a problem. A ventilation hood or fan should be provided in this area. The darkroom is another place of importance: when cleaning the processor ventilation is necessary. This is another good reason to go with digital x-rays to eliminate this concern. The last item is an autoclave that uses chemicals instead of steam to sterilize instruments. These should have filters attached if you continue their use. Because of this, steam sterilizers dominate the market today.

Nonionizing Radiation

This pertains to radiation originating from radio stations, radar equipment, and any other source of electromagnetic radiation. This section does not apply to the dental office.

Hazardous Materials

This applies to several items in the dental office. Bulk oxygen is one of them; if you have central nitrous available in your office, you must comply with storage regulations for the large tanks. Hazardous materials are another—check with your state regulations on disposal of certain items in your office. Examples include amalgam, developing solutions, sharps containers, and any other hazardous chemicals you may use in your office. Proper training of employees in handling and storage of these items is essential. Make sure you have procedures in place in case of any accidents involving these items, including proper protective wear and notification in case of spills.

Personal Protective Equipment (PPE)

In the dental office we consider the following items of PPE: warm-up jackets (long-sleeved, high-necked, and fluid-resistant), masks (these should be selected based on procedures being performed using ASTM ratings), protective eyewear (must have side shields or wrap around face), and gloves (latex, nitrile, or neopreen for dental procedures, heavy duty gloves for cleaning). Masks should be changed between patients. Gloves should be changed and removed when leaving the operatory. These items should be provided to the staff members in order to protect them from possible contamination from body fluids or chemicals. Warm-up jackets should be worn during dental or cleaning procedures *only* and changed daily or when penetrable blood is present. Jackets should not be worn in break rooms or out of the office. The employer is required to launder this item in the office or have it laundered by a professional service. This is the largest protective item we wear. It is also the most exposed. Keep this in mind when training employees about the exposure this item has received throughout the day. Safety glasses are another item that is extremely important but not always worn. Challenge those employees who choose not to wear provided safety glasses to wear them just 1 day and see all the material that accumulates on them. This should be an easy reminder of how important wearing this item is for their safety. The following is the proper sequence to put on and take off PPE:

Put On:

Jacket
Mask
Eyewear
Gloves

Take Off:

Jacket
Gloves
Eyewear
Mask

Wearing PPE is one of the easiest ways we can prevent exposure. As an employer it is your obligation to train employees on the proper use of these items.

Medical and First Aid

Because we work in a health care facility, we usually think that much more is required in this area than is actually necessary. OSHA requires that you provide a basic first aid kit that includes bandages, antibiotic ointment, a one-way valve for CPR, and a compression wrap. You must also provide an eyewash station for employees. This should be properly maintained by checking it on a monthly basis to ensure it is working correctly. Make sure everyone knows the location of the first aid kit and the proper use of the eyewash station. (You must remain under eyewash station for 15 minutes). It is also a great idea to post important phone numbers such as those for the hospital, police, fire, and poison control. Also list the name and phone number of all staff members who have special training. Don't forget to put the number and address of your facility on this list so that it is easily found in case of an emergency.

Fire Safety

Do you have a fire extinguisher? This should be the first question you ask yourself regarding this subpart. Many of the fire safety items were discussed in the Means of Egress subpart. However, having, maintaining, and training your employees on the proper use of the fire extinguisher are the main components of fire safety. You should have the extinguisher inspected on a yearly basis and consult with your local fire station regarding training of your employees on its proper use. The Pull Aim Squeeze and Sweep or P.A.S.S. is the best method to use.

Electrical Safety

This is, again, common sense. Check all cords for frays. Do not alter plugs. Do not overload outlets. Check with manufacturer recommendations on certain equipment items regarding the use of dedicated outlets or circuits. Take care when plugging in items that are near water. Make sure all electrical connections are tight. These should be regular safety practices that we use in our own homes.

Employee Medical Records

Employee records should be kept for the duration of employment plus 30 years. This may seem like a long time, but doing so is in your best interests. These records should include the employees name, Social Security Number and hepatitis B vaccination status. Other items that should be included are the results of medical examinations or lab tests, medical opinions or diagnosis, record of first aid, and employee medical complaints. They should not include wages or reviews. Remember that even though your employee may be a patient, this OSHA record should be kept separate from an employee's individual patient files. Employees can request a copy of these records, and you are required to give them a copy within 15 days of such a request.

Ionizing Radiation

This is the radiation that pertains to x-rays. Each employee using such equipment should be properly trained on its use and should employ monitoring devices such as a badge as your state law requires. Badges are available to monitor employee exposure to radiation. Modern x-ray devices are fairly safe to use. Be wary of any pointed cone x-rays that are still in use. Some states are now opting for regular equipment calibration rather than individual monitors due to the safety of dental x-ray devices.

Blood-Borne Pathogens

This is the subpart that most health care workers focus on and is a very real concern in the dental office. This pertains to all employees that are exposed to blood and other potentially infectious materials. Saliva exposure during dental procedures is on this list. The most serious viruses are HIV and hepatitis B, although other hepatitis strains such as A and C are becoming more prominent in the population.

The Exposure Compliance Program is an important part of this subpart. This includes providing all employees with the hepatitis B vaccination. If they choose not to receive this protection, they must sign a declination form. Also, it is necessary to provide care to any employee that might be exposed during work. This could include a needle stick or instrument poke. Instrument pokes are more common and should not be treated lightly. You must send any employee who is exposed to the proper health care facility. Check your area for facilities specializing in worker issues. Also, you must receive proper follow up from that facility. Record keeping is vital during this situation. Refer to the flow chart provided on the American Dental Association website www.ada.org/prof/resources/topics/osha/flowchrt.asp for specific details.

The use of standard precautions is vital in protecting ourselves from these diseases. The definition of standard precautions is that we treat all patients as if they are carrying an infectious blood-borne pathogen. This is very important since many patients are unaware of diseases they might be carrying. Health histories are important but should not be a trusted means of protection because of this fact.

Infection control is the best way to prevent exposure incidents from happening. Work practice controls such as hand washing, use of proper PPE, and employee training are one of the best ways to avoid incidents. The approval from the CDC of hand sanitizers in the last few years has made compliance much easier and more effective. The other is engineered controls such as needle recappers, sharps containers, and cassettes. These items are made to eliminate your chance of exposure. Again, training on the proper use of these devices is crucial. Finally, cleaning, sterilization, and disinfection of the work area and instruments are vital to stop exposure. Please keep in mind the following areas that exist in your office:

Critical: An instrument that is used to penetrate soft tissue or bond *must* be sterilized or disposed of. This critical category includes anything that goes in the mouth.

Semicritical: Instruments that come into contact with mucous membranes, but do not penetrate, must at least receive high-level disinfection. This disinfectant must be able to kill hepatitis B and should be left on the recommended time to do so. This area is approximately a 3-foot area around the mouth. Anything in this area can also be sterilized or thrown away.

Noncritical: If there is no contact or penetration with any mucous membrane on an item or surface, it can be treated with intermediate-level disinfection. A household disinfectant is sufficient for this purpose. This area is the rest of the operatory.

The use of barrier covers should also be considered in the operatories as these will eliminate the need for difficult areas to be cleaned between patients. These should be replaced with every patient. Instruments should be in a covered container when being transferred to the processing area.

According to CDC recommendations, sterilization areas should be organized in order of the receipt of the instruments—dirty, clean (debris removed), and sterile. Please keep in mind that in cleaning instruments, ultrasonic cleaners are considerably more effective than hand scrubbing and alleviate the risk of exposure. Sterilizers should be tested on a weekly basis using a spore test. Positive spore tests could indicate sterilizer failure or user error. Retest immediately if spore test is positive. Upon second positive test, recall all instruments and re-sterilize with properly working sterilizer. All sterile instruments should be stored in the packages used for sterilization in a cool dry area away from contaminated areas.

This subpart may be the most important one for any health care facility, but it is not the only one. Remember, OSHA is for worker safety, not patient safety. It is a positive outcome that our patients are safer because our workers are safer.

Hazard Communications

Chemical inventory is your first step in compliance with this section. This is simply an alphabetical list by product name of all products requiring an SDS (safety data sheet) used in your office. Ask your supplier representative to help you with this.

This list should be posted for all employees. Next is the SDS book. This is the most misunderstood item in the office. It is simply a copy of each SDS for each item listed on your chemical inventory. It should be arranged the same way: in alphabetical order by product name. Use your chemical inventory list as a table of contents. Remember that with both the chemical inventory list and the SDS book, discontinuation of a product does not mean it is removed from the office. You must maintain your SDS sheets for 30 years. Each item you purchase that requires an SDS sheet will be sent to you with a copy of the sheet. Many companies are now sending these or making them available electronically. You need to keep only one copy in your book. However, if the chemistry has changed, you must maintain both. It is advisable to have two SDS books: one for discontinued items and one for currently used items. This can be overwhelming to an office that does not keep its book current. However, if you keep it current from day 1, it should be a simple matter requiring minimum time. When you introduce any new products into your practice, you should post the SDS sheet for your employees to review. Make sure all employees know how to read the SDS sheets. They should understand the 16 part format, signal words (danger or warning) and pictograms. Please refer to the Quick Card   https://www.osha.gov/Publications/HazComm_QuickCard_SafetyData. html for training on SDS sections as well as the Quick Card https://www.osha. gov/Publications/HazComm_QuickCard_Pictogram.html for training on pictograms.

Labeling is another area that is widely misunderstood. You must label any-thing that is not in its original container except items for immediate use. In most offices, the main items that require labeling are the cold sterile container, the ultrasonic machine, and the film processor. I recommend that for any surface disinfectant you use manufacturer-labeled spray bottles. GHS (Global Harmonization System) compliant labels are available from most dealers and are easy to use. A simple tip is to make a copy of the first label you make and keep it with your SDS book, and then when that label is destroyed you don't have to look up the information again.

This is the most overwhelming part of OSHA for most dental offices, but if kept up, it can be simple and not as time-consuming.

Workplace Violence

This is not a new part of the standard and is advisory in nature. Each industry faces a different risk. As an employer you should be aware of this as a part of OSHA and should provide a violence-free workplace.

OSHA Compliance and Inspections

Following the recommendations in the above subparts should go a long way in making any office compliant. It is recommended that you purchase an OSHA book. These are available through the American Dental Association (www.ada.org), the Dental Resource Center (http://drcdental.com/index.asp, then click on View All Titles), and various other organizations. Make sure when you purchase one that it is as complete as possible. Many of the available OSHA books provide forms for incident reports, emergency action plans, and so forth. It will save you a lot of time and headache to use these forms instead creating them yourself. Why reinvent the wheel? Proper state and OSHA forms must also be posted in your office. These forms are available for sale or free at www.osha.gov.

Inspections from OSHA in the dental industry are rare but do happen. You could face substantial fines for noncompliance. Inspections can be triggered by some of the following situations: imminent danger present, catastrophes and fatal accidents, employee complaints, and programmed inspections. OSHA uses the "worst first" system of inspections. This is not meant to scare anyone, but you should always ensure your facility is compliant.

Yearly training of all employees is the biggest component to OSHA. All existing employees should attend OSHA training on a yearly basis, and new employees should be trained upon starting employment. Training should consist of review of all subparts. This can be done by an outside source, you, or an employee whom you have designated as the OSHA officer in your practice. However, if you decide to provide it, this training is required and is part of your compliance.

Further questions and information on the OSHA regulations can be answered at www.osha.gov.

Sexual Harassment

While outside of the regulatory/legal domain of OSHA, sexual harassment represents a serious problem in the workplace and should not be taken lightly. You should consult training manuals and reliable websites to understand this subject more fully. Here are three of many websites: http://www.eeoc.gov/laws/types/sexual_harassment.cfm, http://www.state.gov/s/ocr/c14800.html and http://www.nwlc.org/our-issues/employment/sexual-harassment-in-the-workplace. Sexual harassment can happen to anyone at any time, and may take a variety of forms. As an employer you should be knowledgeable about and prevent sexual harassment involving dentists-owners, team members, patients and vendors. Chapter 22 discusses preventing sexual harassment in more detail.

What Is HIPAA?

With the increase of electronic data interchange within the health care industry, lawmakers needed a way to protect patient privacy and security of patient records. Because of this, HIPAA was created. There are two main components involved in HIPAA: HIPAA Privacy Rule and HIPAA Security Rule

Your first step to compliance is to assign a HIPAA coordinator in your office. In a small office this person may also take on the responsibilities of transaction compliance officer, privacy officer, and security officer. As the practitioner, you should remain the practice executive unless your office is quite large. As with OSHA, a HIPAA compliance book is recommended as well. There are a lot of forms required for HIPAA so ensure your book includes these that can be customized. Some companies such as Dental Enhancements will provide customized forms for you.

HIPAA Privacy Rule

A major goal of the Privacy Rule is to ensure that individuals' health information is properly protected while allowing the flow of health information needed to provide and promote high-quality health care and to protect the public's health and well-being. The rule strikes a balance that permits important uses of information, while protecting the privacy of people who seek care and healing. Given that the health care marketplace is diverse, the rule is designed to be flexible and comprehensive to cover the variety of uses and disclosures that need to be addressed.[1]

All health care providers, health care clearing houses, and health plans must comply with this rule as well as business associates in your office that would have access to patient information. All business associates should sign a HIPAA business associate contract that you should keep on file. This may include accountants, attorneys, business consultants, computer consultants, dental suppliers, dental service technicians, or temporary employment agencies.

Protected health information (PHI) is considered anything that is stored electronically, on paper, or orally discussed. This includes a lot of information that we deal with every day. All employees should be trained in the proper use of this information and how it should be transferred in your office that allows your patients to be protected. The patient's PHI can only be disclosed as follows: directly to the patient; to carry out/provide treatment, payment, or health care operations, generally accompanied by a consent form; in compliance with a patient authorization form; upon informing a patient in advance of proposed disclosure, when the patient can agree or disagree; when disclosure is required by law or for public health reasons.

The greatest practical implication for staff regarding this standard is this: limit access to patient records by not leaving them unattended, not discussing PHI outside the office, not removing files or patient records from the office, restricting employee access to records except for assigned business needs, and storing historic records similarly. Some activities that may be affected by this law are sign-in sheets (names only are allowed), schedules that contain anything other than patient names, and oral communication of PHI. A special effort to provide privacy for each patient should be enacted.

Notice of the HIPAA policies must be provided to your patients and their acknowledgement of these policies must be stored in their file. Any updates to the HIPAA policies must be provided to the patients as well and their acknowledgement of those updates must also be stored.

Data safeguards should be put in place to protect patient records. These can include shredding, password access to computers, time outs on monitors that are not being actively viewed, and limited access to certain employees.

HIPAA Security Rule

A major goal of the security rule is to protect the privacy of individuals' health information while allowing covered entities to adopt new technologies to improve the quality and efficiency of patient care. Given that the health care marketplace is diverse, the security rule is designed to be flexible and scalable, so a covered entity can implement policies, procedures, and technologies that are appropriate for the entity's particular size, organizational structure, and risks to consumers' e-PHI (electronic protected health information.[2]

As with the privacy rule all the same entities are covered. The covered entities are required to secure e-PHI against reasonable threats using available technology. Because

---

[1] Taken from www.hhs.gov.
[2] Taken from www.hhs.gov.

technology is changing, these procedures can change with the current threat, so it is imperative for you to consider variables such as hardware, infrastructure, and potential risks when selecting practice management software and computers for your office. Chapter 11 discusses technological issues in practice. You must keep patient record security in mind as well as functionality. You should regularly review these items as well.

Other considerations are facility access and control as well as workstation and device security. Proper storage and back up of your computer information is vital. Consider using cloud-based backups or onsite server backups and not sending information home with employees. Also verify that any entity that you send e-PHI to is also in compliance.

HIPAA compliance is required for all facilities no matter what size. Make sure whatever practice you end up in is compliant. Fines and penalties can be high for noncompliance and unlike OSHA, HHS can and will do spot inspections. Patient complaints are probably the biggest reason for inspections, so ensure your patients feel that you take their health information security seriously.

CDC Guidelines

From time to time, the CDC issues updated guidelines for dentistry to help stop the spread of disease. These guidelines do become part of the OSHA standard, so compliance should not be optional. They also keep everyone safer.

The latest guidelines for dentistry were released in December 2003 and are as follows:

1. Developing written comprehensive policies and programs
2. Not refilling your soap bottles without washing and drying them first
3. Using sterile gloves with surgical procedures
4. Keeping fingernails short, and no artificial nails or extenders
5. Changing masks between patients
6. Allowing packages to dry before they are handled to avoid contamination
7. Designating a central processing area into distinct areas: receiving, packaging, sterilization, and storage
8. Transporting instruments in covered containers
9. Using chemical indicators on the inside of the bag
10. Wrapping of all instruments that are not being used immediately
11. Examining wrapped packages of sterilized instruments before opening them to ensure the barrier wrap has not been compromised
12. Avoiding the use of carpeting and cloth-upholstered furnishings in dental operatories
13. Meeting Environmental Protection Agency regulatory standards for drinking water (500 CFU/mL) for routine dental treatment
14. Advising patients to not close their lips tightly around the tip of the saliva ejector

Government Agencies Unraveled

In the end, the best approach to any regulatory agency is to analyze it piece by piece and make it work for you. Many people are overwhelmed by the idea of OSHA or HIPAA, but when you break down the compliance issues, they are entirely manageable. Compliance can even make your practice better. By providing a safe workplace for your dental team, you are more likely to retain them. Given the average, short duration dental assistants tend to stay in a practice, retention of staff remains very important for practical and economic reasons.

References and Additional Resources

Health Professions Training Consultants. 2001. HIPAA Unraveled. Available at http://drcdental.com (accessed 2006).

The ADA HIPAA and OSHA Compliance Kit. 2013. American Dental Association. Chicago, IL. 2003. *OSHA Compliance Manual.*

www.ada.org. ADA (American Dental Association) website; (www.ada.org/goto/hipaa, www.ada.org/prof/resources/topics/amalgam.asp).

http://www.cdc.gov/oralhealth/infectioncontrol/guidelines/index.htm

http://www.hhs.gov/regulations/index.html Health and Human Services website

www.osha.gov OSHA (Occupational Safety and Health Administration) website.

Learning Exercises

1. Use your current classroom and create an emergency evacuation map.
2. Find and analyze at least two SDS sheets for items you use in the clinic.
3. Create a label for one of the items you found the SDS sheet for. Use http://www.msdsauthoring.com/msds-safety-data-sheet-chemicals-samples-msds-examples-sds for example labels.

References and Additional Resources

Listening Exercises

Chapter 16
Understanding Embezzlement
David Harris

Introduction

Embezzlement is a problem that will afflict the majority of practicing dentists eventually. This chapter will discuss how and why embezzlement happens, the limits of conventional protective strategies, what really is effective in controlling the problem, the investigation of embezzlement, and what happens to victims and perpetrators afterward.

As someone who is probably looking at becoming the owner of a practice within the next few years, it is important to increase your understanding of this topic and how it affects dental practices.

What Is Embezzlement?

The Merriam-Webster online dictionary defines embezzlement as "to appropriate property entrusted to one's care fraudulently to one's own use."

In a dental office context, this equates to staff members (or possibly independent contractors) stealing from the owner or owners of the practice.

Embezzlement is a scourge that afflicts far more dentists that many realize. Surveys of dentists consistently return results suggesting that between 50% and 60% of those surveyed have already been victimized. Because an unquantifiable amount of embezzlement never gets detected, and a further amount is detected but not reported, the true prevalence of dental office embezzlement is indeterminable. However, it is clear that the majority of dentists will be victims at some point in their careers.

Sometimes embezzlement is of a minor nature—it may involve taking pens or toilet paper. In other situations it involves hundreds of thousands (or in rare cases a million or more) dollars. While it is sometimes tempting to dismiss low-value theft as more of an irritant than a real crime, the words of Steve Albrecht, a highly respected fraud investigator, should be borne in mind: "that there are no small frauds; just large frauds that are caught early." People who steal low-value items have already found a way to rationalize dishonesty; we should expect that it is only a matter of time before they graduate to bigger theft.

Dental Practice Transition: A Practical Guide to Management, Second Edition.
Edited by David G. Dunning and Brian M. Lange.
© 2016 John Wiley & Sons, Inc. Published 2016 by John Wiley & Sons, Inc.
Companion Website: www.wiley.com/go/dunning/transition

To contextualize the amounts stolen, the last time we studied our own case files, the average amount stolen was slightly over $109,000. The Association of Certified Fraud Examiners (ACFE), which in addition to providing training and certification to fraud examiners, also conducts considerable research into embezzlement, states that the median occupational fraud loss (across all industries, and not limited to dentistry) is $141,000.

However, dollars only tell part of the story. I have seen embezzlement force dentists to lose their practices or declare bankruptcy. Some dentists are forced to postpone their retirements (which may also affect you as a student dentist—fewer practices on the market increases the price of those actually available to buy). Some dentists have voluntarily left the profession as a result of embezzlement, and embezzlement was the root cause of at least one murder when, in 2012, Shantay Joiner Hickman pled guilty to murdering Maryland dentist Dr. Albert Ro, from whom she had been embezzling.

Embezzlement touches every corner of dentistry; it affects both general dentists and every dental specialty. Proprietorships, group practices, multioffice organizations, and large dental service organizations are all victimized. It takes place in urban practices and small town offices. Some of the perpetrators are newly hired employees with "baggage" that isn't identified; others have worked in the practice for many years and have unblemished records when something causes them to start stealing.

Many embezzlers work in front desk or office management functions, but we also see clinical staff, bookkeepers, associate dentists, and outside parties such as accountants embezzle. And it is more common than many realize to find dentists in group practices embezzling from their colleagues, or the husband, or wife of dentist stealing from their spouse.

Embezzlers employ a dizzying array of techniques. We have seen hundreds of different methodologies used, and sometimes the creativity of thieves is startling.

So Who Are These People and Why Do They Steal?

One of the most frequent comments I hear once the identity of an embezzler is confirmed is that he or she is "the last person I could imagine stealing." Their surprise is understandable. We all have preconceptions about how criminals look, dress, speak, and act. Our mental image of the criminal is shaped by what we see on the news, TV dramas, and by direct observation in our own communities.

Embezzlers do not fit this stereotype; many of them remind me of Sunday school teachers (which, in fact, some of them are). The explanation for why embezzlers don't fit the preconception is simple—you would never hire someone who you think looks like a criminal. So as an employer, you have already eliminated certain people because they haven't passed your personal "smell test," whereas everyone you hire has.

Criminologist Donald Cressey probably had the greatest influence on the development of our current understanding of economic crime. In his landmark 1973 book *Other People's Money*, he proposed a framework called the Fraud Triangle. Cressey theorized that there were three necessary preconditions for fraud: pressure, opportunity, and rationalization. I revised Cressey's original model as depicted below in Figure 16.1, substituting "Motive" for "Pressure" and adding "Embezzlement" at the center of the triangle.

Motive

Motive can be either financial or emotional, and we sometimes label embezzlers with these characteristics as "Needy" and "Greedy," respectively.

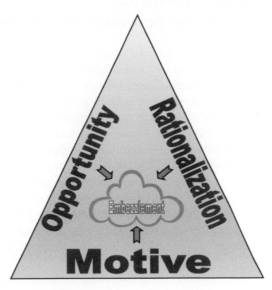

Figure 16.1. The Embezzlement Triangle.
(Adapted from Cressey, 1973.)

Needy embezzlers steal to address financial needs; some event has created a long-term financial imbalance, and this deficiency has threatened their ability to keep themselves afloat. They steal to fund necessities like rent and mortgage payments. There are many possible triggering events. Some common ones are divorce, a spouse losing their job, or a gambling or substance addiction.

In contrast, Greedy thieves steal to address an emotional deficit. In many cases, they feel that society (represented by you, their employer) has failed to recognize the true value of their talents, and they steal to address this perceived inequity (and to prove how truly smart they are). They may, perhaps even with justification, look at you as an intellectual peer. They conveniently forget the outlay you made to acquire your education and the financial and emotional burdens of practice ownership, and in their simplified worldview it seems unfair that you earn ten or twenty times what they do. To make it worse, many have an imperfect understanding of your finances because they aren't aware of all of your costs, so they overestimate what you take home, which increases their perception of inequity.

There are also those who derive physical pleasure from the act of successfully taking a risk; they are somewhat analogous to the "celebrity shoplifters" we occasionally hear about. A spectacular example of this is one of our "alumnae" who had been stealing from her doctor for several years when she won a $3 million lottery prize. After her big win . . . she continued embezzling. Clearly, at that juncture, stealing was being done to address emotional, and not financial, pressure.

One of the differentiating characteristics of Greedy thieves is how they spend their money. Greedy thieves spend conspicuously, and normally on luxury items that would otherwise be unaffordable; we have seen $140,000 automobiles, yachts, and in one notable case the chartering of a plane to take friends on a shopping trip.

A question I am often asked is whether embezzlement is more common when the economy is booming or in recession. Economic conditions affect our two groups differently. Tough times create more situations of financial desperation, and therefore more Needy thieves. When the economy is good, the perception that their friends are getting ahead more quickly than they are motivates some people to join the ranks of the Greedy.

Although embezzlement could take place at any point in a dentist's career, I think that new dentists are particularly vulnerable. This isn't because dishonest people specifically target new dentists; an employee's decision to become dishonest actually has relatively little to do with you, and is far more related to their own needs and wants. I would describe someone's decision to start embezzling as a statistical "random walk." It is correlated with almost no other factors, including your age or stage of career.

What is different about young dentists who are new owners of practices is that their business skills are still developing, and they face a large number of distractions—young families, the pressure of trying to achieve both clinical mastery and business competence, and often a crippling combination of business, personal, and educational debt. It is this combination of developing skills and competing priorities that makes it far less likely that a young dentist will notice that they have a problem, and their debt burden gives a young dentist far less capacity to absorb a financial "shock" than a mid- or late-career dentist.

What isn't often understood is how powerful the motivation to steal is, and how the combination of determination, cleverness, and knowledge of how your office operates creates a climate where embezzlement can be successfully carried out, at least for a time.

Rationalization

In addition to feeling some form of pressure, an embezzler needs to decide that stealing from you is an acceptable way to address the pressure that they are facing. I often explain rationalization as an ethical "bar" that a thief must be able to jump over before stealing.

Increased pressure motivates an embezzler to jump higher, and (probably without realizing it) you may do various things that lower this bar. For example, if staff members see you cutting professional ethical corners or cheating on your income tax, or if you do something that a staff member interprets as rubbing your relative affluence in their face, you are making it much easier for them to justify stealing from you.

I remember a doctor taking his entire team to a conference in an exotic location—great idea, except that the doctor purchased first class tickets for himself and his wife, while the rest of the office was on the same plane in coach. Another doctor used to complain to staff about how expensive repairs were to his Mercedes; you can imagine the animosity this could cause since the car cost more than the annual salaries of every staff member in the office.

At a minimum, this kind of behavior shows the doctor to be insensitive; it can also "lower the rationalization bar" to the point where a would-be embezzler feels comfortable jumping over it.

Opportunity

The final precondition for embezzlement is opportunity, and opportunity exists in every practice.

The biggest misconception I encounter, and I think a major enabling factor for embezzlement, is the belief that policies, procedures, and "checks and balances" can prevent, or reduce, the likelihood of embezzlement. Unfortunately, this misunderstanding afflicts not only practicing dentists, but also the large community of those advising dentists.

To be clear, the misunderstanding is an honest one; most of us understand other types of crime better than embezzlement, and there is a tendency to assume that what is effective in controlling other criminal activity will also control embezzlement.

Most people correctly believe that a burglar alarm installed in a house or business dramatically reduces the chance of burglary. Locking your car doors decreases the probability that your car's contents will be stolen. We assume that the same approach (i.e., increasing the perceived difficulty of stealing) will reduce the likelihood of being embezzled, and that is where we have misapplied the analogy.

What is being overlooked here is that the alarm and locked car doors do not *prevent* crime; they simply *divert* it to some other, less protected, victim. A burglar who spots your alarm doesn't abandon their plan to rob *someone*; they simply find a less defended target and victimize your neighbor instead of you. So control measures do not convert thieves into honest people, they simply channel the actions of thieves away from a specific target.

However, embezzlement is different because diversion isn't possible. In contrast to other types of economic crime, in embezzlement the victim is predetermined—it's you. No one feeling the pressure to embezzle (and I'll repeat that this is a powerful pressure) will decide that since you are too difficult a target, they should quit their job with you, find a new job and invest the time that will be needed to learn the systems sufficiently in their new office to embezzle. That process would take far more time than most embezzlers believe that they have.

What embezzlers can control, and therefore what you can influence, is not their choice of *victim*; it is their choice of *methodology*. If you block an embezzler's first idea for stealing from you, they will move on to their second, third, or twelfth choice until they find something that works. And with dental offices being highly porous in this respect, thieves have lots of options.

So relating this back to Cressey's Fraud Triangle, I view Opportunity as a binary factor—it either exists or it doesn't. For embezzlement, more opportunity does not correlate with increased probably of embezzlement, and reducing (but not eliminating) opportunity does not decrease the likelihood. Let's assume that you have a motivated thief in your office who knows you well—what are the chances that the thief will be unable to find some method of going through or around your controls?

The Relevance When Purchasing a Practice

There are two possible implications of embezzlement when purchasing a dental practice. The first is that you purchase a practice where the seller is unaware that embezzlement is taking place, and, when you discover that embezzlement is happening after you buy the practice, you end up dealing with it at your expense.

The second possibility is that you buy a practice where no embezzlement is taking place at the time of the purchase, but that one of the employees who you acquire as part of the purchase starts stealing afterward.

While embezzlement could take place at any time after you buy the practice, the first year or two is particularly vulnerable. On the one hand, your inexperience with running a practice creates opportunity, and on the other, employees may not feel the same loyalty to you that they did to the former owner. You may be considerably younger than some of the staff, and most new owners want to put their own stamp on the practice by making some changes. These factors may result in a weaker bond between you and the staff than was enjoyed by the previous owner, thus facilitating rationalization.

Controls Are Ineffective

There are other reasons why controls are ineffective against embezzlement. The first point I will make is that there is an inherent trade-off between controls and operational efficiency. Division of responsibilities between front-desk staff is often advocated as a means of reducing vulnerability to embezzlement. For reasons previously discussed, I don't believe this to be the case, and like almost every control, division of duties can be expected to increase staff workload and therefore may increase costs.

Second, many controls and procedures are not performed by the doctor personally; they are really directions given to staff about how to perform their duties. Embezzling staff are normally able to selectively apply these procedures.

I vividly remember speaking to a large audience about how embezzlers steal checks. Many doctors believe that it is difficult for a thief to cash a check payable to the doctor, and I was outlining how easy it actually is. One doctor put his hand up and informed me that theft of checks would never happen in his office, because the backs of checks are stamped with the words "for deposit only" to a specific bank account number.

The question I asked him, which caused him to squirm (and those around him to snicker), was whether he stamped the checks himself. The tone of his reply suggested that he was a "saver of teeth" and not a "stamper of checks." So I asked him why an embezzler, who by definition does not feel compelled to follow society's rules, would be expected to follow his, when doing so would cost the embezzler money. Obviously, he had no good answer to my question.

Let's accept that in a dental office it is impossible to remove *all* opportunity for embezzlement without making it impossible for staff to do their jobs. Furthermore, reducing opportunity carries a financial cost, and since reducing opportunity does not commensurately decrease the probability of embezzlement, spending money for this purpose does not produce a return.

A Crime of Navigation

Every budding embezzler starts the same way—they begin by studying their environment. They are aided in this process by how well they know you and your habits. Specifically, they are very aware of what you do and don't monitor in your practice. I've often described embezzlement as a "crime of navigation" where a thief plans a methodology of stealing that will skirt around your scrutiny.

So, for example, if you are someone who pays close attention to the "daysheet" generated by your practice management software at the end of each day, the thief will certainly be aware of this and therefore will not do something that results in embezzlement indicators on your daysheet. They will instead choose a methodology of stealing that keeps this report pristine. How closely you monitor your practice's bank account, whether you periodically review receivables, the scrutiny you give to adjustments and write-offs—these are all inputs into the thief's decision process on how to steal.

If you change your pattern, the thief will simply adapt in response.

Daily Balancing Is Impotent

At the core of every practice management software is an activity known as "daily balancing." Daily balancing involves printing a "day end report" from the software, and a comparison with the report to what is deposited in the bank. Many dentists believe that, as long as their day end report balances to the bank deposit, they are safe from being embezzled. There are two mistakes underlying this reliance: many dentists assume that output from their computer system must be true and they concurrently underestimate the motivation and creativity of embezzlers.

If the report does not balance to the bank deposit, clearly there is a problem (which may be embezzlement, or something more benign, for example, an addition mistake on the bank deposit); however, the reverse isn't necessarily true. While a discussion of how it is done is beyond the scope of this chapter, many dentists have found out the hard way that it is relatively easy for a thief to "cook" the day end report so that it conceals theft.

Is Embezzlement Therefore Inevitable?

Notwithstanding that many articles have been written outlining how to "prevent" embezzlement, in my experience trying to deter an embezzler from their planned course of action is impossible. This is simply an acknowledgement of the limited ability of humans to influence the behaviors of others, particularly when motivations are strong.

This does not mean that you are powerless against embezzlement; on the contrary you can do a lot to ensure that the impact that embezzlement has on you is minimized. However, this requires a major shift in thinking for most dentists; with one notable exception, they need to let go of the idea that they can prevent embezzlement, and instead focus on detecting it.

Avoid Hiring Mistakes

The one place where dentists have a clear opportunity for prevention is to improve their hiring process so that somebody with the wrong kind of experience does not get a job in your office. Most people who get fired for embezzling respond by looking for a job in other dental offices. They are aided by two factors; the criminal justice system moves with glacial slowness and it is often years before they are charged, let alone convicted of a crime. In this period of legal limbo, thieves are constitutionally entitled to the "presumption of innocence." The second factor is that most dentists do not approach the hiring process with sufficient skepticism, and this allows "serial embezzlers" to successfully conceal their backgrounds from prospective employers.

I've come to realize that most dentists thoroughly detest the hiring process. The making of decisions based on very incomplete information, the regulatory minefield of employment law, and the fact that hiring is often done under some time pressure to replace a departing (or departed) employee makes this a task that most dentists dread. When an applicant looks perfect for the job and can start right away (which describes most embezzlers who just got fired for stealing), the dentist is often so happy to be able to escape the process that the healthy amount of skepticism that should exist seems to vanish.

I will mention that less than 15% of the embezzlement we find is committed by people who have embezzled elsewhere (in other words, the biggest danger to most practices is someone who is already working there, as opposed to the person that they are about to hire). However, it is relatively simple to change your approach to vetting applicants so that your chances of spotting someone with baggage are drastically increased.

Avoiding embezzlement is far from the only reason for carefully screening applicants. In addition to being the public face of your practice, employees have access to Protected Health Information (protected by the very complicated provisions of HIPAA) and have the means to access controlled medications. With one in four U.S. adults having a criminal record and an estimated 53% of resumes having at least some falsified information,[1] the potential for several types of disaster exists if employees are not properly screened.

I'm certainly no expert on how to select the right people for your office; this topic is covered in Chapters 22 and 23 of this book. My interest in this topic is limited to helping you uncover the things that a job applicant doesn't want you to know.

The following are some of the checks that can be done to close the "information gap" between an applicant and you:

1. When checking a resume, any falsehood or inconsistency should disqualify the applicant. Start by comparing the resume you have received with the one available online—most people don't think of this, but the social network LinkedIn maintains a resume on everyone who has a profile there. So, if an applicant has a LinkedIn profile, compare dates, job titles, and employers with what the applicant gave you. And while you are at it, have a look at what the applicant posts on Facebook and Instagram as well. Many people will make pejorative comments about their boss or workplace on social media sites. I'm not questioning their right to freedom of expression, but I would not hire them. Also, other antiwork activities like gambling or excessive partying may become evident through this screening, and allow you to avoid a future problem.

2. Applicants with "baggage" normally have at least one former employer who they do not want you to speak with, and they use various methods to prevent that contact. One common technique is to simply omit that job from their resume, and to instead claim that they were "home with children" or "travelling in Europe." Instead of simply accepting such a claim at face value, you can request (third party) documentation to substantiate such a claim; for example, someone who really was travelling through Europe can normally produce a passport with entry and exit stamps. Someone who was home with children can show you an income tax return (and the assessment of the return by the IRS) showing no income for that period.

3. It astounds me that to get a job driving a truck or virtually any government job I would need to pass a drug test, whereas I could get hired by almost any dental office without one. Especially given that employees of dental offices have access to prescription pads, I cannot understand why most dentists do not consider what happens in their office important enough to screen out people with addiction issues.

4. Other external screening that I think should be routinely done is a credit check and a criminal records check. I will mention that less than perfect credit should not

---

[1] http://www.statisticbrain.com/resume-falsification-statistics/.

necessarily disqualify the applicant; many single parents, for example, have blemishes on their credit history. You are looking for extreme or unexpected money problems; the couple living in an expensive house who appear to be well off but have poor payment history may be a danger sign.

5.   Please note that most types of background checking require the written consent of the applicant, and that you may need to enlist the services of a human resources advisor to ensure that the screening process follows the rules.

6.   Calling "references" is pointless. What some carefully selected acquaintances (e.g., someone's 7th grade science teacher or former gymnastics coach) think of the applicant isn't of much interest to me. The only people I am interested in speaking with are former employers. So, I recommend ignoring "character" references and focusing on former employers. I make a point of calling all former employers over the last 5 years, whether or not the applicant has listed them as "references."

A few pointers for calling former employers:

a.   Know with whom you are speaking. Ignore any phone number given to you by an applicant, and get the phone number of a former employer from an independent source like an online search engine. We have seen many cases where a doctor called a phone number given by an applicant but was unknowingly calling the cell phone of a friend or relative of the applicant who was pretending to be a former employer.

b.   Speak with the right person. If the applicant worked for a dental office, speak with the dentist unless it is a very large office; in that case the office manager might be a better source of information. If calling a nondental business, make sure that you are speaking with someone who was a direct supervisor of the applicant, not a coworker or subordinate.

c.   Ask the right questions. Ask the former employer to provide the exact dates of employment and job title and compare this information with what the applicant claimed on the resume. Any discrepancy should cause disqualification. Another technique for making a job disappear from a resume is to "stretch" the dates of other jobs to cover the gap. Also, ask the former employer who the employee worked for before being hired with that employer, and where they went after leaving the job you are checking on. Compare any answers you get from this "continuity check" with the resume.

d.   One question that should always be asked of former employers is this—"if you had an opening and this person was available, would you re-hire them?" Former employers are often reluctant to divulge unfavorable information about employees, such as the cause of termination, out of a concern over being sued by the former employee. However, even if an employer is reluctant to discuss job performance or the reasons the employment relationship ended, many will find this question a safe one to answer (because it is simply an expression of future intentions, and really does not require the disclosure of any fact-based information, which is where a former employer could get into trouble), and a "no" answer to this question is certainly a huge danger sign. If the former employer is being forthcoming, I'd also ask whether the employee quit voluntarily or was let go, although there is a good chance that this question does not get answered.

e.   Another technique used by someone who has recently been fired is to pretend that they are still employed, and to ask you not to contact this employer because "they don't know that I am leaving." Because this request is frequently made for legitimate reasons, many dentists accept this claim at face value, with potentially dire consequences. I've seen suggestions that you get someone to call what is claimed to be the current employer and ask to speak with the applicant. I don't recommend this because it is duplicitous (and definitely awkward if the applicant is the one who answers the phone). A better approach is to tell the applicant that you are prepared to delay the conversation with the former employer until all other screening has been done and a conditional offer of employment has been made to the applicant, with having a conversation with the current employer being the only condition. This should make applicants having valid reasons for you not contacting their employers sufficiently comfortable for them to now allow you to do so. Those who are hiding something, once they realize that your making contact with this employer is a necessary precondition for employment, will likely abandon the application process.

So, in summary, a certain amount of skepticism is necessary and healthy when hiring. It isn't difficult to do a much better job of weeding out undesirable applicants, and defending against this particular danger than most dentists normally do. And the benefits extend well beyond preventing embezzlement.

What About Existing Employees?

Notwithstanding that many dentists believe that hiring mistakes are the biggest contributor to embezzlement, the statistics do not uphold this. The Association of Certified Fraud Examiners, which produces some of the most authoritative research on embezzlement, states that the vast majority of fraudsters are first-time embezzlers, with only 18% of embezzlement being committed by thieves who have been terminated by a previous employer or punished previously for fraud. So, while it is relatively easy to scrutinize prospective employees better, doing so will have impact on only a small corner of the embezzlement problem.

For most dentists, a far greater danger is posed by existing employees than the one you are about to hire. The burning question, then, is how to address the other 82% of embezzlers.

Expense Fraud

As discussed, a dental office represents a bountiful opportunity for a larcenous employee. Some employees manipulate expenses, and somehow trick you into paying out money that you shouldn't. Payroll and bonus tampering are the most common, but there are many other options available involving fictitious suppliers overpaying existing suppliers and misappropriation of tax and other regulated payments.

Theft of Revenue: The Biggest Problem

Far more common than expense fraud is "skimming," which involves the theft of a portion of a practice's revenue. Once again, there are many possibilities for accomplishing this kind of theft. I have seen dentists try to self-audit to spot irregular transactions, but the number of possible modalities of embezzlement, plus the sheer number of transactions taking place even in a small practice, makes this a daunting task. Most types of practice management software keep an "audit trail" of transactions, and a number of pundits have suggested that dentists periodically review this information. However, the volume of information collected is daunting—the audit log for a one-dentist one-hygienist practice will normally be 2,000 pages or more for a single year. Without some technological assistance to winnow down this mass of data into something useful, looking for embezzlement there is a truly daunting job.

How Embezzlers Act

I've had many dentists tell me that they wished that there was a better approach.
And in fact, there is.
One of the things studied closely by the Association of Certified Fraud Examiners is how embezzlers behave. And the ACFE's research on behavior reveals something that it both startling and encouraging.
Many of the behaviors symptomatic of embezzlement are well known. Embezzlers are reluctant to take vacations. They arrive early, stay late, or come to the office on weekends to "clean things up." They may come into the office on their days off.
Most thieves are more comfortable performing the work to cover up their stealing when they are alone in the office; there are too many interruptions when the office is open (and too large a chance for discovery) for the liking of most thieves.
They resist the involvement of outside advisors like practice management consultants. They are pretty convinced that they can fool you, but an experienced consultant poses a far greater risk to them, so they try to convince you that spending money on consulting is wasteful.
Often they try to exert control over who provides IT services to your practice, or who sells it dental supplies. I'm not suggesting that members of the "team" picked by the thief are necessarily involved in the embezzlement (although they may be). However, people profiting financially from their relationship with a thief are far less likely to question that person's activities (or report them to you) than they might be if their loyalty was to you instead of the embezzler.
More subtly, they may do things like resist upgrades to your practice management software. This is out of concern that upgrades to the software being used may disrupt whatever methodology of stealing is taking place.
A very common behavioral indicator is to offer the promise of "clinical utopia." Virtually every dentist I have ever met wishes that their office would run itself, freeing the doctor to deliver high-end dentistry, without being drawn into the minutiae of managing a business. Embezzlers, for reasons that aren't completely appreciated by their doctors at the time, have a common interest in having you uninvolved in your front office, so they work hard to convince you that the management of your practice is well looked after.
There is both good and bad news here. The good news is that behavior pointing to embezzlement is difficult to conceal. For example, I mentioned a reluctance to take vacation; this is driven by a need on the part of embezzlers to control the flow of information, and to handle patients who call the office to discuss the inconsistencies in their financial accounts that are a frequent by-product of embezzlement. So, even if a

thief knows that "vacation aversion" is a symptom, they quickly decide that the risk of taking vacation (and the possibility of their actions being discovered when they are gone) exceeds the risk that their actions cause the doctor to realize that someone has their hand in the doctor's pocket.

The bad news is that, at least superficially, many of the symptoms of embezzlement also look like the kind of behavior displayed by ideal employees, and for many dentists, differential diagnosis is a challenge.

The ACFE's contribution to the discussion is this: Its research suggests that more than 90% of embezzlers display at least one behavioral trait consistent with embezzlement, and that over 60% show two or more such characteristics.

This is entirely consistent with a 2007 survey performed by the American Dental Association, which studied the clues that led victims to realize that they were being embezzled. While the study did not evaluate the causes exactly in these terms, my company's reanalysis of the findings revealed something quite interesting—68% of embezzlement was unearthed as a result of some telltale behavior on the part of the thief, with the remaining 32% being revealed based on some kind of financial irregularity.

However, I suspect that most dentists believe that the way to discover embezzlement is to look for financial irregularities, not behavioral ones, and then become discouraged because of how burdensome and complex this kind of monitoring can be.

One of the things that makes this statistic even more remarkable is that, for the most part, the dentists discovering embezzlement through behavioral indicia do so without the benefit of any particular tools or training in this area—imagine how much more effective they could be if their process were a bit more structured.

I'll also mention that our work on the survey also revealed that 81% of embezzlement was uncovered by some form of chance occurrence, with a piddling 19% being uncovered by some type of system or control, which reinforces my earlier comment about the systemic overvaluation of controls for the purpose of preventing or detecting embezzlement.

Can My CPA Find Embezzlement?

Interestingly, external accountants, who many dentists consider to be quite important in their system of defenses against embezzlement, found less than 9% of the embezzlement in the ADA survey. This is roughly consistent with the ACFE's research (which covers all industries, and is therefore not specific to dentistry), which found that accountants identify less than 3% of embezzlement nationwide.

Most dentists expect their CPA to be on their "front line" of embezzlement protection, but the numbers show that most dentists overestimate the embezzlement protection provided by the accounting relationship.

Before you reach the conclusion that CPAs are letting the dental community down (and as a CPA myself, I feel some obligation to defend the accounting profession), let me explain some of the elements of the relationship between dentist and CPA that you might not have considered.

Many dentists deal with "generalist" CPAs, who do not specialize in dealing with dentists. While the generalists can bring valuable perspective to your situation, they may not have the basis for comparing your practice to others that a "dental CPA" can.

CPAs can perform three different levels of scrutiny and analysis when doing your work. The highest level of assurance is provided by an "audit." In an audit, your CPA will do sufficient analysis and independent verification to obtain "reasonable assurance that the financial statements are free from material misstatement." An audit's primary focus is financial statement integrity, not embezzlement, and while an audit increases the chance of embezzlement detection, this is not the primary focus of an audit. Even so, audits can be expensive, and for that reason, most dental practice owners elect for a lower level of scrutiny; either a "review" or compilation.

In a review, the accountant normally performs ratio analysis to obtain "limited assurance" that your statements do not need modifications. In a compilation, which is the most common engagement for dental practices, the CPA simply turns your raw information into financial statements, without any particular scrutiny.

So, it isn't that the accountants are asleep at the switch; it's that most dentists aren't prepared to pay for any scrutiny of their information from their accountant. And even if they did, there are some further limitations you should consider.

Most accountants aren't well equipped to think like criminals. For most of what they do, this is hardly a character flaw. However, it reduces their ability to spot embezzlement.

Furthermore, accountants have limited ability to navigate through your practice management software. Most embezzlement happens inside your software, with a much smaller amount taking place outside your software (such as stealing funds out of your bank deposit), without making a "concealing" entry in your practice management software.

Accountants typically have a strong seasonal pattern to their workflow, and most dentists interact at their CPA's busiest time of year. This may limit the amount of mental energy and proactivity that your accountant can offer you.

We have the privilege of working with some truly excellent CPA firms, and I am quick to defend the accounting profession against the sometimes unrealistic expectations of its clients. The lesson here is to ensure that you and your accountant understand each other; accountants are happy to accept a mandate to provide higher assurance about your financial statements, but you have to mandate them to do so and be prepared to pay for it.

Many of the behavioral indicia of embezzlement closely resemble what you would expect from ideal employees—thieves work extra hours, often display considerable attention to detail, and are usually willing to accept extra responsibility, both to expand their range of opportunities and to further embed themselves in your life.

Prosperident developed a tool to assist us in triaging calls from dentists who have embezzlement concerns. It is called the Embezzlement Risk Assessment Questionnaire, and it is designed to help a dentist capture and analyze behaviors displayed by staff members and to differentiate between ideal employees and thieves. The questionnaire is available, at modest cost, at www.dentalembezzlement.com/eraq.

What to Do (and What Not to Do) If Embezzlement Is Suspected

Let's assume that tomorrow, possibly on the basis of what you have read in this chapter, you begin to think that embezzlement may be happening at your newly purchased office. What actions should you take? Most dentists in this situation experience a flurry of emotions, after which their minds, quite logically, turn to what should be done about the problem. In my experience, dentists tend to be action-oriented people, and they will have a fairly strong desire to do *something*. Unfortunately, as some dentists have learned the hard way, what their instinct tells them to do next often isn't the right step to take.

I'll start by telling you what not to do. This is simple: If you suspect embezzlement, do not let the suspect (or suspects) know that you think they may be stealing. There are a couple of reasons for this. The first one is obvious—if the employee is, in fact, not stealing, letting them know that you don't trust them will irreparably damage the future working relationship.

On the other hand, if they are stealing, telegraphing your concerns may result in them trying to escape punishment by destroying your records, or worse. There will be an appropriate time to confront a suspect, but this is well past the "suspicion" stage. A basic observation about human behavior is that the normal restraints on all of us tend not to apply when someone believes their liberty to be jeopardized, and as has been demonstrated, this is when a white collar criminal can become violent.

Confronting an employee is a deliberate tipping of your hand. However, many dentists end up communicating their suspicions by accident. In an effort to stop the stealing, they will make sudden procedural changes. Sometimes they ask staff members for additional reports from the practice management software or start questioning transactions that they haven't queried before. Some will sequester themselves in their private offices for hours talking on the phone with their CPAs.

Procedural changes are unlikely to stop an embezzler; instead you will create a situation where the motive and rationalization to steal still exist, and all the thief needs to do to continue enjoying the act of, or financial rewards from, stealing is to find another opportunity. And they will succeed.

Sudden procedure changes also create the risk that the embezzler will fear being caught. Thieves continually scrutinize you and your behavior for any evidence that you are on to them.

Also, the suspicion stage is not the time to involve police. Something that we sometimes forget is that it is not the responsibility of law enforcement to determine what has been stolen; this is the job of the victim. The police's role is to confirm who did it, and then place the thief in the justice system. No police agency in the country has the technical knowledge and available manpower to properly investigate a dental embezzlement. Involving law enforcement prematurely forces them to open a file that they will be unable to progress, at least until your investigators finish their work, and law enforcement agencies detest "stuck" files. Similarly, there is no benefit, at this point, to contacting dental insurance companies that might be affected. I always encourage dentists in this situation to keep the circle of those in the know as small as possible— usually the dentist, the investigators involved, and possibly the dentist's attorney and the dentist's spouse. Having more people in the know simply increases the chance that the secret gets out.

So, it is important to involve as few people as possible, and to allow the investigators working with you time to complete their work.

And What If I Catch a Thief Red-Handed?

They should be fired immediately. The activities involved in firing a suspected thief need to be thought out carefully, both to make the process go smoothly and to prevent the employee from destroying evidence of their crime or otherwise harming the practice. In addition to having proper termination paperwork prepared, the dentist also needs to have locks changed, computer access revoked, website updated, and to gain control over the employee's office voicemail and email accounts.

Many employees fired for theft will try to claim unemployment insurance, even though they normally do not qualify. In order to avoid the costs that this will create, the dentist will be required to contest the application.

Another issue that you will quickly face if you fire someone is that you will begin to get "job reference" requests from other offices where this person is now seeking work. To avoid a legal backlash, these calls need to be handled carefully. Guidance should be sought from your attorney or employment law advisor.

Investigators

On the subject of investigators, if you need one, what are the attributes you are seeking? I think there are four things that make a good investigator. First, they must understand dentistry, and if you are a specialist, they must have an understanding of the business process involved for your specialty. This is particularly true with oral surgery and orthodontics; we have found that investigators who are very competent at doing general dentistry files often struggle when working in these two types of offices, so we use investigators with backgrounds in these types of practices for oral surgery and orthodontic investigations.

Second, you need someone who has experience as an investigator. This person will need to design and follow an investigative program, report their findings, work with law enforcement agencies, and possibly testify as an expert witness in court. Acquiring these skills typically takes several years. I have seen many investigations botched by someone with great intentions, and possibly a good knowledge of the practice management software in use, simply because they did not possess the skills required of an investigator.

Formal investigative qualifications are an asset to an investigator. The most recognized in this field is CFE (Certified Fraud Examiner), but this is a generalized qualification (i.e., not specific to dentistry) and, like any certification that is exam based, there are people who do well on the exams and gain the certification without understanding much about embezzlement and embezzlers.

As if it isn't challenging enough to require someone having both an understanding of how a dental or specialty office works and the skill sets needed of an investigator, I'll throw in one other attribute. When we hire investigators, the most important attribute we look for is an ability to think like a criminal. Our most able investigators are able to spot opportunities in a situation in the same way that an embezzler will. Of all of the things that an investigator needs, this is the most difficult to cultivate—in my experience, it is either there or it is not.

So, when you are facing an embezzlement issue and considering hiring a friend or relative who used to work in a dental office to assist you, give some thought to what is really needed to effectively investigate this complex, sophisticated crime and act accordingly.

Unless the suspect is no longer working in your office, a further requirement is that your investigator needs to have the skills and technological support to be able to work stealthily; parking themselves in your office for days or weeks is probably a bad idea.

Maximizing "Net Recovery"

Net recovery refers to how much money is recovered minus the cost of investigation and recovery. Maximizing net recovery should be the focus of an embezzlement victim.

One factor that is often overlooked in maximizing net recovery is that the "scope" of an investigation needs to be well thought out, and possibly adjusted. Transactions for a brief period of a few months might be examined, or an investigation could look at several years. Obviously, examining a longer period, or looking at a broader scope of transactions increases the cost of investigating, so it is important that the scope be set, and adapted if necessary, to optimize *net* recovery.

Many doctors initially tell us that they want us to find "every dime that was stolen." We normally propose an alternative approach—since in most embezzlement, the possibilities for recovery are limited (see discussion in the following section); curtailing our efforts once recovery has been exhausted normally produces optimum results. Put another way, it makes no sense for a dentist to pay for additional investigation if the results of that work can't possibly yield additional recovery, because doing so will increase his or her costs, but with no increase in benefit.

Sources of Financial Recovery

Let's assume that investigation confirms that money has been stolen. How do you get it back?

In general, there are four possible recovery sources. The first is the thief himself or herself. I can tell you that it is a rare occasion when we obtain any meaningful funds from a thief; most of them are spending money at least as quickly as they are stealing it. It is common for thieves who have been convicted in criminal court to be ordered to make "restitution" payments, but in many cases they would never live long enough to repay. As an example, an embezzler who stole $260,000 from one of our clients is paying restitution of $150 per month. Full repayment would therefore take 144 years, without applying an interest factor to the money stolen.

The second possibility is that there is someone close to the embezzler who wants to minimize damage to the thief. In one case we worked on, the thief's father was the city's mayor and would pay almost anything to avoid a scandal.

The third (and probably most utilized) repayment avenue is "employee dishonesty" insurance that is built into the business insurance policies that most dental offices have. The default amount of coverage for employee dishonesty in most policies is $25,000; while recovering this amount is welcomed by dentists who have been defrauded, based on what I have told you in this chapter, on average it will allow a dentist to recoup less than 20% of his or her losses.

It is surprisingly cheap to increase this coverage—many of our clients report that the extra cost of bumping this coverage to $75,000 per embezzlement is about $20 per month. Given the prevalence of embezzlement and the amount stolen this represents a major bargain.

The final source of recovery is perhaps less obvious than the others. It surprises dentists to find out how easy it is for a thief to cash checks from patients or insurance companies that are payable to the dentist. If theft takes place in this manner, the bank cashing these checks has done something it shouldn't have and therefore bears some responsibility. The legal issues are complex and discussion is beyond our scope, but we have had good success at recovering funds stolen in this way from the banks improperly cashing the checks. While most thieves are impecunious, their banks are certain to have money.

The Justice System

Civil Court: Lawsuits

Broadly speaking, there are two kinds of courts that may deal with embezzlement matters. The first is Civil Court. When you "sue" someone you are making use of the civil portion of the justice system, and normally the recourse available to you is "damages," which really means financial compensation for losses that you have incurred. Civil courts do not have the power to incarcerate someone—their role is to restore an aggrieved party to their previous position.

But here is the important part—when you sue someone, you pay the cost of your attorney (and any other costs, such as the cost of hiring an expert witness). The court may order the losing party to pay some or all of the victor's costs, but this is really relevant only if the loser has the money to pay.

As discussed earlier, most of our thieves are insolvent, or close to it, and being unemployable and having to pay legal bills certainly won't help their financial position. Therefore, there is a good chance that while your lawsuit against an embezzler is successful, you will be unable to collect, and you will have incurred considerable legal bills that you are also stuck with.

For this reason, we see very few embezzlers taken to civil court.

Criminal Justice

The place where more embezzlers end up is criminal court. There are both state and federal criminal courts in the United States; most embezzlers are tried in state court for breaking the state's laws. There are also federal laws that may be transgressed by an embezzler (the most common are referred to as the "mail fraud" and "wire fraud" laws), but it is uncommon to see a dental embezzler in federal court unless their offences are monetarily quite large.

The primary roles of criminal justice are deterrence and punishment; assisting with the financial recovery of a victim is also a secondary objective, but clearly takes a back seat to the first two.

I am asked by many new clients whether they should "press charges" against an embezzler, which isn't how the justice system works. However, it is understandable, and probably reassuring, that the knowledge of most dentists about the operations of the criminal justice system is limited. In contrast to the civil court system (where victims "own" their matters), in the criminal system the responsibility for obtaining justice belongs to the government whose laws were broken. Your role as a victim is limited to making a complaint to police; the investigation of that complaint, the decision of whether or not to charge the offender, and responsibility for moving the case through the court system, all belong to the appropriate state or federal government.

The good news is that the (often considerable) expense of this process is paid by the state or federal government. The downside is that victims often have far less influence over this process than they would like to, and the fate of an offender is often influenced by factors that have nothing to do with the crime or victim. For example, a state where the prisons are already overcrowded is unlikely to incarcerate a first offender for a nonviolent crime such as embezzlement.

Most victims are probably disappointed by the level of punishment their embezzlers receive.

The other thing that surprises victims is the painful slowness with which the justice system operates. Many victims expect, on making a complaint, the police to immediately appear at their office or the suspect's home and remove them in handcuffs. What actually happens is quite different.

Before they arrest someone, the police need to investigate. In a complex white-collar crime such as embezzlement, no police department has the expertise to analyze transactions conducted in practice management software, so they normally wait for us to complete our investigation and provide them with a report. Using our report as a starting point, they will conduct their own investigation, which might include questioning the suspect, interviewing witnesses, and possibly compelling banks to supply information on transactions through the suspect's account.

Every police department exists in a climate of limited resources, so it must determine its priorities. As you might expect, public pressure to deal with violent crimes often diverts resources away from nonviolent crimes such as embezzlement. As a result, it might take 6 months or more *after* you have made a complaint before a detective is assigned, and then several more months before their investigation is complete. Then the detective will review his or her findings with their supervisor to make a decision about whether there is sufficient evidence to meet with the District Attorney or U.S. Attorney about moving the case into the court system.

Discussions of the details of the court system are beyond the scope of this chapter, but it is a safe generalization that nothing moves quickly through that process. As a result, it may take a year or so after police work is complete before an accused steps into a courtroom and an equal amount of time for someone to be tried, convicted, and sentenced. So the entire process may take 3–4 years to conclude, and as I mentioned, first-time offenders may receive seemingly light sentences. While I share the frustration of many victims about the speed and end results, I also understand the reasons why the system functions as it does, and how unlikely these factors are to change.

Conclusion

Purchasing a practice is a challenging process. The possibility that embezzlement is already taking place, or might in the future, requires the purchaser of a practice to have an awareness of the dangers posed by embezzlement and the warning signs that embezzlement is taking place.

References and Additional Resources

American Dental Association. 2008. *2007 Survey of Current Issues in Dentistry: Employee Termination and Embezzlement*.

Association of Certified Fraud Examiners. 2014. *Report to the Nations on Occupational Fraud and Abuse*. Available at http://www.acfe.com/rttn/docs/2014-report-to-nations.pdf.

Donald R. Cressey. 1973. *Other People's Money*. Montclair: Patterson Smith, p. 30.

Learning Exercises

- Why are controls ineffective at stopping embezzlement?
- Why is a new practice owner particularly vulnerable?
- Which is more common—theft of revenue or expense theft?
- How can embezzlement be taking place even if a practice's day end report balances to its bank deposit?
- What is the most successful approach to determining if embezzlement is taking place in a practice?

Part 4
Marketing and Patient Communication

Chapter 17
External Marketing
Darold Opp

The New Economy

Statistically, the "average dentist" today can be described as follows:

- 54 years of age
- $225,000 in net worth (assets – debts = net worth)
- 67% dislike their profession
- 47% have abused alcohol or drugs during their career
- Have endured three career lawsuits
- Have only 1.5 days of hygiene per week in their practice
- Have a 91% collection rate
- Have a 42% recall rate
- Produce a little over $425,000/year with overhead of 67–74%
- Net pay is around $60.00/hour—average pay of a plumber!

L.D. Pankey said it best: "The average dentist is the best of the worst, or the worst of the best." Charles Schwab added, "The hardest struggle of all is to be something different from what the average man is." No one has ever left dental school hoping to become an "average dentist." So, how do we beat the syndrome? How do we stack the odds in our favor? You begin by having a different mind-set! Not one taught in any dental school. Not even one taught by any of the dental practice management consultants in America today. You look for guidance where business principles are tested every day: in corporate America.

Before we dig deep into what the corporate business world can teach dentists, we need to explore further the challenges facing dentistry in the new economy. An article in the October 2012 issue of *Dental Economics* by Roger Levin listed the eight permanent game-changers that are affecting dentistry:

1. The Great Recession and uninspiring recovery
2. Changes in consumer spending habits
3. Opening of many new dental schools
4. Higher dental school student loan debt

Dental Practice Transition: A Practical Guide to Management, Second Edition.
Edited by David G. Dunning and Brian M. Lange.
© 2016 John Wiley & Sons, Inc. Published 2016 by John Wiley & Sons, Inc.
Companion Website: www.wiley.com/go/dunning/transition

5.   Decrease in insurance reimbursements
6.   Expansion of national corporate dental centers
7.   Fewer associateship opportunities for new dentists
8.   Dentists practicing 8–10 years longer

Dr. Roger Levin, a well-recognized practice management consultant, added more insult to injury when he reported recently in his *Insight* newsletter that after reviewing hundreds of practices, 75% have declined in the past 4 years! One of the greatest challenges facing dentists today is finding enough patients to fill the hygiene schedule. Competition has increased, and patients are harder to come by. Even once-loyal patients have reduced or stopped twice-yearly hygiene appointments due to economic hardship, higher out-of-pocket costs, or loss of dental insurance. A paltry 1.5 days of hygiene per week for the "average dentist" is not the road to profitability and financial freedom.

So, why have all these changes happened at once? Insurance companies have been cutting reimbursements and reducing coverage throughout the past decade. The impact of lower reimbursements hit dentists even harder as they scrambled to deal with the fallout from the previously stated game changers. A chain reaction of events occurred including the stock market crash, which decimated the retirement savings of many older dentists. This forced dentists not only to work more years but also to incur the need to bring in additional support personnel such as an associate. With fewer associate positions available and higher student loan debt, younger dentists joined dental support organizations. Many consumers who were faced with layoffs or declining home values curtailed spending drastically, which resulted in fewer visits to the dentist. Dr. Levin concluded his analysis with this provocative statement: "To operate a successful practice in the future, dentists will have to immerse themselves in the *business of dentistry*."

Has Dentistry Slowly Evolved into a Commodity?

Businesses of all sorts, regardless of the size or nature, are being caught in what we call the "The Commoditization Trap." Probably the best description of this trap comes from a book published in 1999 titled *The Lexus and the Olive Tree* by Thomas L. Friedman:

> A commodity is any good, service, or process that can be produced by any number of firms, and the only distinguishing feature between these firms is who can do it the cheapest. Having your product or service turned into a commodity is no fun because it means your profit margins will become razor thin, you will have dozens of competitors, and all you can do every day is make that product or service cheaper and sell more of it than the next guy, or die.

For the sake of not missing the point here, let's rephrase the above statement and personalize it to our profession of dentistry:

> A commodity is any dental service that can be produced by any number of dentists private or corporate, and the only distinguishing feature between these dental offices is who can do it the cheapest and/or accept the lowest insurance reimbursement. Having your dental service turned into a commodity is no fun because it means your profit margins will become razor thin, you will have dozens of other dentists fighting for the same patients, and all you can do every day is accept lower fees and hope to do more procedures than the next guy to keep your business afloat, or close shop!

Here is the reality of what has just been said, and Dr. Howard Farran, editor and founder of *Dentaltown Magazine*, had this to say about our new economy in the January 2012 issue of his magazine: "I live in Phoenix, Arizona—one of the most saturated markets in dentistry—and I could give you the names of almost 100 dental offices in my backyard that have gone under." Dr. Farran went on to say, "It is time we all realized that we are in this [new economy] for the long haul and we need to remember to return to our core competencies . . . and make it a point . . . to lower your costs, increase your marketing, add something new to your dental armamentarium and lower your fees."

I have been in dentistry for 31 years, and I have seen a few things in my career. When I started, I worked with only one insurance company, and it paid at the 100th percentile of my fees. As I currently speak with dentists from across the country in my consulting business, the alphabet soup of management care (HMO, PPO, etc.) has a stranglehold on everyone, including yours truly! The day of getting paid by insurance companies at the 100th percentile is vain imagination. Here is the stark reality, and it comes from one of my consulting clients and his conversation with the head of a major insurance carrier. The insurance carrier CEO made this statement: "Dentists today need to accept the fact that generous reimbursements are a thing of the past. Dentists are going to have to work harder and smarter for less because this is the new economy that we are living in!" Ladies and gentlemen, we are not in Kansas anymore. Dr. Farran is right; we need to get back to the basics, but I contend we need to take it a step further. We need to go nontraditional, beyond outside the box. Glean from the best of the best in corporate America. Go where no other dental office has gone before!

And that is exactly what I did in 2008.

SmilePalooza Is Born!

About 10 years ago, I came under the tutelage of an entrepreneur many consider the "world's greatest marketer and millionaire maker," Dan Kennedy. In the first few years, I attempted to absorb all the marketing knowledge that I could get my hands on. It was in one of Dan's publications in 2008 that I read something that instantly struck me with that eureka moment. There, in fine print, Mr. Kennedy shared one of his top secrets for adding new referrals to any business. I took that secret, and a free, public appreciation event named SmilePalooza was birthed. Mind you, not just any event, but one that the local newspaper dubbed in a major headline "South Dakota's version of Disneyland."

In the years 2008–2014, inception to current, we had over 30,000 people attend this event. We were unprepared for the 3,000+ that attended in 2008, and thinking it was a fluke, we repeated it in 2009. We were so overwhelmed by the results. In the process we committed a critical marketing error. We failed to capture personal information on the attendees. This information would have allowed for instant marketing follow-up. With information gathering in hand in 2010 and beyond, you can see the incredible financial reward from a once-a-year, 3-hour, external marketing campaign:

- 2010: 147 new patients and $165,588 in direct revenue
- 2011: 172 new patients and $181,425 in direct revenue
- 2012: 230 new patients and $206,116 in direct revenue
- 2013: 232 new patients and $397,594 in direct revenue

Why the huge increase in new patient direct revenue in 2013 over the previous years? We created a new, customized, pre-event and post-event marketing campaign. This focused marketing nearly doubled our previous profits.

A number that few dentists appreciate and yet the corporate world watches very closely is the lifetime value (LTV) of a customer. LTV of a customer is defined as the total dollars flowing from a customer over the entire relationship with that customer. LTVs can have a very diverse range depending upon what dental services are rendered in the practice. Since I do not perform a lot of high-fee dental procedures, my LTV is low, at around $2,700 per patient. Nevertheless, when you total the new patient numbers from 2010 to 2013, 781 (new patients) × $2,700 (LTV) = $2,108,700 (total LTV of SmilePalooza-produced new patients), the financial windfall is astounding!

As we shared in the introduction, the average dental practice in America is producing $425,000 per year. What practice would not want the financial momentum of $2,000,000+ in future revenue? Do the numbers with SmilePalooza get any crazier? Yes! Though we did not gather this information at the SmilePalooza event itself, we ask each new patient coming into our office this question: Whom can we thank for referring you? In 2008 and 2009, 549 new patients said SmilePalooza! With this information in hand, our total LTV of new patients from the SmilePalooza event from 2008 to 2013 is a staggering $3,591,000.

Do not minimize the concept of LTV of the customer! Stanley Marcus, an early president of Neiman Marcus, shares this insightful story in his book *Minding the Store*:

A woman bought a ball gown fashioned of handmade lace. She took it home, wore it once, and "clearly abused it; it looked like she had wrestled in it." Then she brought it back to Neiman Marcus and said she wanted her money back.

Stanley gave it to her—cheerfully—reasoning that it would cost a lot more to replace that customer than the $175 (remember this was 1932) the dress cost him. He was right. "Over the years," Stanley writes, "this woman spent $500,000 with us."

In 1984, after I graduated from dental school, my wife and I moved back to Aberdeen, South Dakota, to begin our entrepreneurial dream. We purchased a practice that we thought was viable. After all, the dentist who owned it was so confident in his professional accomplishments through the years that he said there was no need to open the practice books and disclose any financial information. Being naïve and too trusting, I bought in to his logic. Long story short, I paid $20,000 for a total of 50 patients of record! All the equipment was antiquated and was respectfully donated to the University of Nebraska Medical Center College of Dentistry's museum. Did I get a bad deal? I thought so! This last month, two of the original 50 patients from 1984 were in my office for their regular annual dental visits. Like Stanley Marcus, I calculated the LTV of just these two patients alone, and each one contributed over $20,000 to the practice!

In a landmark study on customer satisfaction in the *Harvard Business Review*, it was discovered that companies could improve profits by 25% just by reducing customer defections by 5%!

Here is the lesson that needs to be learned: You invested time, money, and energy to get customers inside your dental office. Do whatever it takes to close the back door and keep them there!

Why the unprecedented success with such a simple concept as a SmilePalooza event? We need to look no further for that answer than one of the top social psychologists in the world, Dr. Robert Cialdini. In his classic book *Influence: The Psychology of Persuasion*, Dr. Cialdini writes about six principles of influence that permeate every society.

The first principle is reciprocation: If you do a kindness for another, that person will feel an obligation to return the favor. The incredible success of SmilePalooza in securing new patients was simply the principle of reciprocity at work. Families were returning the favor with their feet and their pocketbooks!

So, what makes SmilePalooza such a unique event? First of all, no one else is doing anything similar. When we began the planning process to host an appreciation event for our patients, I did exhaustive research both offline and online, and I could not find anything like it outside or inside dentistry. That was frustrating. How in the world would I even begin to try planning such an endeavor? But as they say in business, you are either a pioneer who paves the way or you are a settler who reaps the benefits of others' sweat equity. We were not given a choice. Our long history of working with children in the office and creating innovative ideas that gave us staying power in the community was in our favor. We already knew what kids and their families enjoy. So we became event pioneers!

SmilePalooza was created to be a one-of-kind, fun-filled family extravaganza. Imagine with me an afternoon in the park where 4,000 people gather to see Super Heroes and Disney Princesses come to life, the Tooth Fairy and Tooth Man welcoming old and new friends, multiple inflatable bounce houses, 20-ft.-tall walking puppets roaming the park, and the world's largest toy bubble tower filling the sky. Plus we have fire trucks, clowns, circus animals, live music, dance contests, horse races, celebrities on stage, crazy activities for all ages, shirt cannons, snacks and drinks, and tons of prizes. And the best part is all the laughter, all the screams of joy, all the pictures, and all the family memories are FREE! Still not convinced? Go to YouTube and type SmilePalooza 2014 in the search bar and witness for yourself the No. 1 free kid's event in dentistry today.

Here is where it gets really interesting. Although I understood the psychology behind the success of the event, I didn't fully comprehend why it touched such a chord with moms in particular. Then I read an article by Dr. Howard Farran in the January 2011 issue of *Dentaltown Magazine*. His editorial was titled "Getting to the Heart of Mom." Dr. Farran queried all readers as to why they were not doing more in the dental office to appease the No. 1 decision maker in the household. Beyond the decision making, 92% of dental appointments are made by, you guessed it, Mom!

Sally Hogshead in her book *Fascinate: Your 7 Triggers to Persuasion and Captivation* writes about a study in which more than 1,000 people were asked this question: "What is your No. 1 fascination in life?" An astounding 96% responded with "my children." This newfound information combined with Dr. Farran's comments and Dr. Cialdini's research on reciprocation finally brought it all home for me! Serendipitously we stumbled upon a marketing juggernaut—SmilePalooza.

Differentiate or Die

So, what secret strategy from the corporate world paved the way for my dental practice success? The answer lies in a concept that Jack Trout outlines in a chapter of his book *Differentiate or Die: Survival in Our Era of Killer Competition*. Trout shares what Rosser Reeves in 1961 called the unique selling proposition (USP) (Reeves 1961). Find a competitive advantage and exploit it to the maximum! Dare to be different! Alan Ashley-Pitt www.goodreads.com/author/quotes/5362099. Alan-Ashley-Pitt had this to say about carving your own trail in business: "You have two choices in life: You can dissolve into the mainstream, or you can be distinct. To be distinct, you must be different. To be different, you must strive to be what no one else but you can be."

Here is the prevailing problem with the challenge of being different. What will other people think? After all, I am a dental professional, and I have an image to consider! What if I fail? Bob Lutz, ex-president of Chrysler, wrote a book titled *Guts: The Seven Laws of Business That Made Chrysler the World's Hottest Car Company*. One chapter in the book is titled "When everybody else is doing it, don't." Mr. Lutz said that being different often requires "going against" traditional thinking. The late, great Zig Ziglar would have said regarding the fear of failing and the "what if" syndrome, "Get that stinkin' thinkin' out of your mind immediately."

Listen to this thought-provoking story from a person to whom we owe a debt of gratitude. Christopher Columbus was challenged by critics after discovering the Americas. They claimed that this was really no great accomplishment and that in a country like Spain, abundant with great and knowledgeable men, many could have experienced the same discovery on such an adventure. Instead of responding to the comments, Columbus asked for a whole egg to be brought to him. Upon receipt of the egg, he challenged the men present to make the egg stand on its end. All tried, and all were unsuccessful. Columbus took his turn and gently tapped the egg on the table, breaking it slightly. With this, the egg stood on its end. The confounded men exclaimed, "Anyone could have done that!" "Yes," said Columbus, "anyone could have, but only I did."

I had to ask myself these sobering questions in 2008: Is there anything in dentistry that is unique to me? Is there anything that makes me stand out from the crowd? In the "sea of sameness," what separates me from any of the other eighteen dentists in the Aberdeen community? If I get a new piece of equipment and the dentist next door does the same thing next week, does that distinguish me? If I take this new, hotter than ever continuing education course and the dentist next door follows in step, does that create a USP for me? No! Unfortunately, this keeping up with the Joneses trap is promoted by well-meaning sales people who don't always have the dentist's best interest in mind! Yes, we need to keep abreast of what is new in our field of endeavor, but somehow we need to find something within that area of interest that will differentiate us from the crowd.

Rosser Reeves in 1960 said that your USP must meet three critical criteria: (1) It must provide a specific benefit. (2) It must be something that the competition cannot, or does not, offer. (3) It must be so strong that it can move the masses.

How did SmilePalooza meet all three criteria of a killer USP? Let's carefully analyze each demand.

Did we indeed provide a specific benefit? First, we need to ask the critical question that all great marketing must address. What is the difference between a feature and a benefit? Simply stated, a feature, in the mind of the consumer, asks the question "So what?," whereas a benefit challenges the consumer with the affirmative statement "Tell me more!"

In 2008, the year of our first SmilePalooza, getting the word out to the public about a new, free, fun-filled family event happened two weeks prior to the premiere. Frantically, we purchased 900 hot dogs, thinking 300 people at best would attend and three dogs per person would be more than enough! We went through those 900 hot dogs in the first 30 minutes, and we were scrambling to feed the multitudes thereafter. Was the promotion of free food the obvious primary benefit? No! The following six events were not held over the dinner hour and the so-called meal was eliminated, but the crowds still appeared. What was the prevailing benefit? Families (grandparents, parents, and their kids) spending valuable time together and having the time of their lives! In a very small sense, we were replicating what Disney does every day of the year—providing a "memorable experience"! We were emulating Disney's definition of marketing: Do what you do so well that people can't resist telling others about you. That was the foundation of the event being successful year after year.

Did SmilePalooza offer something other dentists in my community did not offer? Yes! We were first and entirely unique! Al Ries and Jack Trout in their iconic book *The 22 Immutable Laws of Marketing: Violate Them at Your Own Risk!* have this to say about being first in the marketplace: The Law of Leadership allows you to create a category that you can be first in. Getting into the consumer's mind with a new idea, product, or service trumps coming behind and trying to convince that consumer you have something "better." Case in point: What is the name of the first person to fly the Atlantic Ocean solo? Charles Lindbergh, right? What is the name of the second person to fly the Atlantic Ocean solo? Not so easy to answer, is it? Bert Hinkler. Bert was a better pilot than Lindbergh—he flew faster, he consumed less fuel, yet who has ever heard of Bert Hinkler? In today's competitive environment, the leading brand in any category is almost always the first brand into the prospect's mind. Look no further than Coca-Cola in cola and Hertz in rent-a-car.

Were we able to meet the third criteria of a killer USP by moving the masses? The community I live in has a population of roughly 26,000 people. To have over 30,000 people attend our event over the past 7 years with some people travelling hundreds of miles just for the free entertainment validated what Dr. Robert Cialdini calls the influence of "social proof." The principle states that we determine what is correct by finding out what other people think is correct. The principle applies especially to the way we decide what constitutes correct behavior. We view a behavior as correct in a given situation to the degree that we see others performing it. The tendency to see an action as appropriate when others are doing it normally works quite well. As a rule, we will make fewer mistakes by acting in accord with social evidence than by acting contrary to it. Usually, when a lot of people are doing something, it is the right thing to do.

The Battle for Your Mind

In 1981, Jack Trout and Al Reis wrote a book titled *Positioning: The Battle for Your Mind.* The authors assert the following points about the human mind:

1. Minds are limited—they can only remember a small number of points.
2. Minds hate confusion—they are attracted to simplicity and order.
3. Minds are insecure—which is why they are so easily swayed by convincing authority.
4. Minds rarely change—they find changes so difficult.
5. Minds can lose focus—they are easily distracted and confused by vague communications or images.

Harvard psychologist George A. Miller (psychclassics.yorku.ca/Miller) conducted research on how many units of thought the average mind can retain, commonly called "The Law of the Ladder." He concluded that seven is the maximum number for most individuals. (If you are not on one of the top three rungs, you won't even be considered when prospective patients are deciding where to go for the service you offer!) In this same study, Dr. Miller revealed that 71% of people surveyed could not name a chiropractor and 52% couldn't name a dentist! My friend Dr. Mike Abernathy said this to me recently, "If you do not become remarkable in what you do in dentistry, eventually you will become invisible!" I believe Dr. Miller's research is an incredible wakeup call to all of us in the dental profession!

Build Your Brand

Brand strategy, USP, value proposition, and positioning all have their place in a total marketing strategy. Here is a definition of each and how they apply to my practice:

Positioning: Place reserved in a customer's mind for your product. Steven Van Yoder in his book *Get Slightly Famous: Become a Celebrity in Your Field and Attract More Business with Less Effort* talks about the power of your position statement. Here is the critical question: Can you tell another person in 30 seconds or less "What business you are in"? Here is my ultra-simple statement: We have created a very unique dental office experience where moms think they are at a day spa and kids think they are in the comfort of their own home!

Value proposition: The features of your product or process that can be considered as valuable for your consumer. Over 50% of Americans avoid the dentist out of fear! By creating a dental experience whereby people look forward to coming to see you (we have many testimonials that validate this) and are unhappy to leave the office because it is too enjoyable (kids having too much fun), you have an incredible value proposition!

USP: The unique feature of your product. It dictates why people buy your brand and not another brand selling the same product. SmilePalooza, Heart of Mom, and all the community involvement of our dental practice create a synergistic competitive advantage difficult to rival.

Brand strategy: All the associations you want to be made with your brand. (The combination of positioning, USP, and value proposition define our brand.)

Branding is nothing more and nothing less than helping people buy what products or services do for them! When successful, branding allows you to be the first business people think of when they need your type of service.

Here is the million-dollar question: Can you be No. 1 in another person's mental real estate? Can you be No. 1 on that mental ladder as Dr. Miller's research alluded to earlier?

David Ogilvy is one of the greatest marketers of our generation. This is what he had to say about building a brand: Any damn fool can put on a deal, but it takes genius, faith, and perseverance to create a brand. (www.azquotes.com/quote/521181). Those who dedicate their advertising/marketing to building a favorable image, the mostly sharply defined personality for their brand, are the ones who will get the largest share of the market at the highest profit.

In 2008, I unintentionally decided to create a brand that would reach out to moms and their kids. After the early success, it became very clear that to emulate Disney and even McDonald's with their focus on kids and their families was a no-brainer.

In 2011, after reading the editorial "Getting to the Heart of Mom" by Dr. Howard Farran in *Dentaltown Magazine*, I created and sold a DVD called Heart of Mom to other dentists interested in creating their own specialized kids niche. What SmilePalooza was to our external marketing USP, Heart of Mom (twenty secrets to creating a kids-focused practice moms talk about) became our internal marketing USP.

Chuck Mefford in his book *Brands Formation: How to Transform Your Healthcare Practice into a Great Local Brand* asks the following questions regarding brand creation:

- Is your brand compelling?
- Does it tell me who you are and why I should trust you?
- Does your brand show passion?
- Does it show passion for what you do?
- Is it memorable?
- Does your brand fill a need or solve a problem?

Like Disney and McDonald's, are we able to give our customers the ability to become our fans through our brand? Here are some keys:

1. *Friendliness factor:* Chick-fil-A employees say "my pleasure" as opposed to "you are welcome." Are your receptionists trained in the proper phone etiquette? Do they always answer with a smile?
2. *Go the extra mile:* One of our recent new patients wrote in her exit interview survey that she was so impressed to see one of the receptionists go out of her way to help an elderly person into the office. Her closing comment in the survey said: "That act of kindness solidified that I chose the right office for years to come."
3. *Do things others are not:* In our office, warm paraffin hand wax treatments are complimentary along with dental chairs that offer heat and massage. Kids get to write on the magical wall, receive twisted balloons, observe magic by the team, and often see Super Heroes and Disney Princesses walking the hallways.
4. *Follow-up phone call:* "Dr. Opp was wondering how you are feeling today?"
5. *Create a powerful workforce of brand believers:* TEAM (Together-Everyone-Achieves-More) players unite to create an ongoing WOW experience in the office that carries into the community.

In 2007, *Harvard Business Review* adopted the term "touchpoint" to describe instances of direct contact between a customer and a service. Branding creates expectations. Your brand is your promise. Touchpoints are the vehicles that help you deliver on your promise.

A downloadable PDF version of all the potential Touchpoints can be found at www.brandsformation.com.

"A brand is not built overnight. Success is measured in decades, not years." —Al Reis

The great football legend Vince Lombardi said it best: "The difference between a successful person and others is not a lack of strength, not a lack of knowledge, but a lack of will."

Find your brand. Constantly develop it. Stay the course!

Key Online Brand-Building Strategy

Web 3.0—What is it? Web 3.0 is a term used to separate user-centric designs from static website designs and systems used in the past.

At its heart, 3.0 is about giving users access to information and allowing them to share it. This is what makes it so incredibly valuable to you and your practice. It is also about attracting attention through different means.

There are quite a few different components to this topic as well, including the following:

- SEO (Search Engine Optimization)
- Paid Search and AdWords
- Local Search Optimization
- Social Networking and Marketing
- Mobile Marketing
- Blogging

Do yourself a favor and contact Colin Receuver at www.smartboxwebmarketing.com. He will send you information free of charge to get you up to speed on Web 3.0.

What can a focused 3.0 system do for your dental practice? Here are some results from my dental practice:

- Organic traffic increased by 179% since new website launch
- Paid traffic increased by 563% since new website launch
- Overall traffic increased by 62% since new website launch

Getting traffic is the key, but how you handle the traffic makes all the financial difference in the world. It is rare that a first-time viewer will see you online and schedule that first office appointment. Trust has yet to be established, and therein lies the strategy of "drip marketing."

Drip marketing is a method of staying in contact with your potential prospects by keeping a persistent drizzle of high-quality materials flowing to them. Information materials may come in the form of automated messages, free offers and bonuses, social network communications, and so on.

Greg Mortenson and David Oliver Relin wrote a book titled *Three Cups of Tea: One Man's Mission to Promote Peace—One School at a Time*. This is an important statement from their work: "The first time you share tea with a Balti, you are a stranger. The second time you take tea, you are an honored guest. The third time you share a cup of tea, you become family . . ."

The process of becoming familiar, and also trusted, is the goal of high-quality marketing. You introduce yourself in an official and appealing manner, and if you do well you are more than welcome to "visit" or communicate again. After a while, you are a familiar "friend" whose communications are appreciated, trusted, and respected.

If you keep dripping good information and offers for your dental services and products in front of prospective patients (and even with existing patients), you are going to create a relationship based on trust and value. This will result in the "conversion" from prospect to paying patient.

A successful drip marketing campaign is found in being persistent and consistent. The National Sales Executive Association (NSEA) found that it can take up to twelve times of contact or communication before a consumer decides to do business with a particular individual or group. (www.aa-isp.org/inside-sales-answer.php?id=246)

Glenn Fallavollita, CEO of Drip Marketing, Inc., published a study in 2010 showing that medium- to high-value sales take 15–30 "cups of tea" (telephone conversations, face-to-face meetings, voicemails, letters, emails, and so on) before a cold prospect will be converted into a paying patient. (Mortenson and Relin 2014)

Lesson learned: A static business card website has no place in your marketing arsenal. Do it right or don't waste your money!

Top Offline Brand-Building Strategies

Here are six offline ways to build your brand:

Newsletters

Newsletters are one of the best ways to stay in front of your current patients. According to Shaun Buck of Newsletter Pro, newsletters can help your business and bottom line grow in the following eight ways:

1. Increase the length of time your average customer does business with you and, in turn, increases your profits on every new and existing customer.
2. Stay top of mind.
3. It is far easier to sell more to existing customers than it is to find new customers.
4. Build your expert/celebrity status.
5. Build relationships with newsletters.
6. Newsletters help build your brand.
7. Newsletters have staying power.
8. Newsletters have pass-around value. (www.amazon.es/Newsletter-Marketing-English-EditionShaun-ebook/dp/)

Card Campaigns

From thank you notes to birthday cards, the key here is to be creative. A program that I currently use in our office is a unique strategy I borrowed from one of the top restaurant marketers in America, Rory Fatt. The birthday card we send out is custom made with a special gift to the recipient. The gift is a free dinner at a local restaurant. I do not pay for the dinner; the restaurant is more than happy to offer this incentive because it too is looking for ongoing customers. It truly is a win-win-win for all parties involved. We do a similar campaign for the children, and the free meal is at a kid-friendly restaurant. Try this concept. I guarantee you will like it!

Public Relations Enhanced Through Press Releases

I had the pleasure of working with a branding agency (Nanton Agency) in the past, and I discovered the power of targeted press releases. From local newspaper attention to television media coverage, it was a new frontier that really helped develop my TOMA (Top of the Mind Awareness) within my community.

Radio Show Host

I do not have any experience in this arena, but I know of two dentists who have cornered this market in their respective locations, Dr. Sean Tarpenning in Eau Claire, Wisconsin, and Dr. Scott Westermeier in Buffalo, New York. Reach out to them if you have the opportunity to delve into the radio spotlight.

Speak at Seminars

I had the opportunity to speak at my first seminar in October 2013. Dentist Office: Impossible was a collection of some of the top marketers in dentistry and the corporate world. I had the privilege of sharing the stage with Fred Catona of Bulldozer Digital. His marketing firm propelled Priceline.com into the fastest growing billion-dollar company in the history of business in this country. The time with Mr. Catona was absolutely special. In April 2015, I held my first 2-day solo seminar in the same location as Dentist Office: Impossible 2013. It gave me an opportunity to teach other dentists how to brand their business and recession-proof their practice for years to come!

Write a Book

In 2014, I had the privilege of coauthoring a book with one of the top sales trainers in the world, Brian Tracy. The same month *Transform Your Life, Business & Health* was released, and *The Definitive Guide to Dental Practice Success: Time-Tested Secrets to Attract New Patients & Retain Your Existing Patients* was coauthored with my good friend Jerry Jones. The coolest part of all this is to see your book page on Amazon. That is a great feeling of accomplishment.

External marketing is so much more than I can share in these pages. It is my hope that you not only learned something new, but you also were challenged by all the possibilities that await you!

Here is my parting wisdom: Wherever you amble in this life, fellow dentist, whatever be your goal; keep your eye on the donut, not the donut hole!

Continued success in your journey!

References and Additional Resources

Cialdini, R. 2007. *Influence: The Psychology of Persuasion*. New York: HarperCollins Publishers.

Farran, H. 2011. Editorial. *Dentaltown Magazine* 1: 12–14. Available at http://www.dentaltown.com

Farran, H. 2012. Editorial. *Dentaltown Magazine* 1: 16–18. Available: http://www.dentaltown.com.

Friedman, T.L. 1999. *The Lexus and the Olive Tree*, New York: Picador. Available at http://www.picadorbookroom.com.

Hogshead, S. 2010. *Fascinate: Your 7 Triggers to Persuasion and Captivation*. New York: Harper-Collins Publishers.

Levin. R. 2012. Eight permanent game-changers for today's dentist. *Dent Econ* 10. Available at http://www.dentaleconomics.com.

Levin, R. 2013a. Time for a mid-year course correction. *Dent Bus Rev* 5/6: 1. Available at http://www.levingroup.com.

Levin, R. 2013b. Explaining the new dental economy to Wall Street. *Dent Bus Rev* 7/8: 1. Available at http://www.levingroup.com.

Lutz, R. 1998. *Guts: The Seven Laws of Business That Made Chrysler the World's Hottest Car Company*. New York: John Wiley & Sons, Inc.

Marcus, S. 1997. *Minding the Store*. New York: Little, Brown & Company.

Mefford, C. 2008. *BrandsFormation: How to Transform Your Good Healthcare Practice into a Great Local Brand*. Argyle, TX: Lighthouse Communications.

Mortenson, G. and Relin, D.O. 2014. *Three Cups of Tea: One Man's Mission to Promote Peace—One School at a Time*. SmartBox Web Marketing.

Reeves, R. 1961. *Reality in Advertising*. New York: Alfred A Knopf, Inc.

Ries, A. and Trout, J. 1994. *The 22 Immutable Laws of Marketing: Violate Them at Your Own Risk!* New York: HarperCollins Publishers.

Ries, A. and Trout, J. 2000. *Positioning: The Battle for Your Mind*. New York: McGraw-Hill.

Trout, J. and Rivkin, S. 2008. *Differentiate or Die: Survival in Our Era of Killer Competition*. New York: John Wiley & Sons, Inc.

Yoder Van, S. 2007. *Get Slightly Famous: Become a Celebrity in Your Field and Attract More Business with Less Effort*. Charleston, S.C.: CreateSpace Independent Publishing Platform.

Learning Exercise

Create Your Own Unique Selling Proposition (USP)

You just purchased your first dental practice. There are eighteen other dentists in your community. You now understand that it would be incredibly strategic as a dentist/entrepreneur to create your own USP for your practice. The concept of "riches in niches" makes sense!

1. Where would you logically begin your research?
2. How do you discover what USP is available and most viable?
3. It is possible for a USP to occupy more than one practice niche?
4. How can you bring your USP and your niche together to create an ongoing brand?

Chapter 18
Internal Marketing and Customer Service

Amy Kirsch

Marketing your practice in today's tough marketplace is challenging. Many practitioners are confused about what kind of marketing (internal, external, and/or advertising) will work for them. In my experience as a dental practice management consultant throughout the United States, it is rare to meet a dentist who is "closed" to new patients. Even the busiest of practices still needs new patients to meet production, collection, and cash flow goals.

As we all know, the best new patients are those who have been referred to us by others. With a focus on internal marketing and customer service skills, you and your team will be able to separate yourself from other practices and ensure a healthy new patient flow every year. Our goal in this chapter is to give you techniques and communication skills to:

- Increase quality internal referrals as a result of the "WOW" factor
- Implement and enhance the internal marketing program in your practice
- Implement high-level customer service skills
- "WOW" each and every patient from the initial phone call through the greeting, treatment, and dismissal
- Learn skills to ensure each patient is treated like a "guest" in your practice, not a bother in your workday

Marketing and Customer Service: How Do They Relate?

Where does marketing end and customer service begin? Marketing (internal or external) is the way we attract and retain patients to our practice. Customer service skills are part of the marketing plan. Marketing and customer service skills in dentistry are closely intertwined. Without customer service skills, the marketing plan will fail. Without a marketing plan, the customer service skills may not be a priority for all of the team.

Interestingly enough, most of us in dentistry have not received any specific training or education on marketing or customer service skills. If you worked for a high-end

Dental Practice Transition: A Practical Guide to Management, Second Edition.
Edited by David G. Dunning and Brian M. Lange.
© 2016 John Wiley & Sons, Inc. Published 2016 by John Wiley & Sons, Inc.
Companion Website: www.wiley.com/go/dunning/transition

bank, restaurant, or retail store, you would receive extensive training in customer service skills before working directly with the public. Not so in dentistry.

As in any service industry, we distinguish our practices in how we communicate and how we deliver our services. To your patients, the best marketing you can do is internal marketing by providing a high level of customer service. It is low cost and has the biggest impact on patient retention, treatment acceptance, and referrals.

It is very important to be able to deliver what you promise. If you talk "quality service," you need to be able to back it up with your communication skills, facility, and technical skills. Inconsistency between your promises and the product you deliver can lead to low trust as well as decreased patient referrals and poor patient retention. Many practices that struggle with adequate new patient flow have not spent enough time on the internal marketing and customer service side of the practice and have many dissatisfied patients who do not refer and often leave the practice.

Internal Marketing

As we have discussed, many of the best patients in your practice have been referred by other patients. They already have a certain level of trust in you and your team. This trust is based on the recommendation of a friend or family member whose opinion they value. They have a higher level of treatment acceptance and retention because they were referred to your practice and did not pick your name from a list or from the internet.

Although you may need to belong to a reduced fee dental plan or have a direct mail campaign to help your practice grow, you will be able to reduce your costs and time spent recruiting new patients with a strong internal marketing plan in place. You want all patients, regardless of their referral source, to experience a high level of service, so they in turn will refer patients to the practice. A good internal marketing program has the following marketing ideas in place:

- Greet the patient (by name if possible) as he or she enters the office. If you have not met the patient before, shake hands and introduce yourself. You may come around the counter to collect any forms or insurance information from the patient.
- Eliminate any sign-in sheets you may have at the front desk.
- Be honest with your patients and let them know how long they may have to wait if there is a delay in getting them seated. Always check back with them after 10 minutes so they will not feel neglected. If you checked them in, you are responsible for following up if the clinical team is running late.
- Try to address patients by Mr., Mrs., Ms., or Dr. until they give you permission to do otherwise.
- To speed up the patient checkout, the paperwork should be completed prior to escorting him or her to the business area. Most patients have printed the necessary forms from your website and already completed them prior to the appointment.
- If a team member is busy checking out another patient, the clinical staff member should go to the next staff member for the patient's dismissal; no patient should ever be standing in line for a checkout if there is a business staff member available. It does not matter what anyone's job description is; if there is a patient who needs to be dismissed, whose payment needs to be collected, or who needs to be scheduled, any business staff member should help.

- The "90-10" rule: God gave us two ears and one mouth for a reason! We should be listening to our patients and letting them talk 90% of the time, and we should only be talking about ourselves 10% of the time.
- Use the "second question technique" to keep the patient talking. The more the patient talks, the more you get to listen. The more you listen, the more trust you build. Example: "Tell me about your trip to Hawaii. What islands did you visit? Would you go there again?"
- If you have kept a patient waiting, always say, "Thank you for your patience. I know that your time is valuable."
- Wear nametags 100% of the time. Your patients want to know your name!
- Always be on the same eye level with the person with whom you are speaking. That means not talking to patients when they are reclined or when you are behind them.
- Utilize "quality statements" about the doctors, referring doctors, and other staff members. Examples: "Jenny is an expert at dealing with insurance. Let me go get her for you." "Dr. Hite is a perfectionist and an artist when it comes to his cosmetic dentistry." "You will love Dr. Cleeves. He is an excellent oral surgeon and has a very warm personality."
- Each team member should have his or her own business card and give it to a few patients each day. Each team member should also carry several business cards and give them out in the community to friends and family.
- Weekly, each team member should write a thoughtful note on the office card stationery to a patient he or she felt a connection with or felt should receive a card for an occasion (retirement, death in the family, graduation, illness, birth of a baby, etc.)
- So that everyone can give the patient his or her full attention, no cell phones should be on at work. Personal phone calls from family and friends should be limited, and internet usage should be limited to business issues.
- The doctor should write a handwritten thank you note to referring patients.
- Gift cards should be sent to patients who refer more than one new patient into the practice. (Check with your individual State requirements regarding the legality of rewarding patients for referrals.)
- Document all referrals in the patient records and software systems (who has referred them and who they have referred).
- Complete a telephone information slip for each new patient.
- Send a "Welcome" Email or Text to each new patient prior to his or her first appointment.
- Document personal comments on each patient record (babies, pets, vacations, etc.).
- 100% postop calls for difficult cases/appointments should be made by the doctor or hygienist.
- Each team member and doctor should target a quality patient and ask him or her to refer to the practice.
- Tell each and every patient, "It was a pleasure seeing you today."
- Have lunch with one specialist (or general dentist) per month to develop a better professional relationship and to increase referrals.

The Three Levels of Patient-Friendly Customer Service

In any service industry, there are three common levels of service: minimum service, exceeding standards, and outstanding standards. For example, think of a large "box" store where you have recently shopped. You probably received (and expected) minimal service. This trip probably involved buying some basics for the office or your home, did not cost very much, and was a quick trip. You chose this store primarily because of cost and convenience and probably had low expectations for customer service. You were satisfied because your needs in shopping there were met. This is the level of minimum service.

In a dental practice, by providing minimum patient service and by meeting the patients' basic needs and expectations, patients get what they expected and are not disappointed. However, it is not a "WOW" experience. This patient will return but probably will not refer friends and/or family. As a matter of fact, patients may leave at some point because of a change in insurance, location, or one "bad" appointment. They feel no loyalty to the doctor or the team because they probably chose your office based on cost or convenience or their insurance plan.

Here are some of the basic examples of a practice that is providing minimal patient service:

- Clean facility
- Running on time
- Good telephone techniques
- Smooth-running appointments

Now think of a hotel where you have stayed that exceeded standards. It was probably a "chain" hotel at a moderate price range. They may have had chocolate on your pillow, fluffy towels, and room service. It cost more than the motel down the street, but you were comfortable paying more because you were getting more. You chose this hotel based on quality and maybe some convenience, but not solely on cost. You expected a higher level of customer service and quality and were willing to pay for it. This is an illustration of the exceeding standards level of service.

In a dental practice, the middle level of patient service is exceeding standards by anticipating the patients' needs. The dental team starts to go beyond what is expected when caring for the patient. During the morning huddle and throughout the day, the team discusses and anticipates the patients' needs, even those needs that are unexpressed by the patients. This involves the Golden Rule: "Do unto others as you would have them do unto you." This means putting yourself in the patients' shoes and looking for ways to delight them.

Here are a few of the ways in which to exceed standards and to start building loyalty from the patients in your practice:

- Appointment availability through preblocking the schedule
- Taking the time to actively listen and build rapport with your patients
- Knowing your patients' hobbies, family, vacation, and occupation
- Up-to-date with technology and continuing education
- Strong emphasis on patient education
- Cohesive team
- Complaints are handled within 24 hours
- 100% postop calls for difficult cases/appointments are made by the doctor or hygienist

Finally, what is the nicest restaurant you have ever been to? It may have been on your anniversary, your birthday, or another special occasion; hopefully, you had a "WOW" experience. They anticipated your needs even before you did. It was not cheap, you had planned to be there a while because of the experience, and now you cannot wait to go back! This is an example of the outstanding standards level of service.

In the highest level of customer service of outstanding standards, the dental team is creating loyalty by anticipating the patients' needs and wants. This high level of patient service is based on focusing entirely on the patient instead of on ourselves. This relationship style of customer service is rewarding for the patient and results in an overwhelmingly positive response from your patient. The patient feels valued and will actively refer to your practice.

To create patient loyalty, the team offers special and unique benefits to make the patients feel comfortable in the practice:

- Warm face cloth
- Coffee, juice, water
- Relaxing, up-to-date facility
- Professionally dressed doctor and team
- Documented personal comments in the patient records
- Recognition and rewards for referrals (as allowed by each individual State)
- Thorough and comprehensive new patient exam
- Uninterrupted time with the doctor to establish rapport and discuss dental needs

Now how does this apply to your dental practice? What level of service is your practice offering?

Excellence in Communication Skills

Another way patients judge the quality of care in the practice is how we communicate with them. They cannot judge the quality of the crown or the hygiene prophylaxis, but they do know how they were treated. How we communicate and the words we choose can make the difference in establishing patient loyalty and satisfaction. Here are some of the most important customer service skills to use every day in your practice:

- "I apologize . . ." not "I am sorry . . ." (for placing a patient on hold, keeping a patient waiting, etc.)
- "It would be my pleasure . . . ," "It is my pleasure . . . ," "It was my pleasure . . . ," "My pleasure . . . ," not "No problem," "You bet," "No big deal"
- Say "absolutely" to patient requests
- Avoid the word "policy"; you have "procedures" and "arrangements"
- You have "fees," not "prices"
- Never say "no" to a patient. Always say, "I wish I could, however . . ." or "I would love to be able to, however . . ."
- No discussion of sex, drugs, politics, or religion in the office
- "Discomfort" not "pain"
- No lecturing or placing blame on the patient (respect-based communication versus shame-based communication)

Asking for Referrals

When was the last time a patient called and asked your business team member, "Are you accepting new patients?" (It was probably last week.) It is surprising to all of us how many of your existing patients do not know that you are gladly accepting new patients. Why is this? It is probably because we have not communicated this well to our patients. After all, our reception room is usually full, they wait 10–15 minutes to be seen, and they cannot get an appointment with your hygienist for 6 weeks.

Many businesses (realtors, beauty salons, insurance agents) are comfortable asking clients to refer, but most dentists and their teams are not. It feels like you are begging or that you are desperate for new patients. The key in asking for referrals is targeting who to ask for a referral, when to ask for a referral, and developing the communication skills to ask for a referral. Team members who regularly ask quality patients to refer to the practice see an average of a 20% increase in internal referrals. Here are the four steps in asking a patient for a referral:

Step 1: Solicit a compliment or receive a compliment from a patient. "Thank you for letting me know about how comfortable your injection was today. I will make sure to let Dr. Thompson know." "I am so glad that your cleaning with Julie was so thorough. Thanks for letting me know." "How was your new patient exam with Dr. Thompson?"

Step 2: Statement about the quality or the philosophy of care in your practice. "I am so glad that you let me know how much you like your new bridge. Dr. Thompson is such a perfectionist and an artist with his dentistry. He always strives to make his bridges look as natural as possible." "Thanks for the feedback about your new patient exam today. It is very important to Dr. Thompson that he gets to know you and your mouth before he starts any treatment." "I am glad you liked your cleaning today. It is important to me to be thorough but also gentle at the same time."

Step 3: Transitional statement. "Occasionally, we see patients who were surprised how painless dentistry can really be." "You would be surprised how many patients did not know that a dental procedure could be so comfortable."

Step 4: Asking for referral. "If we are not already seeing your husband we would love to have him as a patient in our practice." "If you know of anyone else looking for this type of dental practice, we would appreciate you referring them to us." "As you probably know, we do not advertise for new patients. Our new patients are referred to us from existing patients. If you work with anyone who is looking for a quality dental practice, we would love to see them."

First Impressions Count

Is your phone answered within three rings by a friendly, unrushed team member? Does he or she have a "smile" in his or her voice? We have all heard the adage, "You only have one chance to make a good first impression." The new patient telephone call is the first opportunity to impress the new patient.

Some of the goals in this important phone call are to impress the caller with your organization and professionalism; to gather pertinent information; to complete a telephone information slip; and to have the patient schedule an appointment. The business team member should follow a script but be flexible enough to answer most of the patient's questions concisely. Here is a typical script for a new patient phone call:

Team:	"Good morning, Dr. Smith's office. Jeanne speaking. How may I help you?"
Pt:	*"I would like to make an appointment to see Dr. Smith."*
Team:	"I would be happy to make that appointment for you. How long has it been since you have seen Dr. Smith?"
Pt:	*"Actually, I have never seen Dr. Smith before."*
Team:	"So you are a new patient? Welcome to our practice! So that I may properly appoint you, do you mind if I ask you a few questions?"
Pt:	*"No, not at all."*
Team:	"Tell me what kind of an appointment you feel you need."
Pt:	*"Well, I just moved here a few months ago and I am overdue for my regular check-up and cleaning."*
Team:	"So you would like to have your teeth cleaned on the first visit to our office?"
Pt:	*"Yes, that would be great."*
Team:	"I would love to schedule that appointment for you. In our office, we have five different kinds of cleanings and we work with two different hygienists. To save you time and money, Dr. Smith would like to meet you first, complete a thorough examination, and then make a recommendation for the type of cleaning that is best for you. How does that sound?"
Pt:	*"It sounds good. Can I have my teeth cleaned at that visit also?"*
Team:	"Absolutely! Just a few more questions before we schedule your appointment. Has any dentist or doctor told you that you needed antibiotics prior to a dental visit?" (You may need to explain the reason you have asked this question.) "Can you tell me when you last had dental x-rays taken? What kind of x-rays were they?" (You may need to explain the different kinds of x-rays.) "Where are they located? Can you call and have them emailed to our office?" (Note: If the x-rays are over 2 years old, they may need to be updated.) "To provide you with a thorough exam, Dr. Smith would like to have some new x-rays. We can take those at the first appointment also. Let's go ahead and schedule an appointment for you to meet Dr. Smith and to have a thorough examination of your mouth and teeth. We will also take the necessary films and schedule an appointment with one of our great hygienists. I have an opening on Monday, April 12, at 8:30 a.m. or Wednesday, April 14, at 11:00 a.m. Which one will work better for you?" (Notice the patient chooses from two options given.)
Pt:	*"Monday at 8:30."*
Team:	"Do you have any dental benefits that will be helping you with your treatment? Do you mind sharing that information with me?" (Note: If you are not a participating member of their insurance: "I wish we were a participating member of ____. However, the good news is that we accept all dental insurance benefits. Do you know if you can see a dentist out of your network? Normally, there is slight cost for the patient to see a dentist out of network. We have a lot of patients who come to see us even though we are not on their list." [Note: Why your doctor is not a participating member: "I wish we could participate with the ___ plan. However, we have found that to provide our patients with the highest level of care, the doctor is uncomfortable with an insurance company influencing the kind of care he provides to his patients."]) "Who may we thank for referring you to our office?"
Pt:	*"Maggie Jones, from my church."*
Team:	"Maggie is great and sends us the nicest patients. We will be sure to thank her. Have you been to our website yet? To save you time at the first appointment, you can print and complete the New Patient forms in advance of the appointment and bring them with you. May I have your email address, home address, and phone number? Is there a cell number or work number that you would like to give us?"

Pt: *"Sure. My address is 155 Main Street, Parker 80111. My phone at home is 303-796-0098 and work is 303-798-7763. I do not use my cell phone very much."*

Team: "Is there anything else you feel I need to know before we see you next week?"

Pt: *"Yes, I am kind of a chicken when it comes to dentistry. Is Dr. Smith gentle?"*

Team: "Yes, he is very gentle and a good listener. Please feel free to share any concerns or fears with him when you see him. He wants you to be comfortable. Thank you for calling our office. We look forward to meeting you next week. In the meantime, if you have any questions or concerns, feel free to give me a call. We look forward to seeing you Monday, April 12th at 8:30 am."

The Welcome Packet

The welcome packet is your second opportunity to impress your new patient with your organization and image. The goal is to allow patients the opportunity to complete their paperwork at home and encourage them to keep their appointment. This packet is emailed to your patient or downloaded from your website in advance of their appointment. A new patient would receive a "Welcome Email" from the office and could include the following:

- The Welcome letter (see Figure 18.1)
- Patient registration form
- Medical history form
- Link for directions to the office

Date
Patient Name
Street Address
City, State, Zip
Dear (Patient Name),

A very warm welcome to you. The entire team would like to thank you for selecting our office to care for your dental needs.

Our goals are to provide you with the highest quality dental care in a gentle, efficient, and pleasant manner, and to strongly encourage prevention of future dental problems.

Generally, the first visit will include a thorough examination and necessary x-rays for proper diagnosis, followed by a consultation of your dental needs (unless you have a particular dental problem requiring immediate attention). Treatment costs will be discussed, and financial arrangements can be made.

Please complete both sides of the enclosed health questionnaire and bring it with you for your first visit. Also, so we may assist you in filing any claims, if you have dental insurance, please bring your completed and signed forms.

Should you have any questions, please call at your convenience. Our team is looking forward to meeting you.

Welcome!

Figure 18.1. Welcome letter No. 1.

Date
Patient Name
Street Address
City, State, Zip
Dear (Patient Name),

  We are delighted to welcome you to our practice, and we are pleased that you chose us to serve your dental needs. It was a pleasure meeting with you on Thursday, February 15, 2008.

  We are serious about providing superior dental care, and we are proud of our dedication to our patients. Our goal is to help you feel and look your best through excellent dental care. We look forward to seeing you on a regular basis.

Sincerely,

Figure 18.2.   Welcome letter No. 2.

Do not include your financial policies, HIPAA forms, hours, or scheduling guidelines. These can become objections to keeping the appointment and may be reviewed after the new patient exam.

After the new patient exam has been completed, a second patient letter or email should be sent. The intent of the letter or email is to thank and encourage your new patient. See Figure 18.2.

Morning Huddle

An important part of internal marketing and customer service is preparing for your day with a 15-minute meeting prior to the start of the day. This all-team meeting allows the team to problem solve, to discuss the schedule for the day, and to follow through with the marketing goals for that day.

The best huddles are facilitated by a business team member who follows an outline. All team members are on time and have reviewed their charts and patients for the day. The huddle also includes a motivational statement to ensure that the day starts on a positive note. Read more about staff meetings in Chapter 24. Here is a typical outline for an effective morning huddle:

- Identify emergency and catch-up times
- Identify patients who have a medical alert or who should be premedicated
- Verify lab/implant cases
- Discuss challenging patients and procedures
- Discuss any changes from routine
- Identify and discuss patients with outstanding restorative needs
- Yesterday's schedule: What went right and wrong?
- Today's schedule: Are there any problem areas?
- Next available major appointment
- Next available minor appointment
- New patient information
- Emergency patient information

- Financial information
- Marketing information
- Yesterday's productivity
- Daily production goal for today: Has it been reached?
- Motivational statement

Periodically, you need to evaluate your morning huddle by asking yourself and writing down the answers to the following two questions:

- What is working well with our morning huddle?
- What do I need to do to improve effectiveness of our morning huddle?

Portraying a Professional Image

How important is the appearance of your office? Do the patients really care and do they even notice? Since patients cannot personally judge the quality of a dentist's care, they often use other criteria to measure the practice, the dentist, and the team.

Patients will judge the appearance and location of the facility. If the carpet is stained, they may feel the treatment rooms are also not clean. If the lamp in the reception room is 20 years old, they may feel that your clinical skills are also not up-to-date.

Patients like to be in a professional, warm, and inviting office. They also want to be associated with a successful practice. This does not mean you should have an over-the-top, high-end, or expensive-looking office. However, it does need to reflect the quality of your care and your commitment to a professional up-to-date practice.

Clutter needs to be reduced in the business office, the clinical rooms, and even in the doctor's office (if patients see it), so as to reflect an organized and professional environment. Posters need to be replaced with artwork, charts need to be taken to the storage room, and the consultation room may need to be spruced up. Maybe a fresh coat of paint and new reception chairs will make a big difference. When was the last time you updated your office?

Another way patients judge the quality of your practice is by the way you and your team are dressed. As a rule, the doctor and the business team need to be dressed one level higher than the average patient. For the male dentists, this usually means nice dress pants, a starched shirt, and sometimes a tie. Do not overlook the nice shoes, socks, and watch (but not an expensive one!). Many doctors wear lab coats over their business causal clothes.

For a female dentist, it is very important to dress for success. Because there are typically many women in a dental office, the female practitioner needs to distinguish herself by dressing differently than the staff. Again, business casual is the recommended style with a lab coat.

For a higher case acceptance, and to be able to gain respect and trust with patients, it is highly recommended for all doctors not to wear scrubs unless they are in a hospital setting.

Business staff members should wear business casual clothes because they are dealing with patient financing and scheduling. They are influential members of the team and need to dress the part.

The clinical team should wear matching uniforms or scrubs with lab coats. Patients love the look of a clinical team when team members are dressed alike.

Guidelines for Dental Dress for Success

Business staff should wear coordinating business attire in the business area of the office. You are a representative of the practice. You deal with patients' finances, treatments plans, and scheduling, and therefore you need to demonstrate a successful and professional appearance.

When there are more than two business staff people, it is recommended that the office manager arrange for the staff to meet with a designated sales person at one or two stores. The staff will be directed as to the appropriate styles that would then be approved by the manager (and/or doctors). Recommended:

- Coordinating jacket, sweater sets, skirts, and/or pants
- "Classic" look and classic colors are preferable
- Closed-toe shoes (dress boots are acceptable)
- Appropriate undergarments (no lingerie showing at any time)
- Skirts no shorter than 3″ above the knee
- Conservative jewelry
- Tops and jackets must cover top of the arm
- Appropriate makeup
- Clean, attractive nails

Not acceptable:

- Tank tops or bare arms
- Low cut blouses (or showing cleavage)
- Short skirts (shorter than 3″ above your knee)
- Sandals of any kind
- Denim of any kind
- Cargo pants
- Corduroy
- Five-pocket style pants
- Sweatpants or sweatshirts
- Midriff showing
- Visible tattoos
- Excessive jewelry (one ring per hand, no more than two earrings per ear)
- No tongue piercing or other visible piercing (other than ears)
- Chipped nail polish

The Significance of the Team to the Patient

We all know that the dentist's best asset is his or her dental team. The dental team is on the front line with customer service and internal marketing implementation. Team continuity is more important to patients than dentists realize. Staff continuity is a valuable indicator in predicting high patient retention and referrals. Hiring individuals who have the willingness and ability to deliver is also vital to an effective and profitable practice. Many dentists hire staff based on skill versus personality and fall short in delivering the best in customer service.

By working with team members in dental practices for many years, we find that the most committed team members are people who are motivated by the following:

- A chance to do something well
- A chance to change the way things are
- A chance to do something that makes them feel good about themselves as people
- A chance to do something worthwhile
- An opportunity to develop new skills
- The amount of freedom that they have at their job
- Peers letting them know they did a job well
- Manager letting them know they did a job well
- Patients letting them know they have given them a great service
- Being compensated well for a job well done
- Appreciation for a job well done
- Being in control of their area or of a certain situation
- Having specific goals
- Having rewards when expectations have been met

Definitions of Patient Service

- The point is to not only satisfy your patients but also delight them.
- Do unto others as you would have them do unto you.
- Total quality in the services you provide and how you deliver them.
- What feels right to the patient?
- Giving the patient what he or she wants.
- Involves willingness to see the practice from the patients' point of view.
- Eagerness to move swiftly.
- Everyone working together while keeping the patient in focus and the No.1 priority.
- Overlooking personal needs for those of the patient.
- Commitment to accuracy, follow-through, and details with all the key systems in the practice.

Dental practices that commit and focus on their internal marketing and customer service skills will see an increase in quality new patients. Creating great first impression with your phone skills, an updated facility and modern technology will start the process of building trust with your patients. The focus on building relationships with your patients and treating them as family will increase referrals and case acceptance.

References and Additional Resources

King, L. 2004. *How to Talk to Anyone, Anytime, Anywhere*. New York: Random House.
Stratten, S. 2012. *UnMarketing*. New Jersey: John Wiley & Sons, Inc.
Timm, P. 2002. *50 Powerful Ideas You Can Use to Keep Your Customers*. New Jersey: Career Press.
Vaynerchuk, G. 2011. *The Thank You Economy*. New York: HarperCollins.
Williams, Bryan. 2004. Lecture comments, *Legendary Service at the Ritz*. Denver, CO, April.

Learning Exercises

1. List five areas of customer service and internal marketing you and your team could implement in the next 30 days.
2. List five areas of customer service and internal marketing you and your team could implement in the next 12 months.
3. Customer service skills "fill in the blank:"
   A. Say _____ not "I'm sorry."
   B. Say _____ to patient requests.
   C. Say _____ not "pain."
   D. You have _____, not "prices."
   E. Say _____ not "no problem."
   F. Never say "no" to a patient; always say _____
      or _____.
4. List five areas you could improve in your facility to enhance the image of the office.
5. How can you ensure your patients have a good first impression of the office?

Chapter 19
Chairside Communication with Patients

David G. Dunning and Brian M. Lange

Goals of Communication

"The single biggest problem in communication is the illusion that it has taken place."
—George Bernard Shaw

Led by the dentist, the dental team must strive to achieve the following three goals in patient communication (Cassell 1985; Dunning and McFarland 2014): (1) educate patients about their health and treatment, (2) assist patients to make decisions in their best health interest in the short and long term, and (3) develop a trust-based patient–provider relationship while also empathetically communicating with patients and minimizing physical discomfort. Foundational skills also include cultural and linguistic competencies as well as identifying and adapting to the patient's level of health literacy.

Communication Strategies

"Think like a wise man but communicate in the language of the people."
—William Butler Yeats

Dunning and McFarland (2014) recommend these communication strategies in order to achieve the three core outcomes highlighted above.

Before Treatment Begins

- Accurately and regularly update the patient's medical history to ensure that no care has contraindications due to other existing health issues.
- Explain dental care in terms understood by patients.
- Discuss treatment options and financial arrangements with patients, including dental insurance coverage if available.

Dental Practice Transition: A Practical Guide to Management, Second Edition.
Edited by David G. Dunning and Brian M. Lange.
© 2016 John Wiley & Sons, Inc. Published 2016 by John Wiley & Sons, Inc.
Companion Website: www.wiley.com/go/dunning/transition

- Utilize visual aids in explaining dental disease and dental care. Visual aids could include models, diagrams, video clips, radiographic images, or images from an intraoral camera.
- Ask the patient about any questions they have (e.g., "What questions may I answer for you about your dental care today?").
- Answer patient questions in terms they understand.
- Discuss patient anxieties about care and offer strategies for managing anxiety.
- Negotiate a nonverbal signal (such as a raised hand) through which patients may suspend treatment momentarily by communicating any unusual discomfort or sensations.
- Ask open-ended questions and listen to patients in a nonjudgmental, curious manner about their goals and expectations, for example, "Ideally, how would you describe how your mouth, teeth, and tissues look and feel 20 years from now?" "What do you expect from me as a dentist/assistant/hygienist?"
- Provide feedback to the patient about brushing, flossing, and other health behaviors related to oral health, and offer assistance in developing related skills and setting goals to achieve these skills. One approach to persuading patients to change is motivational interviewing—a nonjudgmental approach in which patients identify their goals and the provider helps coach the patient in ways to achieve goals. For example, a provider might begin such a discussion by asking the patient, "How would you like your teeth to appear when you are 70 years of age?"
- Ultimately, one criterion used to gauge the effectiveness of communication prior to dental treatment is the question, "Can patients identify the tooth/teeth/tissues involved in treatment and can the patients explain in their own words what care will be provided and why?"

During Treatment

- "Provide informative updates about the progress of the appointment (e.g., "All of the decay has now been removed and we are ready to restore or fill the tooth").
- Forewarn the patient about or at least check on the patient's comfort when performing potentially uncomfortable steps (e.g., pinch for injections, vibration for hand-pieces (drills), pressure when using hand instruments, and so forth).
- Notice and acknowledge during treatment both intentional and unintentional nonverbal messages of discomfort (such as squinting, twitching, "white knuckles").
- Demonstrate empathy to patients through a combination of words and nonverbal communication, acknowledging and attending to discomfort, addressing and offering options for fears, anxieties, and physical sensations.

Acknowledge special communication challenges presented in dental treatment: numbness, use of a rubber dam, and fingers and instruments filling the patient's mouth physically hinder a patient's ability to talk, so much so that a common complaint of patients is that dentists ask patients questions when the patient is physically unable to respond."

After Treatment

- Inform the patient about potential and expected post-treatment sensations and complications (e.g., "Teeth may be sensitive to hot and cold temperatures after being treated; this sensitivity should subside in a few days"). Common procedures such as extractions and endodontic therapy (root canals) have essentially standardized postoperative instructions as would certain types of surgery.

• Call, text, or e-mail patients after particularly difficult or potentially uncomfortable dental care.

Delivery of Bad News

A growing body of research has addressed how to deliver bad news in health care and other settings. Dentists must occasionally deliver news that patients may perceive as "bad": news such as a tooth that cannot be saved and requires extraction, extensive and unexpected needed treatment, the need for endodontic therapy, the need to a biopsy to diagnose unhealthy oral tissue, and so on.

Curtin and McConnell (2012) describe a "SPIKES" model consisting of the following stages: *S*etting up the interview, exploring *P*atient perceptions of their situation, *I*nviting patients to indicate how much they want to know, providing *K*nowledge and information, *E*mpathizing/exploring, and *S*trategizing/summarizing. In a model with similar stages, Guneri, Epstein, and Botto (2013) outline an *ABCDE* model: preparing in *A*dvance, *B*uilding a therapeutic relationship/environment, *C*ommunicating effectively, *D*ealing with reactions, and *E*ncouraging/validating emotions. Both models emphasize the need for the dentist to purposefully utilize active listening and to express empathy in setting the situation (physically and socially), framing the context (asking questions about patient/family knowledge, interest, and awareness), actually delivering the news (being succinct, avoiding the use of jargon, managing under- and overinforming), and planning with patients for their oral health (discussing next treatment steps).

Word Choice

> "By your word you will be justified, and by your words you will be condemned."
> —Jesus

Perhaps it goes without saying that word/phrase choice is foundationally important in chairside communication. The following list of words/phrases to use and avoid with patients has been compiled over the years from thousands of hours of clinical observations, conversations with patients and dentists, classroom sessions, and expert sources such as Miles (2003).

Use with Patients	Avoid with Patients
Numb up your tooth or administer anesthetic	Shot; needle
Extract or remove	Pull/yank
Discomfort/sensitivity	Pain/hurt[a]
Remove decay	Grind; drill
Remove build-up or decay	Scrape
Shape tooth/prepare tooth	Grind; drill
Measure tightness of your gums/tissue	Probe
Protect/strengthen your tooth with a crown used as a as a noun)	Crown (especially when verb or alone
With your permission . . .	Policy requires . . .

(Continued)

Use with Patients	Avoid with Patients
Necessary x-rays	Full mouth series
Restore form and function	Fill tooth/filling/patch
Tooth-colored material	Composite
Silver-colored material	Amalgam

[a] Dental patients obviously do experience pain! Please refer to the next chapter section. The suggestion here is that its use prudently parallel patient experiences such as clinical situations involving an abscessed or infected tooth, perio/gum surgery, or extraction of third molars. Patients with routine dental treatment such as exams, cleanings/prophys, and restorations should typically not experience "pain."

Suggested Scripts

As a foundational step in developing a patient management competency project, Dr. Kate Wolford (at the time a D3 student) developed a series of simple scripts. The scripts have been refined and posted on the website accompanying this book. The scripts provide straightforward explanations of nine common dental appointments. While specific points vary based on the type of treatment being provided, the scripts have four common features: augmenting explanations with visual aids such as procedural animations and intraoral camera images, utilizing "therapeutic" language and word choice understood by lay people, asking patients for questions, and negotiating a discomfort cue. Readers interested in practical application of some of the key points in this chapter are encouraged to review, edit, and utilize the suggested scripts accessible in the supplemental information for this chapter on the companion book website.

Management of Anxious, Fearful, and Phobic Patients

The basic building blocks for reducing anxiety, managing patient fear(s), and helping patients manage discomfort (pain) correlate directly with the communication strategies outlined above. Namely, you fulfill your due diligence responsibilities by preparing yourself and your patient before treatment begins, keeping the patient involved in the treatment process, and providing after care that meets or exceeds patient expectations.

ANXIETY

A simple definition of anxiety is fear of the unknown. Anxiety is worry, apprehension, and somatic symptoms that are similar to the tension caused when an individual anticipates impending danger or misfortune. A patient experiencing symptoms of anxiety over seeing the dentist can be helped by the dentist if the dentist uses the following patient management sequence:

- Meet with the patient prior to beginning the dental examination to determine the reason for the patient's visit. Explain the examination process. Walk them through the examination process. If needed, assure them that all findings and options for treatment will be explained to them.
- When presenting findings, encourage the patient to put up questions. Use the opportunity to educate your patient and explain treatment options, including time,

Table 19.1 Physical symptoms of anxiety.

Heart Palpitations	Trembling
Shortness of breath	Sharp pains or discomfort in the chest
Difficulty in swallowing	Abdominal-stomach pain
Hot or cold flashes	Nausea and vomiting
Fears of losing control or dying	Dizziness—lightheadedness

cost of procedure(s), and benefits of your treatment proposal. Reassure the patient that you want them to understand the rational for suggested treatment and be comfortable with treatment that they choose to proceed with.

- Have them state in their own words why they need treatment, what the treatment will consist of and their expectations when finished with treatment. After they provide you with the above information you can correct any misconceptions prior to treatment.
- Patient participation in their treatment, as outlined above, should remove the unknown and reduce or resolve anxiety surrounding their treatment.

If after following the above suggested process the patient either says he or she is anxious or demonstrates physical symptoms of anxiety (Table 19.1), you will need to differentiate between unresolved dental fear and a dental phobia.

FEAR

Fear is a word used to describe a person's emotional reaction to something that seems dangerous. Fear can also be used as a noun for something a person feels afraid of. According to Milgrom, Weinstein, and Getz (1995), about two-thirds of dental patients relate their dental fear to bad experiences in the dentist's office. Another third have other issues for which the fear of the dentist is a side effect, such as an anxiety disorder, PTSD, substance abuse problem, victims of domestic violence, victims of sexual abuse, and psychiatric disorders.

Management of a patient that is fearful, like treating the anxious patient, focuses on giving the patient as much input and control of their treatment as is possible and still provide quality dentistry. See the "During Treatment" section under "Communication Strategies" above.

Treating anxious and fearful patients is not for all dentists. Some dentists lack the patience, or do not want to allow for the time it would take, to reassure and encourage patients that are dealing with anxiety and fear. You will need to make a conscious decision about the cliental your office will serve. Once you have made the decision of cliental you want to serve, it will help you in building a staff that will help meet your goals and help develop/reinvent your internal and external marketing strategies.

PHOBIA

People with specific phobias, or strong irrational fear reactions, commonly focus on animals, insects, germs, heights, thunder, driving, flying, public transportation, dental or medical procedures, and elevators. Although people with phobias realize that their fear is irrational, even thinking or talking about it can cause extreme anxiety. The fear may not make any sense, but they feel like they are unable to stop it. People having a phobia or phobias can lead a disrupted life because they will go out of their way to avoid the uncomfortable and often terrifying feelings of phobic anxiety (Bourne 2015).

Assuming a phobic patient does not have a dental emergency, it is best to refer him or her for therapy to address his or her phobia(s) prior to attempting dental treatment. Options include mental health professionals that utilize the technique of systematic desensitization to, over time, gradually expose the patient in a controlled environment to the things they fear. This can be an effective form of treatment for dental phobias. Other techniques used by mental health therapists include cognitive therapy and psychotherapy. Another option is to have the patient attend dental phobia clinics, which are offered by some hospitals and some dental schools (De Jongh et al., 1995).

If a person with a dental phobia has been injured or is in severe pain due to dental neglect, your options may be limited to intravenous sedation or general anesthesia. General anesthesia should be administered in a hospital setting.

Pain Management

This section is intended to provide a working definition of pain, from the patient's point of view, and to identify the tools you have as a dentist to help your patients manage dental pain.

Pain is defined as physical suffering or discomfort caused by disease process, illness, or injury. The cause of the pain can be physical and/or mental. Pain defined by a layperson is something that hurts. In other words, pain is subjective and individual.

There are several resources available to help you understand the theory of pain, including factors that contribute to a person's perception and management of pain. (http://www.jn.physiology.org/content/1091/1/5) (http://brainblogger.com/2014/06/23/gate-control-theory-and-pain-management) A review of the factors that contribute to a person's perception and management of pain would be helpful in choosing the best tools to help patients manage discomfort and pain. For example, a person with a history of drug abuse should not be prescribed medications that will reinforce his or her use of drugs or cause a potential relapse. Additionally, if you have a patient with severe rheumatoid arthritis who is on pain medication, you may need to consult with his or her physician to determine the best way to manage any additional pain that is the by-product of any procedure you might perform.

There can be a relationship between anxiety, fear, and pain. The relationship works like this: a person has a bad dental experience, pain during and/or after a dental procedure that he or she was not prepared for or did not expect, and/or he or she perceived the dentist to be insensitive to his or her needs. In the above scenario the mental link between dental pain, anxiety, and/or fear is made in the patient's mind. Going to the dentist now becomes associated with pain, which may lead to anxiety and fear at the thought of having to go to the dentist. Again, the best practice to reduce such anxiety and fear is to follow the communication process outlined above for the pretreatment, during, and after treatment and to give the patient as much input and control during the appointment as is practical.

Management Tools

When you only have a hammer, does everything look like a nail? Some dentists approach pain management like a carpenter with only one tool in his or her tool box. That is, they use only IV sedation or nitrous on all patients. There are so many more interesting and effective tools to use in helping patients manage anxiety, fear, and pain. Our choices can be grouped into the categories of behavioral management, relaxation, sedation, hypnosis, spiritual, and the use of support groups. These tools are most effective if used in combination, and are matched with our patient's psychological or emotional needs.

Behavioral Management

Our first and one of the most powerful tools in this category is the CUE. For our purposes a cue is anything that excites action, creates a frame of mind, or mood, in other words, a stimulus. Cues can be subtle or obvious. For example, subtle cues include location of your office, the arrangement and decoration of your office, background music, the appearance of your front desk staff, the layout of the operatory, and your personal appearance. Obvious cues include the greeting of the patient by your staff, your greeting of the patient, and the presentation of your bill. Unthank design is an example of a firm that can help you create the positive subtle cues to help relax your patients. You and your team must work on developing obvious cues. For example, work with your staff to create a warm welcoming reception for your patients, something beyond "Please update your health and insurance forms while you wait for your appointment." You also must work on greeting patients in a way that creates a positive expectation. For example, rather than "Hi, Mrs. Green. How are you today?" how about "It is really good to see you today. Last time I saw you, you were getting ready to go on vacation. How was your vacation?" or for the anxious child "Hi Emma it is good to have you come in today. Let's take a little tour of the office and then take a look at your teeth. Doesn't that sound like fun?" Using positive cues does help to distract and refocus patients. However, if their anxiety and/or fear level remain(s) high even after your and the staffs' best efforts, you will need to explore further to uncover the source of the anxiety and/or fear.

A fun tool, even for adults, is the show-tell-do approach to presenting the treatment of the day. This approach allows for questions from patients and helps them build a mental image and time line for the treatment they are about to receive. The show-tell-do tool helps reduce anxiety and helps build a bond with the patient.

Another tool is distraction. Distractions may come in several forms. Questions to the patient about something important to them can serve as a distractor. We all like to talk about things we are interested in. Distraction can include listening to music the patient chooses, watching a TV in the operatory, and talking to the patient while giving an injection.

Relaxation

Relaxation techniques are easy for the patient to learn. However, to achieve the best results, practice is necessary. Relaxation can take the form of listening to soothing music, nature sounds, deep breathing, guided imagery and progressive relaxation.

Sedation

Sedatives such as diazepam relax the central nervous system and help people feel calmer and more relaxed. However, sedatives can take 30 minutes to work and the side effects like drowsiness can last for hours.

Hypnosis

The effects of hypnosis are similar to the effects of sedation, without the side effects. Hypnosis may be guided by either the individual (self-hypnosis) or the dentist or the patient's therapist, through the use of suggestions to relax the body and redirect conscious thought, which leads to a relaxed body and mind.

Spiritual

People of faith may use prayer and meditation on the Word of God as a way to focus their mind and priorities. Studies have shown the positive mental and physical results of people that pray and patients that are prayed for. Prayer is often ignored because it is not well understood, the topic makes many people feel uncomfortable to talk about and some care providers fear they might offend patients. Most likely, if your patient is a person of faith, he or she will be praying about his or her treatment and any concerns he or she has with or without your suggestion to pray. If you and your patient are both people of faith, praying together will benefit you and your patient (http://www. webmd.com/balance/features/can-prayer-heal?).

Support Group

Many types of support groups exist to help people overcome or manage a host of issues or conditions. Support groups include people dealing with addictions, grief, weight loss, being a foster parent, spousal abuse and many, many others issues. Support groups exist to help people with anxiety and phobias and can be suggested as an option to help manage anxiety. Support groups are, obviously, intended to provide support, not treatment. Therefore, patients with severe anxiety and/or a phobia also need to be in treatment for their anxiety and/or phobia.

Special Needs Patients

Dental patients with special needs may include the following:

- Aging and elderly
- Individuals with mobility problems
- Individuals with mental or physical disabilities
- Immunocompromised individuals
- People with complex medical issues
- People with mental illness
- Children with behavioral or emotional conditions

Among the accommodations that dental patients with special needs may require include the following:

- An efficient and systematic approach to the examination and treatment so that appointments are short when necessary
- Knowledge of the medical, physical, mental, or behavioral condition in order to best manage appointments and oral health
- More chairside assistance during examinations and treatment to better control and monitor the patient
- Sedation dentistry to promote patient comfort if longer appointments are required
- Flexible appointment scheduling
- Caregiver or case manager involvement in treatment planning, providing instructions and information during treatment, and insuring patient brushes and flosses or has someone who ensures a high level of home oral health care

When considering acceptance of patients with special needs into your practice, you may want to focus on one or two special need conditions. By limiting your treatment to one or two special need conditions, you and your staff can become proficient and reduce the length of appointments and increase patient-caregiver satisfaction. See the following website for more information: http://www.yourdentistryguide.com/special-needs/.

Book Companion Website

The book companion website at www.wiley.com/go/dunning/transition includes additional material for this chapter that is not included in the printed version of the book. Please see *About the Companion Website* at the start of the book for details on how to access the website.

References and Additional Resources

www.adaa/understanding-anxiety/DSM-5-changes.

Botto, Ronald. 2006. Chairside techniques for reducing dental fear. In: Mostofsky, David I., Forgione, Albert, and Giddon, Donald (Eds.), *Behavioral Dentistry*. Ames, IA: Blackwell.

Bourne, Edmund J. 2015. *The Anxiety and Phobia Workbook*, 6th ed. Oakland CA: New Harbinger Publications.

Cassell, Eric. 1985. In: Cassell, Eric J. (Ed.), *Talking with Patients*, Vol. 2. Cambridge, MA: MIT Press.

Curtin, Sharon and McConnell, Mary. 2012. Teaching dental students how to deliver bad news: S-P-I-K-E-S model. *J Dent Edu* 76(3): 360–365.

De Jongh, A., Muris, P., Horst, G. Ter, van Zuuren, F., Schoenmakers, N., and Makkes, P. 1995. One-session cognitive treatment of dental phobia: preparing dental phobics for treatment by restructuring negative cognitions. *Behav Res Ther* 33(8): 947–954.

Dunning, David and McFarland, Kim. 2014. Oral health and dentistry. In: Thompson, T.L. and Golson, J.G. (Eds.), *The Encyclopedia of Health Communication*, Vol. II. Sage, pp. 996–1001.

Guneri, Pelin, Epstein, Joel, and Botto, Ronald. 2013. Breaking bad medical news in a dental care setting. *J Am Dent Assoc* 144(4): 381–386.

Kessler, Ronald, et al. 2004. Prevalence, severity, and unmet need for treatment in the World Health Organization world mental health surveys. *J Am Med Assoc* 291(21): 2581–2590.

Miles, Linda. 2003. *Dynamic Dentistry*. Virginia Beach, VA: Link Publishing.

Milgrom, Peter, Weinstein, Philip, and Getz, Tracy. 1995. *Treating fearful dental patients*. University of Washington, Seattle.

Unthank Design Group: www.unthankdesigngroup.com.

Weiner, Arthur, (Ed.) 2011. *The Fearful Dental Patient: A Guide to Understanding and Managing*. *Ames*, Iowa: Wiley.

Wright, Robin. 1997. *Tough Questions, Great Answers: Responding to Patient Concerns about Today's Dentistry*. Hanover Park, IL: Quintessence Publishing.

Learning Exercises

1. You have a potential patient in your orthodontic practice, Samantha. She is a 64-year-old female in exceptionally good general health. She has longed for 50 years to have a more attractive smile with straight teeth. However, she always lacked the financial resources until now when, due to an inheritance, she can afford orthodontic care. Your initial screening exam for orthodontic treatment reveals questionable periodontal health to serve as a foundation for orthodontic treatment. So, you referred Samantha to the periodontist who confirms without question that Samantha's periodontal health will not allow for orthodontic treatment.

   Describe in writing how you would communicate this bad news to Samantha. How would you set the scene, what steps would you follow, and what specifically would you be watching for and communicating with her about? What would you actually say to her?

2. In written form, identify, step by step, how you will go about managing a fearful patient, including how to identify a fearful patient, what you will say to them, the role of your staff, and the tools you will use to help them manage their fear.

Part 5
Associateships and Dental Support Organizations

Chapter 20
About Associateships

Richard S. Callan

The term "associate" can be used as a verb, an adjective, or a noun. As a verb, it connotes the joining together of two previously separated entities. As an adjective, it substantiates the connectivity of these separate entities while introducing the possibility of one being subordinate to the other. An associate (noun) is a fellow worker, a partner, or a colleague. It is important to recognize how all three forms of this word enhance our understanding of not only what an associateship is, but also on how it is formed, how it functions, and if it can be considered a success.

For the purpose of this chapter, an associateship will be defined as simply the partnering of an owner-dentist with an associate-dentist. The associate, as implied by definition, is in some way subject to the owner but the two are colleagues, with an agreement to work together in some way, shape, or fashion.

Types of Associateships

The types of associateships are categorized by the relationship between the owner-dentist and the associate-dentist. The associate is an employee, someone who will eventually buy into the practice, someone who will eventually buy the entire practice, or someone who is only renting space from the owner-dentist. It is important to note that these distinctions are made for the purpose of explanation and are not to be considered static positions. The employee may eventually buy into a practice or purchase the entire practice at some point in time. It is the initial understanding between the two parties at the time the agreement is made that is important to the "success" of the associateship. Failure rates for associateships differ depending on the source and the criteria determined for success. If both parties achieve their intended goals from the associateship, and the associateship lasts for 2 years or more, then that agreement can be considered a success. The important point is to approach the agreement with a common understanding of its intent and to be true to that understanding.

Dental Practice Transition: A Practical Guide to Management, Second Edition.
Edited by David G. Dunning and Brian M. Lange.
© 2016 John Wiley & Sons, Inc. Published 2016 by John Wiley & Sons, Inc.
Companion Website: www.wiley.com/go/dunning/transition

Purpose for Associateship

The purpose of entering into an associateship agreement will depend greatly on the individual. Whether an associateship can be considered a success will depend on how closely the purpose(s) match the needs and desires of those entering into the associate agreement.

Owner-Dentist

What are some of the factors that would motivate an owner-dentist to seek out an associate?

Too Busy

Many times the dentist is so busy that he or she cannot see all patients in a timely manner. Patients are calling every day with no availability in the schedule. Emergencies are becoming increasingly more difficult to squeeze into an already overloaded schedule. This type of situation can have great potential for success.

Wants to Slow Down

Many dentists reach a point in their careers when they decide they want to slow their practice down to a less demanding pace yet not lose the patient base they worked so hard to create. This may be a good time to bring in an associate, if only on a part time basis. Once again, it is imperative for both the owner and the associate to understand completely the specifics of the proposed arrangement. The owner must consider the impact the decreased hours of production will have on his or her income as well as the number of hours it will take to manage the new associateship. The associate must be clear on the number of hours to be worked and realize his or her responsibility to be as productive as possible in the hours allotted.

Has Space Available

A dentist may have additional, otherwise unused space within the office and wish to bring in an associate to generate income in that space. An independent contractor relationship would exist when an associate- dentist rents that additional space from the owner-dentist. The associate-dentist is responsible for, and makes all decisions concerning this portion of the practice. Otherwise, this associate-dentist would normally have to be classified as an employee. The main consideration in this arrangement is the equitable division of the new patients coming into the practice. Other considerations are staff utilization, equipment and supply costs, and hours of operation.

Transition into Retirement

Similar to the dentist wanting to slow down, many owner-dentists planning for retirement will bring in associates to transition their practice to them. Although generally accomplished over a period of years, this arrangement should be thought through well in advance and put in motion at a predetermined date. Depending on the desires of the owner-dentist and the needs of the associate-dentist, the associate may begin on a part time basis and gradually increase as the patient load develops and/or the retiring dentist continues to decrease time spent in the office. The associate may eventually purchase the practice and hire the previous owner as his or her associate, essentially reversing the relationship. As mentioned in Chapter 7, a dental transition specialist can be of great assistance with the logistics of associate agreements and the eventual sale of a practice.

Mentorship

There are many dentists who have been practicing for a number of years and also desire to pass their experience and expertise on to the next generation of dentists. Their primary motivation for bringing in an associate is to do just that. The personal satisfaction they receive from assisting in the growth of the associate is in many ways greater than the monetary gain from their efforts.

Associate

There are numerous practice options available to dental school graduates; corporate dentistry, the military, public health, solo practitioner, and associateships. The following are some of the reasons a recent graduate may choose to become an associate of an existing practice.

Mentorship

A large number of new dental school graduates are looking for opportunities to become involved in a successful practice to hopefully learn from the experienced owner-dentist both technical skills and the art of operating a small business. As hard as dental schools try to work these skills into their curriculum, there is nothing better than on-the-job training guided directly by the tutelage of a private mentor.

Increase Speed/Confidence

If one lacks the confidence to strike out on his or her own immediately following graduation, it is a good idea to work within someone else's practice for a period of time to help develop the confidence and speed necessary to be a successful sole practitioner. No matter how fast a procedure is completed, if it is completed incorrectly or with poor quality, it has accomplished little.

Make Money

While planning/building a practice, some become associates to make money. The average student debt upon graduation from dental school continues to rise, for both public and private schools. Coupling this with an ever increasing cost of setting up a practice from scratch makes the option of an associateship ever more attractive. The ability to earn money through the associateship allows the associate-dentist to not only decrease their debt but also to save money for future professional plans.

Future Practice Partnership/Ownership

It is not uncommon for an associate-dentist to enter into an arrangement with an owner-dentist with the hopes of eventually buying into a partnership with that dentist or eventually purchasing the entire practice outright. The associate phase of this relationship provides both parties the opportunity to get to know each other, to evaluate their respective roles and communication styles, to determine if there is agreement as to practice philosophy, and to establish a mutually acceptable plan to move forward.

Not Desiring to Own a Practice

It may never be the desire of the associate-dentist to possess his or her own practice. Such individuals may be content to practice their chosen profession without the burden and responsibility of all that is encumbered with ownership of a practice. This may be an individual preference and one definition of success, and is no less valued than any other.

Advantages/Disadvantages

The items listed previously under the section Purpose of Associateship once accomplished can at the same time be considered as advantages to both the owner-dentist and the associate-dentist.

Increased Profitability/Expenses

By bringing an associate into an efficiently operating practice, the owner-dentist can expect an eventual increase equaling approximately 30% of the associate's gross collections. The addition of the associate should be considered an investment into the practice, and like most investments may require some time before dividends are realized. A reasonable amount of time should be allotted so that the associate can acclimate into the practice, develop a patient base for the associate, develop speed, collect on treatment rendered by the associate, and provide time for mentoring. This increased profitability will not be immediate but should be forthcoming.

More Operating Hours/Overhead

Expanding the business hours can help attract additional patients to the practice, resulting in increased productivity and profit.

Fewer Vacation Closings

The office can now be open when the associate and/or owner is either sick, on vacation, or out for any other reason. The practice does not stop unless both doctors are gone at the same time.

Less Emergency Coverage

The more doctors there are in the practice, the fewer days each has to be on call for emergency coverage.

More Free Time/Continuity of Patient Care

Having the associate in the practice can permit the owner the opportunity to be away for periods of time and still have the needs of their patients met.

Opportunity to Specialize

The owner-dentist may want to concentrate his or her efforts in a particular area of dentistry without losing the patients that don't require that type of service. The addition of an associate to perform those other services can allow the owner to devote additional time to that endeavor. Care must be taken not to abuse the associate by not providing him or her the opportunity to learn all aspects of dental treatment the practice has to offer.

Entrepreneurship

Many practitioners have decided to expand their practices to more than one location. Additional dental professionals must be brought on board in order to keep each practice simultaneously operational. Although this type of arrangement may not provide the desired level of mentorship available when both dentists are in the same location, it does represent yet another opportunity for those dentists seeking employment.

Consultation and Fellowship

Dentistry can be a very rewarding profession. It can also be a very lonely profession. The inclusion of an associate into a practice gives both the owner and the associate the opportunity to fellowship with an individual of like mind and interests. Not only can this be beneficial as a second opinion for difficult cases, but also as a sounding board in time of need.

More Efficient Use of Employees

Many of the functions in a dental office are routine in nature and must occur regardless of the number of operatories or providers of care. Having staff members that are crosstrained and able to function in various areas throughout the office can be a huge bonus when an associate is added to the mix.

Purchasing Discounts

An increase in the number of patients seen in an office will likely necessitate a greater utilization of supplies and equipment. Many dental supply companies and manufacturers are willing to offer a discount when things are purchased in bulk. An increase in supplies purchased to accommodate for the increased patient flow may actually result in a decrease in cost per item, without the concomitant problem of long-term storage.

Meet Growing Demand and Provide Coverage in Case of the Unexpected

Many practices are unable to meet the demands of their growing population. The addition of an associate can provide opportunity to see these patients in a timely manner.

Potential Buyer (Death, Disability, or Retirement)

The owner-dentist will likely be comforted by the fact that someone has already associated with the practice and able to take over without advance notice. This is one aspect frequently overlooked within associate contracts. What is to happen if either the owner-dentist or the associate were to unexpectedly become disabled or deceased?

Associate

Initial Income Potentially Higher

An associate in a practice can probably expect to make more money initially than his or her counterpart starting a new practice. The reasons for this are obvious. He or she has no immediate business overhead and should have a source of readily available patients. Although someone purchasing an existing practice would have a patient base and immediate cash flow, there is the expense of purchasing the practice and the overhead of the practice that accompany that option.

Little or No Risk

This statement is only partially true. While there is little financial obligation in being the associate, there can be substantial professional risk. There may also be contractual stipulations restricting the associate from practicing in the area outside of the office(s) of the owner-dentist. This can be a difficult situation once the associate and family are established in community, schools, faith-organizations, and so on.

Little or No Capital Outlay

Generally speaking, the associate has little financial obligation to the practice. Under special circumstance there may be provisions for the associate to purchase certain equipment. This is with the understanding that the equipment be allowed to leave with the associate or considered appropriately if and when the purchase into the partnership, or of the entire practice, is consummated.

Learn/Build

The associate is permitted the opportunity to concentrate on developing the quality skills, speed, and interpersonal acumen required for a successful practitioner. The desire to continue to learn and grow is one that should be evident throughout one's entire career. In essence, associateships offer an "Earn while you learn" opportunity. An associate may earn a living and at the same time see how the dentist-owner developed a practice that is successful enough to hire him or her.

Disadvantages

The dynamics within a dental office change considerably with the addition of a new associate, adding complexity to almost every aspect.

More Sophisticated Management

The addition of an associate into an already busy practice does not, in and of itself, make the practice run more smoothly. Metaphorically speaking, it is like the circus performer balancing the revolving plates on top of thin wooden poles. The inclusion of each additional plate only makes the task more difficult for the performer. The importance of the need for organization and efficiency in the office prior to the addition of another provider cannot be overemphasized.

Autonomy/Decision Making

All decisions made within the practice must now factor in the impact it will have on both the owner and the associate. The freedom for either party to act independently is greatly diminished.

Delay of Building Own Practice

One obvious disadvantage for the associate committed to an associateship can be the delaying of the building of their own practice. One compromise that can, in some instances, be beneficial for both the owner and the associate would be for the associate to work part time for the owner while setting up a practice somewhere outside of the noncompete area specified in the contract. This way the associate can decrease the number of days he or she works in the owner's office as his or her own practice continues to grow. Honest, open communication is the key to making this sort of relationship successful.

Making the Connection

Making the connection between the owner-dentist and the associate-dentist can be a difficult task. How does an owner-dentist looking for an associate find just the right person for his or her practice? How does the associate-dentist locate the practice that best fits his or her needs? Beyond the obvious advertising in the local newspapers, and the numerous internet resources, there are many other avenues in which this connection can be made.

Recruiting the Right Associate (Owner)

How does one find an associate once the decision is made?

This can be a very difficult challenge. When faced with a difficult situation, it is best to envision the perfect answer to the question. What does your perfect associate look like (be realistic)? Where can such a person be found? How can I make contact with this person? What will it take to get him or her to come to my practice?

Finding the Right Practice (Associate)

How does one find the right practice? This question is as difficult as the one asked by the owner looking for an associate. Let's try a similar approach. What does the perfect practice look like? Where can such a practice be found? How do I get in contact with such a practice? What will it take to get into that practice?

The answers to these questions are quite similar for both the owner and the associate.

Dental Schools

A good place for an owner-dentist to begin looking for a potential associate is a dental school. This does not necessarily have to be the school nearest to the practice. As the clinical testing agencies expand their number of participating states and the expansion of states allowing for licensure by credentials continues to grow, many graduates are searching for opportunities beyond their state or region. Many schools handle such inquiries through their alumni affairs office. A number of schools have recently hosted dental job fairs where dentists are invited to set up booths promoting their practices to interested students. Through these meetings, acquaintances are made and conversations are begun, which can potentially lead to the formation of an associateship arrangement.

Dental Supply Companies

Another popular method of making the connection is through the local dental supply companies. Many times these company representatives are the first to know of opportunities available in their area. Both the owner-dentist and the associate-dentist have access to this resource. The contact information for the prospective associate should be given to the owner-dentist so that a convenient time and place can be arranged for them to meet and discuss the potential associateship.

Practice Transition Specialists

The past few years have seen the emergence of the practice transition specialist. These individuals or companies promote their services to help make the connection and direct the transition of the owner to the incoming dentist, be they potential associates, partners, or purchasers of the practice. Recognizing the need for and the potential of this business opportunity, these specialists have evolved into providing services well beyond the simple matching of an associate to a practice. The range of services offered by these specialists differs depending on the expertise of the individual(s), and the desires of the dentist(s). These services may include the locating of the associate for the practice or the practice for the associate, the personality compatibility testing of the interested parties, the development of the transition plan into associateship, partnership and/or sale of the practice, determining the value of the practice, the financial arrangements including purchasing, tax planning, asset protection and retirement planning, and all the legal paperwork associated with each and every step of the process. The value of making sure these activities are handled in a fair and proper manner cannot be overstated. It is of course a cost-to-benefit consideration and one should make sure he or she receives the benefit of what is paid for as these services do not come cheap.

Journals and the Internet

State dental journals can be of some assistance in finding an associate position as many dentists are choosing to list their practices in these widely published periodicals.

In addition, there are an ever increasing number of internet sites promoting practice opportunities. This mode of communication will continue to serve as a valuable resource for many years to come.

Define Success

Traditionally, the "success" of associateships has been defined more in terms of how long they have lasted, with the reported average of approximately 2 years, perhaps less. Time is just one of the factors defining the success of an associateship. The real success of such a relationship is better determined by the purpose(s) of the parties when entering into the agreement. It is therefore, imperative that both parties are clear in their own

Expectations

Associate

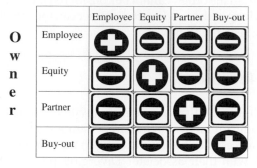

		Employee	Equity	Partner	Buy-out
O	Employee	✚	⊖	⊖	⊖
w					
n	Equity	⊖	✚	⊖	⊖
e					
r	Partner	⊖	⊖	✚	⊖
	Buy-out	⊖	⊖	⊖	✚

Figure 20.1. Expectations for associateships.

minds about what they hope to achieve through this joining together of their professional lives. If the associate is interested in future ownership of a practice and the owner only wants someone to help increase revenue, this could be a recipe for an unsuccessful associateship. On the other hand, if the associate is looking for mentorship and an opportunity to increase skills and efficiency, and the owner is looking to mentor someone while at the same time decrease his or her practice burden, this could be a highly successful associateship relationship. Both examples could last just 1 year with one being considered a success and the other being a failure.

Figure 20.1 reveals the potential of success for varying associate relationships depending on the expressed purpose of both the owner-dentist and the associate-dentist. The pluses (+) indicate a higher potential for success whereas the minuses (−) may be indicative of an associate agreement with a high likelihood of being considered a failure.

As Figure 20.1 indicates, associateships are most likely to succeed when the owner and the associate purposes match in the areas of the associate being an employee, building/earning equity in the practice, becoming a future partner or eventually buying out the practice. Mismatching of expectations is likely to lead to a failed associateship.

There are, of course, many other elements to consider beyond the purpose(s) when determining the success potential of the associateship; but without a clear understanding by both parties of each other's intended goal, the chance of success is greatly diminished. It is recommended that both the owner and the associate write down, individually, what they envision their successful associateship would look like. Include a timetable of perhaps 6 months, 1 year, 2 years, 3 years, 5 years, and so on. Nothing is written in stone at this time, and these are not binding contracts, but it does allow opportunity for each to understand the direction the other is planning to go.

Win-Win

Once identified, it is imperative for both parties to recognize the need to fulfill the other partner's purpose or desire. Seldom does either party get everything he or she wants in a negotiation, but if both recognize the desire of the other to be fair and earnestly seek what is ultimately best for all involved, the chance for a win-win agreement is greatly enhanced. Any arrangement made in haste, that ultimately benefits one side to a much greater degree than the other, cannot be considered a win-win. This type of agreement will last only as long as the less favored partner can tolerate the abuse, and almost never ends amicably. Seek the win-win.

Evaluation of a Practice

Numerous well-intended owner-dentists invite an equally motivated associate into their practices only to end in a premature separation. How can this happen? How can a dentist with a successful practice, desiring to mentor a new practitioner, have such a negative result with their associate? Diverging personalities not withstanding, the problem could be that the practice could not support an additional dentist. There are many factors that need to be considered. The prospective associate-dentist would also do well to take these issues into consideration when deciding whether to join a particular practice or not.

Am I working as efficiently as I could?

Before bringing on another practitioner, the owner-dentist should review the efficiency of his or her current efforts. There is great benefit to be gained by taking a good look at how one is scheduling patients. One might consider block scheduling if it is not already being utilized. If you find that you work better in the mornings than the evenings, then try to schedule the more intense procedures when you are at your best. Hiring an assistant for your hygienist or even an additional hygienist can have a marketed effect on office productivity. An additional assistant may enable you, the dentist, to do more of what your license qualifies you to and less of what an auxiliary is permitted to do for you. Do you have your operatories, sterilization areas, labs, and so on organized in such a manner as to maximize efficiency? Utilize the services of a practice consultant to help identify areas in your office that may be deficient or counterproductive. Many times an unbiased eye will pick up on items that many times go unnoticed to those intimately associated with the process.

This would be a good time to evaluate the amount of unproductive time spent in your office. Are you, or members of your team, talking on the phone to any appreciable degree? Are certain procedures being done during patient care time that could be accomplished during hours when patients are not being seen?

Even if you are in need of an associate, bringing one into a well-oiled machine can only improve the chance of success and maximize the benefit of another provider.

Are there a sufficient number of patients to support the additional provider?

Depending on the type of practice and the variance of procedures being performed, this number could vary greatly. A minimum of 1,200–2,000 active patients is required for the average private practicing individual dentist. In addition, an adequate supply of new patients is required to sustain that population. Although, in most cases, the incoming associate will not initially have the speed to immediately double the patient supply demand, a constantly increasing supply will be required to match the combined need of both providers. What are the current marketing efforts of the office, both internal and external? How can they be improved? It may be tempting to enroll in capitation plans in order to increase your patient pool, but be cautious. If you have not already done so, there was a reason you chose not to participate in these plans. Are you now willing to go against your better judgment in order to provide patients for your new associate, committing him or her to a practice model you decided was not best for you? Is this in keeping with our desires for win-win relationship? If you are participating in these capitation plans, be sure to take this into consideration when computing the compensation for the associate. Otherwise you could be requiring the slowest operator in the practice to work at a pace they are not capable of (while simultaneously providing quality treatment), in order to make a living.

Is the facility adequate for the additional demands?

Once the office is running to maximum efficiency, it must be determined if it can support an additional provider. This consideration involves much more that just another operatory or two. There will be additional traffic flow due to the increased number of patients coming through the office (hopefully). Additional staff will most certainly be required. Both of these will demand an increased number of parking spaces that may or may not be available at your current location.

Some of these problems can be accounted for by adjusting the office schedule and extending the hours of operation. This will work fine until the associate decides he or she is tired of working late afternoon, evenings, and Saturdays so that the owner-dentist can be home by 3:00 p.m.

If staggering of office hours is not the solution, then perhaps a renovation or addition to the existing office is in order. Ultimately, a new facility may be required. Although having the associate purchase the necessary equipment for the expansion is something that might be considered (these can be retained by the associate if things don't work out), requiring the associate to invest in renovations, expansion, and/or a new building is unreasonable unless the appropriate arrangements have been formalized for future ownership, either part or whole.

Is my staff adequate, in both number and makeup?

As mentioned in the section concerning running an effort-efficient office, the appropriate utilization of auxiliary staff will also provide the associate the opportunity to be maximally productive. Again, the speed and ability of the associate must be taken into consideration before the added expense of additional staff is incurred. As the practice continues to grow, it would be unreasonable to expect that additional assistants, hygienists, and front office personnel would not be required.

Compensation Package

How is the associate to be compensated for his or her effort?

Should the associate receive a salary or be paid on commission or both? Is this commission to be paid based on production or collection? And what benefits should the practice provide to the associate?

The purpose of the associateship can be the deciding factor in how the associate is to be compensated. If the agreed upon purpose of the associateship is for the associate to work a couple of years in the practice and then move on to something else, then perhaps the easiest solution to compensation would be to offer the associate a percentage of production, less an proportionate deduction for lab expenses. Market demands may dictate these percentages. Historically, the range can be from 28% to perhaps as high as 40%. The owner-dentist may prefer to pay a percentage of collections in lieu of a percentage of production, claiming that he or she cannot pay the associate if monies are not collected. In addition, what is to stop the associate from providing treatment to patients regardless of the patient's ability to pay for the treatment? I would contend that the owner-dentist is the one responsible for the collections, as he or she is the one that established the collection policies of the office and has also hired the person responsible for maintaining an acceptable collection rate. The caveat to this concept is that the associate cannot begin treatment on a patient until the finances for that treatment have been vetted through the financial officer of the office.

On the other hand, if the purpose is for potential partnership-ownership, then the compensation can become quite complicated. An initial base salary may then be offered with the inclusion of a portion going into an escrow fund to be used later as the down payment. There would be a matching amount placed in the fund by the owner-dentist as a gesture of mutual commitment to the agreement. Guaranteed base salaries vary widely by market and could be as little as $60,000 to well over $100,000. These salaries may or may not be tied to production/collection incentive bonuses in which associate compensation surpasses the guaranteed based when production/collection goals are reached. In order for this to be a true and timely incentive, the production goals should be monthly, not yearly. For instance, if an associate is guaranteed a base salary of $100,000/year, it would be better to calculate that on a monthly basis of $8,333/month. Any productivity over this amount would be subject to the bonus provision as opposed to waiting until the associate produced over $100,000 before paying a bonus.

The possibilities are as numerous as the factors involved in the compensation decision. As an employee, the associate-dentist should be entitled to all that each individual employed in the office is entitled to, and under the same provisions. This could include items such as health insurance, disability insurance, malpractice insurance, retirement plans, profit sharing, vacation time, sick leave, association dues, CE opportunities, and so on. Each item should have a dollar figure associated with it and be considered in the overall compensation package offered to the associate. As with all employees, it is important that the associate understand the total expense related to being employed in the practice. Don't forget to include the monthly unemployment check that must be paid.

Failure

Why do associateships fail? For the purpose of this discussion, "failure" will be defined as the premature dissolution of the association agreement. What this means is that one or both parties did not accomplish what they had hoped through the associateship and is/are seeking to end the relationship.

Lack of Written Agreement

It has been suggested that the number one reason for failure of an associateship is the lack of a written agreement. The ability to seal a deal with a handshake has long since gone away. The English language is imprecise at best, as evidenced by the exponential increase in litigation in our country, and the memory of the individuals involved in the agreement is either conflicting or altogether lacking. It is hard to believe that professionals will enter into an associateship without a written agreement. Putting points of agreement on paper not only records the event but also helps to clarify the intent. Still, all things considered, the success of an associateship has more to do with the people involved than the words on the paper.

Unclear Expectations

The divorce rate in this country is now over 50% for first time marriages. It would be safe to say that certain expectations were not clear at the time of commitment and thus, ultimately unmet. Why would one enter into an associate agreement without first being as specific as possible in expressing expectations? It is difficult for anyone to meet unknown expectations.

Unfair Expectations

Many associateships do not make it through the honeymoon period because of one or both parties not living up to the expectations of the other. The owner-dentist may expect the associate to have a positive financial impact on the practice from the first day. Depending on the individual practice and the investment required to bring the associate into the practice, it may be as long as 6 months before any real profit is realized. On the other hand, the associate may expect to be able to bring home as much money as the owner-dentist within the first couple of months of practice. This, too, would seem to be an unrealistic expectation.

Inability of the Practice to Support the Associate

Despite the good intentions of both parties, a practice that cannot support both the owner-dentist and the associate dooms the associateship to fail. The owner has not done his or her homework in determining the capacity of the practice and the associate did not search for nor find the practice indicators that would warn him or her of impending failure.

Unwillingness to Adapt

Change is more difficult for some people than for others. Neither party involved in an associateship agreement should expect to remain unchanged. The ability of individuals to compromise is imperative to the success of any undertaking, and is particularly important when considering going into an associateship agreement. When the owner is unwilling to accept some changes suggested by the associate or the associate is unwilling to adapt to certain mandates from the owner, the associateship will fail. Open, honest communication is an imperative. No one can think of everything when developing the agreement, but the more that is decided ahead of time, the greater the chance for success and the smoother the road to be traveled will be.

Inadequate Compensation, Inadequate Effort on Part of Associate, and Lack of Mentoring

These topics should probably be best placed as a subheading under unclear/unmet expectations. The total compensation package should be clearly defined before the associate begins to work in the practice. The expectations of the owner-dentist should also be spelled out in detail. What are the production goals for the associate and when should they be met? Are they realistic? What are the extenuating factors affecting those goals (i.e., patient assignment)? What are the consequences of not meeting those goals? These are all questions that should be answered during discussions prior to employment.

One of the advantages of an associateship mentioned for both the owner-dentist and the associate is the ability to mentor and/or be mentored. How does the owner-dentist plan on becoming a mentor, what does that mean to him or her? What does the associate expect from a mentor? New graduates may accept a slightly less lucrative associateship with the expectation of a great mentoring experience. When this experience fails to materialize, the associates may leave, feeling not only disappointed but cheated as well.

Unfair Patient Assignment

The owner-dentist is cheating him- or herself when he or she doesn't maximize the potential of an associate. If the associate understands from the onset that his or her role in the practice is to see only Medicaid patients and/or those participating in capitation programs, and is satisfied with the compensation received for these efforts, then so be it. Can we expect this type of relationship to be a lasting one?

Another aspect of unfair patient assignment is the type of patient assigned to the associate. The owner-dentist may instruct the front desk person to assign all crown and bridge patients to him or her, thus delegating the associate to the role of supporting cast. If the owner expects the associate to be a productive participant in the practice and to someday be a partner or future owner of the practice, then an equitable distribution of all types of patients represented in the practice is a must. To assign the associate a back operatory with the oldest equipment, working with the least experienced assistant is not a recipe for success.

Not Part of Decision-Making Process

Not having the associate be part of the decision-making process of the office can lead to a sense of not belonging with the practice. This can work in both directions; the associate may wish to be part of the process and is not. Or, the owner may want the associate to be part of the process and he or she is not desiring to do so, thus implying a lack of commitment from either or both parties.

Unfair Compensation

Last, but certainly not least on the list of why associateships fail, is the subject of compensation. This is a topic that works in both directions: either the associate feels undercompensated for the work he or she does or the owner feels the associate is overcompensated for the amount of work produced.

Associateship Contracts

A fair associateship contract is one that meets the needs and desires of both the owner-dentist and associate-dentist. The owner-dentist and the associate should spend many hours in preparation of their agreement (or at least points of understanding) prior to obtaining legal council. Although this service is invaluable to the overall process, the basics of the agreement can best be determined by those directly involved with its results. The dentists understand the operations of a dental office and only the individuals reaching the agreement know how important each specific element is to them, and thus how hard a line to hold on what issues. Once the particulars have been worked out, each dentist can enlist the services of a lawyer to review the proposed

Table 20.1 Components of a dental associate contract.

Date entered into
Owner name
Associate name
Services
Term
Duties
Restrictions
Compensation
Employer obligations
Employees obligations
Insurance
Fees
Records
Solicitation of employees
Vacation
Termination
Patient assignment and operations management
Status
Noncompetition
Notice
Indemnity agreement
Purchase
Death or disability
Financial commitment
Mediation/arbitration
Fees and costs
Entire agreement
Amendments
Enforcement of agreement
Assignability
Severability of provisions
Counterpart signatures

contract not only to ensure that its provisions are legal but also to advise them about its shortcomings and potential risks. Every contract should, of course, identify those participating in the agreement and the length of time the agreement will be in affect. An outline of typical components of an associate contract can be seen in Table 20.1. The following section, although not intended to be all inclusive, lists some additional provisions that should certainly exist within every associateship contract. It should also be understood that each contract is an entity in itself, and the handling of each provision is up to the individuals making the contract, not to any prescribed "norm."

Owner/Associate Responsibilities

What the owner-dentist and the associate-dentist are responsible to provide should be clearly spelled out. It is not uncommon for the owner to supply the building, the signage, the telephone listing, the staff, the equipment, and the supplies. The associate-dentist typically is responsible for his or her own insurance (malpractice, health, and disability), dues to professional associations, licensing fees, and payment for any continuing education courses. Some contracts may provide for one or more of these benefits as the market for associateships changes. Once again, it is important for the associate to be aware of the current value of each of these benefits in consideration of the entire compensation package.

Patient Assignment

One of the first questions the prospective associate should ask when reviewing an associateship contract is: "Where are my patients going to come from?" This question can be answered in many ways, but needs to be precisely stated in the contract. Some owner-dentists require the associate to build his or her own patient base over time, through the recruitment of patients, while others are willing to share the current patient population with the associate. The owner-dentist may decide to give all new patients to the associate for a given period of time and then alternate the assignment of new patients. Many patients would prefer to be treated by the new dentist, whose schedule is not yet full, rather than waiting a longer period of time to fit into the schedule of the owner-dentist. However it is handled, both parties should be clear on its intent and be willing to live with the consequences.

Preferred Provider Organizations/Capitation/Medicaid

If the practice does participate in one or more managed care plans, private or public, how these patients are to be assigned must be included in the contract. This is of particular importance when the associate is to be paid according to production. This subject was covered in an earlier section but is mentioned here specifically for its inclusion in the contract. Associates earning income based on collections may have their incomes significantly and negatively influenced by "write-offs" related to managed care plans.

Work Hours

The hours to be worked by the associate should be part of the written contract. This should consist of not only the days of the week, but also the hours of the day. This protects both the associate and the owner-dentist. Any requirements for overtime, evenings, weekends, and emergency coverage should be included. Any vacation time and sick leave must be made available to the associate, within the guidelines provided to any other eligible employee. If the office is closed for a week over the Christmas holiday and everyone else is required to use that time as part of their paid vacation, then the associate is also obliged to do so.

Noncompete/Nonsolicitation

The true intent of a noncompete/nonsolicitation stipulation is to protect the owner from losing his or her patients and/or staff to the departing associate. Such provisions are not recognized by all states and thus are not included in the contract. In the states that it is permissible, it is typical for it to be included. The noncompete and the nonsolicitation inclusions are generally defined by both time and distance; one cannot work in a practice within a certain distance from a specified location for a specific period of time. In most instances, it is more the possibility of the associate taking the patients and/or staff from the owner-dentist's practice that is the real potential insult or harm. It is important to note that some dentists may own several practices at different locations, and that this stipulation may be enforceable from any or all of these locations.

It is also important to be specific when defining "practice." An associate may return to school to receive a specialty degree in hopes of returning to the same area to practice. Upon returning, he or she may still be prohibited from setting up practice at the desired location because of the confines written in the previously agreed upon contract.

Where permitted, noncompete/nonsolicitation provisions are generally enforced. The enforcement of these provisions may be related to the reasonableness of its terms. A 10 mile radius may not be acceptable in a large metropolitan area but yet completely reasonable in a rural setting. Five years may be deemed too long a waiting period and thus nonenforceable. Many contracts now include language addressing the enforceability of the stated terms. A contract can stipulate a buy out of the non-compete/nonsolicitation agreements. These buyouts are generally quite expensive, and justifiably so.

As an aside, similar noncompete/nonsolicitation stipulations should also be included in a sales contract, prohibiting the selling dentist from practicing within a certain distance from a specified location (or locations), within a given period of time. The reader is encouraged to study Chapter 7 on practice buy-ins and buyouts.

Compensation

The means by which an associate is to be compensated for professional service to the practice should be explained in detail. Included in the explanation should be the handling of various associated factors, such as the lab bill, taxes, individually specific supplies or equipment, and any personal expenses incurred by the office. It may be helpful to include an addendum to the contract with an example representing a normal month's compensation calculations. Figures 20.2 and 20.3 show the difference in the bottom line when the lab bill is either taken off the total collections (Figure 20.2) or after the associate's percentage (30%) is already compensated for (Figure 20.3), the later method taking the lab bill out of the associate's percentage of income.

Obviously, it is in the associate's best interest to have the lab bill paid "off the top" of collections rather than "after percentage." In the example, monthly collections of $20,000 with a $2,500 lab bill result in an income difference of $1750 to the associate.

Hygiene

One of the seldom discussed and somewhat controversial issues in associateships concerns what income if any associates receive for overseeing hygiene examinations and services. This would of course apply only in practices with hygienists. Most contracts

Lab fees

Off the top

$20,000
$- 2,500$
$17,500
.30
$5,250

Figure 20.2. Lab fees "off the top."

Lab Fees

<u>**After percentage**</u>

$20,000

___.30___

$6,000

__$2,500__

$3,500

Figure 20.3. Lab fees "after percentage."

are silent on the issue, meaning that, by default in almost all cases, associates receive no income related to hygiene production. This default position builds in considerable profitability for the dentist-owner if the associate is assigned oversight responsibility in the hygiene area. Some contracts specify that associates overseeing hygiene activity are to receive $10 per hygiene examination or perhaps up to 30% of hygiene production. Other contracts may specify which dental care will result in associate income from hygiene (for example, credit for examinations but not for prophies). As with all other pivotal aspects in a contract, it is critical that the owner and the associate understand and agree upon this hygiene production issue from the outset.

Insurance

The type (claims-made or occurrence) of malpractice insurance and the amount of coverage required by the associate should be established within the associateship contract: The decision as to which type of insurance may be determined based on the overall goal of the associate agreement and the philosophy of the practice toward malpractice insurance. Provisions should also be stipulated for additional tail coverage, if necessary with claims-made policies.

Noncompliance

It is important to include statements pertaining to the consequences of noncompliance on the part of either the owner-dentist or the associate-dentist. This can be done for each item of the contract individually or for the contract as a whole, whichever is deemed most appropriate. What happens to the associate if he or she decides to take a week off with no notice? What happens if the owner changes the associate's schedule to 3 days/week instead of the agreed upon 5 days? If the contract is subsequently dissolved due to such unacceptable action, is the noncompete/nonsolicitation provision also no longer in effect? The answer to that question would depend on who may be asked, the owner or the associate.

Termination

Many contracts include a description of certain offenses that, if committed by the associate, would result in immediate termination. The owner-dentist must have the ability to protect his or her practice and patients. I would recommend that this section of the contract be looked at very closely and discussed to whatever extent necessary to establish the specific intent of its meaning. "Action unbecoming a professional" is a broad concept and open to much interpretation. This should not be a vehicle by which the owner-dentist dismisses the associate simply because things are not working out as planned.

Death or Disability

Few contracts include provisions concerning the associate in the event of death or permanent disability of the owner-dentist. Without such provision, the associate may be forced to relocate his or her family and start all over again. A first right of refusal or first right to purchase for the associate for the purchase of the practice might be one suggestion. A term life insurance policy on the owner-dentist, sufficient to cover the cost of the practice, can be purchased on behalf of the associate. The cost of the premium for this policy could be split by the associate and the owner, with the assignment going to the owner's beneficiaries. There are many ways to manage this unfortunate possibility. The important thing is to plan ahead, be prepared, and pray it never happens.

Provide an Out

Every contract should provide a means by which the associateship can be terminated. It is wise to recognize the fact that all agreements do not always work out as planned. It is also wise to have a plan if your particular agreement does not work out.

Conclusion

Certain assumptions have been made in the writing of this chapter. One assumption is that the owner and the associate are being honest in their dealings with each other. A poor contract agreed to by honest individuals seeking what is fair to both parties has a greater chance of success than the best written contract made by dishonest, egocentric individuals. The other assumption is that the owner and the associate have sought individual counsel/representation before signing a legal document. It is difficult for anyone to give equal and fair consideration to two parties, particularly when being compensated, perhaps unequally, by both parties.

Student indebtedness upon graduation from dental school has reached an all time high. Real estate and construction costs continue to rise. The proportion of women in dentistry continues to increase, and fewer women as a percentage seem interested in opening up their own solo practices. Further, so-called "corporate dentistry"/dental service organizations are certainly exerting influence on the changing paradigm of associateships (see Chapter 21). These and many other factors are contributing to an increase in the number of dental school graduates seeking associateship positions in the United States. The need for a clearer understanding of the mechanics of this dynamic relationship has never been greater. The appreciation of its complexity and respect for its importance, are absolute requirements for the ultimate success of these relationships.

Acknowledgments

The information presented in this chapter represents years of knowledge gained from various sources. Much of the same information is shared between many of the contributors, making it difficult to site one particular source for its content. Many of these individuals I have spoken to personally and/or listened to their presentations, while others I have just read from their publications. Still I am sure there are facts that were obtained from sources long since forgotten.

I would like to recognize the following individuals for their contributions to the content of this chapter:

Dr. Arthur (Ron) Croft
Mr. Rick Willeford, CPA
Dr. Earl Douglas
Dr. Gene Heller
Dr. Bill Adams
Dr. Richard Ford
Dr. David Griggs

References and Additional Resources

Griggs, D. 1997. *Successful Practice Transitions*. Tulsa, OK: PenWell Publishing Company.
Halley, Meghan, Lalumandier, James, Walker, Jonathan, and Houston, James. 2008. A regional study of dentists' preferences for hiring a dental associate. *J Am Dent Assoc* 139(7): 973–979.
Ramsey, D. 2003. *The Total Money Makeover: A Proven Plan for Financial Fitness*. Nashville, TN: Thomas Nelson Publishers.
Stanley, T. and Danko, W. 1996. *The Millionaire Next Door*. New York, NY: Simon & Schuster, Inc.
Wilde, J. 1996. *How Dentistry Can Be a Joyous Path to Financial Freedom*. Hamilton, IL: The Novel Pen.
Wurman, R., Siegel, A., and Morris, K. 1990. *The Wall Street Journal: Guide to Understanding Money & Markets*, New York, NY: Access Press.

Learning Exercises

1. List four types of associateship arrangements.
2. List five reasons an owner-dentist may desire an associate.
3. What are five reasons a person may seek to be an associate?
4. List ten potential advantages the owner-dentist may realize by having an associate.
5. List five potential advantages the associate may realize by entering into this arrangement with an owner-dentist.
6. What are some potential disadvantages to an associateship arrangement?
7. How can you find the right associate (associateship)?
8. What is your definition of a successful associateship?
9. List four questions the owner-dentist should answer prior to bringing an associate into his or her practice.
10. Describe how the compensation package for the associate can vary depending on the purpose of the associateship.
11. List ten potential causes of a failed associateship.
12. List ten provisions that should be stipulated in every associate contract.
13. Describe the difference between the "nonsolicitation" and "noncompete" provisions of an associateship contract. What are the determinants of their enforceability?

Chapter 21
Dental Support Organizations
Rick Workman

As you may have noticed, dental support organizations (DSOs) have become more and more prevalent in the dental industry over the past few decades. Today, these organizations support an estimated 8,000 licensed dentists practicing in 5,000 dental offices who, in turn, serve more than 27 million patients across the country each year. Despite this growth and expansion, many dentists and dental professionals still do not fully understand how DSOs operate.

To give you a general overview, DSOs support the nonclinical responsibilities dental offices face so that dentists and team members can focus on providing high-quality care. Instead of finding time to market their office, complete payroll, hire new team members and other administrative tasks, supported doctors and team members can gain access to a variety of professional teams specialized in these different areas. In addition, many dental support organizations offer continuing education opportunities to help support dentists and team members advance their clinical and communication skills.

My entrance into the DSO world stemmed from my own experience as a practicing dentist. After graduating dental school in 1980, I looked for a job that paid at least $25,000, but couldn't find one. Instead, I soon started my own basement dental office. After years of building up this office, as well as advancing it to a multilocation group practice, the rigors of spending 50 hours a week at the dental chair and 25–30 hours on the business side of dentistry began to take its toll. Although my group practice was successful, I was quite stressed and other aspects of my life were negatively affected. From working with 20 doctors in multiple locations, I saw new dentists repeat the same mistakes I had made. I knew that if I was witnessing these struggles, countless other dentists were more than likely experiencing the same thing. From that, I worked to create a system of support that in 1997, would officially become Heartland Dental— now the largest DSO in the United States.

I wasn't alone in my ambitions. Over the years, many other dental support organizations have been founded, such as Pacific Dental Services, Aspen Dental Management, Inc., Dental Care Alliance, Affordable Care, Inc., and many more. DSOs are different from one another in many ways but all share the same goal—to support dentists so they can provide the best patient care, which will positively affect our industry and the dentists that it is comprised of.

Dental Practice Transition: A Practical Guide to Management, Second Edition.
Edited by David G. Dunning and Brian M. Lange.
© 2016 John Wiley & Sons, Inc. Published 2016 by John Wiley & Sons, Inc.
Companion Website: www.wiley.com/go/dunning/transition

An Evolving Industry

Identifying these support needs has certainly been a main reason why DSOs have come into existence, but it's not the only reason. Throughout the years, the dental industry has continually changed. Dental support organizations have become more prevalent—due, in large part—to the establishment of this new reality. Modern dentists are encountering a multitude of challenges, including keeping up with technology, increased costs, slowing number of patient visits, government regulation, legal issues, third party payment changes, and so forth. In today's industry, many dentists are unable to transition or share their offices with associate dentists, and young dentists with $300,000 plus in student loans often cannot finance new offices on their own. This has led to a doubling of the number of quality dentists searching for a means to succeed. Other aspects of dentistry have also changed. In previous decades, dentists have predominantly been male, but now dentist gender is almost split even. Forty-five percent of all dental school graduates are now female (Reed, Corry, and Liu 2012). In addition, today's millennial dentists desire to maintain geographic flexibility in terms of practicing. They often don't feel the desire to commit to one area for their entire lives.

A 2013 study released by the American Dental Association discussed several items that have triggered these industry changes. Here are a few:

- Consumers have become much more astute purchasers of health care and seek value for their spending.
- An increasing number of dentists are being trained, but mounting debt load and changing demographics are altering the practice choices for new dentists.
- Commercial dental plans are increasingly using more selective networks, demanding increased accountability through data and performance measures, and pressuring providers to reduce costs.
- With the increased demand for value in dental care spending, practices will need to become more efficient.
- As corporations are forced to increase medical insurance costs, after-dental benefits are being reduced, which decreases demand and revenue for dental offices.

Much of the support DSOs offer is designed to help dentists meet the needs of this ever-changing industry. In terms of new dental school graduates, it's harder to start out on your own these days. Only 50% of new dental graduates currently enter private practice once graduating, according to the ADA. As I previously mentioned, new grads often come out of school with upward of $300,000 in debt, making it difficult to open a solo practice. In quoting Dr. Steven Holm, president of the Indiana Dental Association, "If you are a new graduate the dental landscape looks bleak. And you will be entering the profession with alarming levels of educational debt. In 2013, the average educational debt per graduating dental school senior was $215,145.00. If you went to a private dental school, your average debt was $283,978.00." Some dental school graduates are simply unwilling or unable to take out a loan to finance a new practice on top of already significant student loan obligations.

As the U.S. economy continues its slow rebound, DSO financing provides a viable option at a time when industries are looking for investors and capital and states are looking for new avenues of job creation and increased access to dental services. Many of today's young dentists are also looking for a lifestyle with freedom and flexibility, with the ability to practice at locations of their choice. DSOs can be an attractive option for these new grads because of the flexibility and immediate success offered.

In terms of meeting the needs of today's dental patients, it's not as simple as it used to be. Today's "dental consumers" have more options, information, and education at their fingertips than ever before. With a few clicks of the keyboard and mouse, people can learn more about the dentist or service they are searching for, identify hundreds of clinicians who provide that service, and pinpoint the right price that fits their budgets. Patients can access countless social media and review and rating sites (Facebook, Google+, Yelp, Angie's List, etc.) with office recommendations (and oppositions) left by other patients. As they are now more knowledgeable and savvy than ever before, it's necessary for dental offices to adapt to their needs.

This shift isn't necessarily a bad thing, as it creates many opportunities to positively impact the health and livelihood of more people, stay ahead of changes, and advance your office in terms of marketing, community involvement, and patient communication. This is another reason why many dentists choose the DSO route. DSOs are equipped to help dentists succeed in these areas, such as marketing, public relations, social media, communication methods, and so on.

In terms of experienced dentists, industry changes are having some considerable effects as well, especially to solo practitioners. To quote Dr. Richard T. Kao, "Effective practice management has become progressively more difficult for solo practice owners. Increased government regulations, rising supply costs and competitive labor markets have made practice overhead difficult to contain." The ADA's Health Policy Resources Center has concluded that the rate of solo practitioners is falling. In 2010, 69% of dentists were solo practitioners compared to 76% in 2006. By comparison, group practices, many supported by DSOs, have increased 25% from 2009 to 2011. Does this point to the extinction of the solo practitioner? No, I don't believe so. I think solo practices will always exist in the dental industry. But I do think because of the reasons described above by Dr. Kao and other developing trends (rising technology costs and reductions in employer-sponsored dental insurance coverage, to name a few) more and more dentists are turning to DSOs for support.

Unfortunately, another current element of our evolving industry is limited access to care for patients. Dentistry—as is the case with healthcare services in general—is often in short supply across the United States, and certain areas of the country have very limited or even no access to dental care due to geographic and socioeconomic factors. According to the ADA, more than 181 million Americans did not visit a dentist in 2014. More than 47 million people live in places where it is difficult to access dental care and nearly 9,500 new dental providers are needed to meet the country's current oral health needs (HRSA's *Shortage Designation*, 2012). In other healthcare fields in the past, professionals have found ways to resolve such issues. For decades, physicians and other healthcare professionals have formed or engaged entities such as management services organizations (MSOs) for assistance. As stated by the American Health Lawyers Association Physicians and Physician Organizations Law Institute, MSOs assist with the "administrative challenges associated with running their business. MSOs take advantage of economies of scale to provide the practice with a heightened level of expertise and to help the practice obtain better results at lower cost." In a similar fashion, DSOs address the *nonclinical* aspects of practice management so that dentists are able to focus on the *clinical* side of their practices.

As financial barriers create a larger separation between the public and dental care, administrative support provided to dentists by DSOs—like those provided to physicians by MSOs—can be a beneficial option in ensuring the long-term financial viability of dental practices. By spending their time more efficiently on providing dental care, dentists who are supported by DSOs (like their MSO counterparts) are able to increase the amount of time available for providing dental services and at lower prices, thereby increasing the accessibility of dental care to wider segments of the communities in which they practice.

To summarize this evolution, no matter what level of experience you possess, whether new graduate or seasoned professional, I'm sure you have felt the effects of these new industry trends. Dental support organizations have set themselves up in the industry to be an advantageous option for many in overcoming these challenges.

As a reminder, Chapter 20 explores the dynamics and variables related to associate-ships, and much of that content is applicable to understanding and potential employment in dental offices contracted with DSOs.

DSO Models and Processes

As I mentioned, DSOs are aligned under the same goal of supporting dentists, but not all DSOs operate under the same business model or utilize the same branding strategy. In terms of models, there are several different ways DSOs experience growth, such as coordinating the opening of brand new offices for client PC owners, recruiting new dental school graduates and tenured dentists looking for new opportunities within PC owned practices, and supporting additional dental offices that associate with client PC owners. Some DSOs utilize all these methods to expand their support, while others only apply some of these methods. In terms of location, many DSOs do concentrate on supporting offices in certain regional locations. However, there are DSOs who are expanding nationwide as well.

In terms of branding, some DSOs use an encompassing brand approach, where all supported offices are branded under one name. For example, all Aspen Dental Management, Inc.-supported offices are branded Aspen Dental. Some others use more of a multibrand approach. At Heartland Dental, each supported office retains its own name, logo, and brand. A few other DSOs use a combination of both methods— Dental Care Alliance supports many offices that are each branded under different group names, such as Advanced Dental Care, Main Street Children's Dentistry & Orthodontics, Manatee Dental, and others. Some DSO-supported offices are primarily focused on Medicaid patients (DSO-supported offices are well equipped to handle Medicaid's low reimbursement rates and heavy paperwork requirements, allowing them to efficiently provide Medicaid care). Other supported offices are focused on providing more episodic or emergency care. Some DSOs are focused on supporting specialists who handle complex cases, such as ClearChoice and dental implants. Heartland Dental supports upscale general dentists as well as specialists.

When it comes to models and branding, there is no standard method that a DSO must choose. Each organization implements processes that best fit their specific mission and goals. However, there are certain elements of DSO service that affect all DSOs across the board, especially with ownership and what services can be offered to dentists.

Misunderstandings Regarding Ownership

DSOs are often connected with the "corporate dentistry" or "private equity" stigma when referenced or discussed. With these phrases, detractors infer that dental practices give up control—that in choosing to be supported by a DSO, they illegally transfer all clinical decisions and duties made in their practices to DSOs.

However, in the structure of a DSO-supported office arrangement, a professional corporation or other professional entity owns the supported dental office. In compliance with state law, the shareholders of this professional corporation are licensed dentists. Therefore, the supported office is owned entirely by licensed dentists. The professional corporation or entity then contracts the dental service providers, so all dental care responsibilities are controlled by the shareholder dentist(s) or dental service providers in that office. The professional corporation or entity then contracts with the DSO to provide administrative services to that office. At all times, dentists are responsible for patient care and clinical decisions.

This arrangement is the same as many sole practitioner arrangements. DSOs do not directly employ dentists or provide dental care. Dentists are, instead, employed by the professional corporation or entity that, in turn, contracts with the DSO. As a result of these factors, the term "corporate dentistry" in no way describes a dentist's use of a DSO any more than a physician's use of an MSO. The same philosophy of managed healthcare that pharmacy, medical, and optical have adopted applies to this contractual agreement between dental offices and a dental support organization. The service level that dentists provide their patients doesn't decrease. The prices that their patients pay don't increase. Actually, the costs and productivity enabled by DSOs often help supported offices lower fees for patients. Stock ownership opportunities and other retirement benefits may be available to supported dentists depending on the DSO involved.

As with the term "corporate dentistry," detractors often attempt to vilify DSO-supported dentists by noting that many DSOs are owned by "private equity" or other investors that attempt to claim control on dentists and the dental care performed. Actually, over the past few years, there has been a false narrative disparaging private equity financers. Private equity typically consists of funds (similar to, and including, mutual funds and pension plans) in which many investors pool their monies to invest in companies that are not listed on a national stock exchange. The investors in private equity funds include people from all walks and stations in life—such as a teacher's union pension plan that recently invested in a DSO. I should point out that some of the largest hospital groups in the United States are "for profit" and are backed by private equity. Most companies in the United States are not listed on public stock exchanges, although private equity funds may also invest in publically traded companies. In other words, many Americans are invested in funds that have investments in DSOs that detractors attempt to misconstrue.

Mandates in the Affordable Care Act, state laws, as well as the innovative nature of dentistry in general are moving the profession to invest in electronic health records, CAD/CAM technologies, digital x-rays, and so on, all of which benefit patients. New, fully equipped dental practices often require start-up capital in excess of $700,000. Unless a dentist is independently wealthy or has the means to afford bank loans to fund these investments, both the dentist and his/her patients may have to do without these new technologies. This is yet another reason DSOs and their employees strongly feel they assist dentists in improving dental care.

With the support of DSOs, dentists can bridge the access-to-care gap by offering new technologies and the development of new practices, on terms that even new dentists or dentists with limited credit can now afford. These financial resources help level the access-to-care playing field to the benefit of patients and dentists alike (and without relying on tax dollars). Private equity represents a free-market solution within the dental profession at a time when government reimbursement for dental care is significantly lower than general healthcare services. It should be noted that private equity has played a similarly vital role in supporting organizations across the full healthcare spectrum including hospital companies, pharmaceutical and life sciences companies, home health and hospice providers, ambulatory surgery centers, medical device manufacturers, behavioral healthcare providers, and other groups that also face the pressures of rapidly escalating technology costs.

A Clear Division of Clinical and Nonclinical Support

For decades, health professionals, such as physicians, pharmacists, and optometrists, have successfully utilized outside sources for nonclinical responsibilities, for example, MSOs and other outsourced administrative support. This setup has worked well and different models (private practices and MSO-supported practices) have coexisted with one another. For example, in sectors such as optometry, independent optometrists continue to operate individual practices, even with the popularity of companies such as LensCrafters. Countless other sources of nonclinical support also exist that provide options to these health professionals. This evolution has taken place because the laws of medical boards have been continually modernized to fit the current needs of these health professionals. With this modernization, a clear distinction between clinical and nonclinical services has been made with regard to these healthcare sectors.

It can be argued that within the dental industry, the laws and regulations of dental boards have not been as modernized to accommodate new industry trends and shifts. Many of these laws were created even before World War II. So in many circumstances, their relevancy and application in contemporary dental practice (meeting technology advancements, increased costs, work–life balance needs, and transition options) can be questioned. In relation to that, it can also be argued that there has not been a clear separation made between clinical and nonclinical tasks carried out in dental offices. Because of that lack of definition, the relationship between client dentists and DSOs is often misinterpreted in comparison to MSOs and other healthcare sectors. This misinterpretation doesn't necessarily stem from whether the DSO model is right or wrong, but more from lack of education about what DSOs actually offer.

How dentists choose to handle their practice's administrative needs is their decision. Some dentists may choose to outsource all or a portion of their administrative needs (to one or more contractors), while others may choose to address these tasks internally, either by themselves or by team members in their practice. Such needs include bookkeeping, accounting and tax preparation, payroll administration and processing, billing and collections; banking and financing; creation and placement of dentist-approved advertising, promotion (social media), marketing; information technology; and human resources, general office management, property management, house-keeping and risk management, including legal and regulatory, and compliance and insurance. Regardless of how dentists choose to address these nonclinical administrative needs of their practice, the fact remains that the decision has no bearing on how they address clinical matters in the practice. Dental practices that contract DSOs to handle their administrative needs remain *dentist owned and operated*.

Scrutiny or misinterpretation of clinical versus nonclinical often arises because DSOs can offer all of these nonclinical, administrative tasks in one comprehensive suite. Critics often claim that because DSOs support so many aspects of a dental office, this has the potential to influence clinical activities of a dental office as well. But with changing demands taking place in the dental industry, more and more dentists are needing a comprehensive suite of support such as this, rather than seeking nonclinical assistance from ten or fifteen different sources. These industry changes are the reason DSOs exist. DSOs have simply identified these market changes and created turnkey options for dentists in an evolving industry.

DSOs also see the need to document the distinction between clinical and nonclinical responsibilities. These organizations have a great understanding of what support they offer and don't offer, but this understanding needs to be more widespread across the industry. According to Dr. Quinn Dufurrena, "DSOs are very supportive of the need of clearly stating the things which they have no involvement with, but should be allowed to support the non-clinical areas that so many dentists struggle with."

DSO Success Stories

Over the last several decades, many dentists from all career levels and backgrounds have benefited from choosing a DSO as a means to support their nonclinical tasks. Here are a few examples:

- Marvin Berlin, DDS, McKinneyDentist.com in McKinney, Texas: In 2010, McKinneyDentist.com was already an extremely successful independent practice with forty-two employees on staff, including four doctors, and an average of two hundred new patients per month. With success, though, comes more challenges and more responsibilities. Dr. Berlin and his team chose DSO support and were able to extend their success even further—opening a new state-of-the-art facility, advancing themselves personally and professionally with continuing education and gaining work–life balance. Today, Dr. Berlin is a clinical director and mentor at a DSO and is helping other dentists advance their level of care and leadership skills.
- Jade DeSmidt, DDS, Valley Park Dental Care in Valley Park, Missouri: While attending the University of Minnesota School of Dentistry, Dr. DeSmidt contemplated her options after graduation. She knew she wanted to move to the St. Louis, Missouri, area. However, not being from the region, networking for an associateship there proved difficult. Opening an office by herself, though a tempting idea, seemed daunting when she thought about all of the management work and numbers. So, when she was first exposed to what DSOs offered in her third year of dental school, she welcomed the additional option. Now a DSO-supported dentist, she is leading her own team right out of dental school in a new state-of-the-art office while receiving beneficial education and support.

Now that I've discussed some the benefits and advantages DSO-supported dentists have experienced, let's dive deeper into the specific methods DSOs use to further expand their support.

Supporting New Office Openings

One of the ways that dentist-owned professional corporations (PCs) grow their practices is by adding new dental offices. DSOs often have beneficial data and experience with this process that PC owners can utilize. In many cases, this first starts with locating ideal construction sites to purchase or lease. Different criteria exist when it comes to choosing these sites, but the goal is typically to support the construction of offices in areas that are demographically ideal for both dentists and their patients. For instance, at Heartland Dental, we utilize an outsourced provider to help us with demographic information to make sure we support offices in locations that have a need for a dentist. So we know that supported offices' patients in the Midwest, for example, will drive 19 minutes on average to visit their dentist.

These scratch-start (De Novo) offices are designed with the best interests of supported dentists, their team members and their patients in mind. DSOs consider many factors during this process. Typically, the largest considerations involve supporting offices that are patient-friendly and patient-oriented, but that also support the daily needs of dentists and teams. This also alleviates dentists from having to negotiate with vendors and implement equipment—DSOs can handle this for them.

These beautiful new offices are designed to be comfortable and functional for patients, dentists, and team members. Implementing the right technology and planning for ideal work space to advance efficiency also plays large roles in this process. By doing the necessary due diligence and utilizing patient satisfaction measurement methods, DSOs attempt to determine what features will work most effectively.

Supporting the implementation of cutting edge technology and equipment is certainly a focus, but this equipment needs to be proven and effective. DSOs recommend equipment that will be beneficial rather than costly and unnecessary in the long run. There are countless new dental technologies emerging constantly, but rather than implement every flash in the pan, all technology options available are researched and evaluated with supported dentists to determine pros and cons. Then, DSOs can negotiate optimal prices for recommended equipment. Dentist feedback is extremely important during this process. Sharing ideas helps create "best practices," which help DSOs support dentists more effectively.

Recruiting Dentists

Once new offices are constructed, doctors and team members are needed to bring them to life. That's where the recruiting side of DSO growth takes place. Each DSO has its own means for recruiting dentists for supported offices, but most have a recruiting team that specializes in communicating with possible recruits and working with them through the recruiting process. These recruiting teams connect with dentists through a number of ways, such as major dental trade shows and dental school presentations. Most DSOs also list available opportunities for dentists on their websites with different ways of inquiring. It should be noted, the client dentists (PC dentists) always make the final decisions with regard to employment of joining dentists.

If you were interested in a position, the recruiting teams would guide you through the interview process, which varies by DSO, but typically consists of several stages of phone and face to face interviews to discuss. They would also be available to answer any questions or concerns you had. As far as tips on the interview process, DSO-supported offices look for the same qualities that most other professionals seek. Here are a few suggestions for success:

- Bring the right materials. You must not face an interview empty-handed. It's a good idea to bring copies of your resume, especially if you've accomplished something new since the last time you sent the office your resume. You may be interviewing with more than one person, so have a few copies to share. You may find it helpful to bring your own copy to refer to as well. You should also bring copies of your dental credentials, as well as any certifications you have.

- Dress in professional attire. This should go without saying, but always dress for an interview in business professional clothing. Your appearance will be the very first thing the employer notices, so you want to make a strong first impression. Dressing professionally lets people you meet know that you are serious about the position and can be viewed as a professional.
- Know exactly what you have to offer the dental office. While it is impossible to know the exact questions you will be asked, you can still think through responses for predictable scenarios. You can expect to discuss your own philosophy on dentistry, and how it reflects the office's mission and goals, your leadership style, your ability to work with a team, strengths and weaknesses, past experience, explanation of your specific certifications, and specialties and overall knowledge of dentistry and procedures. Bring your own questions too! In addition, your body language and tone are equally if not more important as the questions you will ask and answer.

As this process continues, you would have the ability to visit the supported office to see where you would be practicing. From there, if you were determined to be the right fit, you would be offered a contract with full benefits and salary. Again, contract details and doctor compensation models vary among DSOs.

A sometimes repeated myth about DSOs is that they only seek to recruit young dentists and new dental school graduates. This is simply not the case. While many new graduates do choose DSO support, DSOs recruit dentists from all backgrounds and experience levels. In fact, at Heartland Dental supported offices, the average age of recruited dentists is 33. The criteria of choosing candidates actually focus on goals, personality, and passion, rather than age or experience. DSOs look for recruits who are open, positive, and mentally flexible.

I also touched on this previously, but there are many reasons why dentists who are looking for new opportunities choose DSO support. Along with the relief from administrative tasks, a big reason is the flexibility offered. Depending on the DSO, opportunities exist all over the country, so interested dentists have the option to practice in a location of their choice. Once they begin practicing, they also have the option of transferring to another location later on if they desire.

Another attractive aspect of DSOs is the continuing education opportunities available. Many DSOs offer supported dentists a variety of courses to help advance themselves, not only clinically, but with their leadership and communication skills as well. While these opportunities are available and beneficial to dentists of all experience levels, young dentists and recent dental school graduates may especially benefit. Although curriculum in modern dental schools continues to progress, there are still many important things dental students are not learning involving leadership, communication, and the business side of dentistry. Young dentists are often ill-equipped to deal with all the complexities of a dental practice. They may not be able to manage people, time, and money the way a profitable practice requires. Many are facing all the challenges of starting a family. And what's more, the average new dentist today is burdened with $200,000 in debts from dental school (Diringer, Phipps, and Carsel 2013).

I reference another report created by Dr. Paul Homoly, president of Homoly Communications Institute, in conjunction with Pacific Dental Services titled *Developing Young Dentists into Providers of Excellent New Patient Experiences*. In this white paper, Dr. Homoly explains, "Young dentists know it's important to offer every new patient an excellent experience on their first visit. The problem is, what they believe constitutes an excellent experience is often not what the new patient thinks. While every dental student is consciously learning the technical aspects of dentistry, they are unconsciously learning to communicate in the language of the profession. As a result, they receive an intentional education in dentistry at the same time as they receive an accidental education in how to communicate to patients."

In succeeding right off the bat, young dentists need to be quality leaders and communicators in addition to outstanding clinicians. The educational opportunities offered by DSOs can provide this base knowledge and help them develop into well-rounded dentists. Not to mention, these young dentists can connect to a network of colleagues who can offer guidance and advice.

Supporting Existing Dental Offices

Another way some DSOs extend their support and growth is to affiliate with existing dental offices. In addition to recruiting teams, DSOs also often have affiliation teams, made up of representatives who communicate with dental offices nationwide to find ideal fits. As with the recruiting process, affiliation teams work on behalf of the PC owner dentists to facilitate growth. These affiliation teams communicate with dental offices in various ways, such as attending major trade shows across the country to speak with dentists.

If you are a practice owner and were interested in exploring your options of becoming supported by a DSO, here's how the process will typically go. First, you will communicate with the affiliation team to discuss your needs and ultimate goals, as well as address any questions or concerns you may have. You and the team or representative will also confidentially discuss your operational and financial information to determine if affiliation is the right option.

If moving forward, you would meet in person with the affiliation team or representative to discuss the terms of affiliating. Each DSO is different with regard to what offices they look to support. For instance, PCs that Heartland Dental supports recommend that offices have more than $800,000 in annual revenue, are located in well-populated cities and suburbs, have five chairs or more, and can commit to transitioning with the office for at least 2 years after affiliation. However, like with recruited dentists, having an open, positive, and flexible personality means more.

I have discussed how DSOs alleviate administrative tasks to create work–life balance for dentists, but I can't emphasize enough what this truly means for dentists. Practice management relief is a significant demand in our current industry. Recent research confirms this. In November 2013, the Dental Economics/Levin Group 7th Annual Practice Research Report noted that, "One-third of survey respondents indicate that their greatest challenge is finding ways to increase practice production and profit. Another third of dentists report that inefficient practice systems are the primary barriers to success." The survey also reported that more than a third of general practice dentists utilize the assistance of consultants or coaches for assistance in practice restructuring and development. As this shows, many practice owners are searching for guidance on how to practice more efficiently and handle nonclinical responsibilities. DSOs are poised to help meet these needs.

In addition, dentists are retiring later in life than previous years. This is occurring for many reasons including this main one—lack of transition options. If you are nearing retirement, what will you do with the practice you've worked so hard to build? How will you get your equity out? Should you walk away? Should you sell to an associate?

Should you sell outright? Many dentists in this situation look at transition strategies with DSOs in order to get value and retire on their terms.

DSO Models versus Group Practice Models

Like DSO growth, there are a growing number of "group practice" models in today's industry. In these models, one or more dentists own a number of dental practices typically within a set regional location and directly employ associate doctors. Some of these group practice models also offer some administrative support to employed doctors. While there are some similarities between these models and DSO models, there are still many differences. Compared to DSOs, most group practice models have a smaller amount of supported offices and are positioned in a set region, while many DSOs now have a more expansive positioning throughout the country. In terms of administrative support, most DSOs offer more expansive support options compared to most group practice models. While group practices can offer some nonclinical support (which is outsourced to other businesses in many cases), many DSOs have complete teams housed in one location for services such as accounting, marketing, education, information technology, human resources, and so on. As already mentioned, in most group practice models, associate doctors are employed by the doctor(s) who owns the group practice. DSO-supported doctors are not employed by DSOs.

The Present and Future of DSOs

Despite common misunderstandings of what DSOs actually do, I think with the needs of today's dentists—particularly older, established dentists—the future is bright for DSOs. Over the next 20 years, I believe the number of dentists practicing at DSO-supported offices will at least triple. In a 2014 report from Levin Group, Dr. Roger Levin states that DSOs held 5% of the dental services market in 2006. By 2018, he reports that DSOs will have 20% of the dental services market.

The biggest challenge these organizations will continue to face is settling differences between organized dentistry and dentists who are supported by DSOs. Like I mentioned previously, I believe the majority of dentists share common ground. Yet DSOs are often blamed for inhibiting others to practice solo or own offices. This opposition from organized dentistry has caused many DSO-supported dentists to consider (traditional) industry positions to be out of touch or even hostile toward these said DSO-supported dentists. Some feel this is why membership in the ADA is declining, especially with DSO-supported dentists. Many within organized dentistry understand this, yet others disagree. Time will tell, but the trend is clear.

Changing of traditions is difficult for many. But through education, I do believe DSOs will be accepted for the benefits and advantages they create. Over the past several years, a group made up of DSOs and DSO management teams has been formed to accomplish that very goal. This organization is known as the Association of Dental Support Organizations, or ADSO.

The ADSO is an industry trade organization that currently represents over fifty separate DSOs in forty-six states, as well as in Canada, Australia, New Zealand, and the United Kingdom. Supporting over eight thousand dentists, the mission of the association is to enthusiastically represent to the dental community the powerful advantages that dental support organizations offer dental professionals in improving the quality of dental care for patients and the quality of life for those dental professionals. ADSO members collaborate closely to introduce new technologies, business processes, and patient services. This supports delivery systems that improve effectiveness, efficiencies, and enhance the quality of services to all ADSO constituents, including dental professionals, dental manufacturers, industry providers, and ultimately, the supported dentists' patients.

The ADSO Code of Ethics specifically outlines six principles of member company conduct that are consistent with a dentist's responsibility. These include the following:

- Act with integrity.
- Focus on meeting the needs of dentists.
- Never interfere with dentists' clinical decision-making and treatment services.
- Employ qualified staff and use proven methods to deliver effective support.
- Provide a variety of business support services to meet the needs of dentists.
- Support dentists as they meet needs at home and abroad through charitable activities.

Most of the founding members of the ADSO (myself included) have known each other for 10–20 years. Originally made up of ten DSO management teams, our group met throughout each year at the meetings of other professional organizations. As this became a regular occurrence every year and our numbers continued to grow, we soon realized that all of us were trying to accomplish the same thing and were facing the same challenges. From this group, the ADSO was initiated in 2007 with thirteen-member groups. Although it can be argued that we are business competitors, our group shares more common problems and opportunities than actual "competition." We are all seeking to advance the personal and professional livelihood of supported dentists and to positively impact the dental industry as a whole. Similarly, we are all facing the same opposition.

As time has passed and the number of DSO-supported offices has continued to grow exponentially (the ADSO has experienced a 15% annual membership growth), different outside entities, often feeling threatened by DSO model success, have tried various tactics to suppress or eliminate DSO support or growth (often the detractors I previously spoke of). The past couple years have been particularly active as it relates to proposed anti-DSO legislation or regulation. As discussed, one of the biggest misconceptions is that the administrative support offered by DSOs interferes with the clinical decisions of dentists. However, those supported by DSOs still lead their offices and make decisions regarding their patients and teams. From that standpoint, there is really no difference between a DSO-supported office and a solo office.

Many other highly regulated business sectors have previously faced the same challenges the ADSO faces today and have succeeded. Their innovative ways of creating effective results have eventually become valued. Dentistry is one of the last business models to transform the way it evolves in the marketplace relative to medicine, pharmacy, and vision care. But we are confident that in the future, the benefits DSOs provide to supported dentists will be looked back upon with amazement that these benefits were not universally available. This will be measured when organized dentistry and DSOs can reach agreement on how the roles and responsibilities of each can work together for the advancement of our industry.

With declining patient numbers to dramatic increases in both education and practice start-up costs, the dental industry faces significant challenges while the United States contends with a national oral healthcare crisis. Dental support organizations offer vital assistance in the fight against oral disease and access to oral healthcare, providing dentists with a multitude of administrative support and development resources, training, financing, and other nonclinical services that would otherwise involve numerous vendors or hours of a dentist's valuable time.

As the dental industry evolves, many dentists will continue to choose solo practice. But we know that solo practitioners spend an average of 10–15 hours a week on nonclinical/business responsibilities (a material percentage of them increasingly struggle with these business aspects), and that a large amount of dentists want an option to focus on patient care. If this describes your situation, whether you are an experienced practice owner or recent dental school graduate, the ADSO strives to ensure that the option continues to be a reality.

References and Additional Resources

American Dental Association. 2012. *2010 Survey of dental practice characteristics of dentists in private practice and their patients (updated 2012)*. Available at http://www.ada.org/~/media/ADA/Science%20and%20Research/HPI/Files/10_sdpc.ashx.

American Dental Association. 2014a. *ADA explores growth of large group practices*. Available at http://www.ada.org/en/publications/ada-news/2012-archive/april/ada-explores-growth-of-large-group-practices.

American Dental Association. 2014b. *Action for Dental Health, Year One: 2014, A Report to Congress*. Available at http://www.ada.org.

American Dental Association. 2014c. *A Proposed Classification of Dental Group Practices*.

Anderson, G.D. and Grey, E.B. 2013. *The MSO'S prognosis after the ACA: a viable integration tool?* American Health Lawyers Association Physicians and Physician Organizations Law Institute. Available at http://www.healthlawyers.org/Events/Programs/Materials/Documents/PHY13/B_anderson_grey.pdf.

Association of Dental Support Organizations. 2014. *Toward a common goal: the role of dental support organizations in an evolving profession*. Available at http://www.theadso.org/professional-resources.

Association of Dental Support Organizations. 2015. http://www.theadso.org/about.

Blaes, J. 2013. Solid Recovery Offset by Outdated Systems. Dental Economics/Levin Group 7th Annual Practice Research Report.

Cox, C. and Foster, S. 1990. *The Costs and Benefits of Occupational Regulation*.

Diringer, J., Phipps, K., and Carsel, B. 2013. *Critical trends affecting the future of dentistry: assessing the shifting landscape*. Prepared for the American Dental Association. Available at http://www.ada.org/~/media/ADA/Member%20Center/FIles/Escan2013_Diringer_Full.ashx.

Holm, S. 2014. House of Delegates Address. Available at http://www.indental.org/About-IDA/Leadership/Officers/Holm-Speech.

Homoly, P. and Feldsein, J. 2014. *Developing young dentists into providers of excellent new patient experiences: a special report for leaders of dental group practices*. Homoly Communications. Available at http://www.theadso.org/resources/DevelopingYoungDentists.pdf.

Health Resources and Services Administration (HRSA). 2012. *Shortage designation: health professional shortage areas and medically underserved areas/populations*.

Kao, R.T. 2014. Dentistry at the crossroads *J Calif Dent Assoc* 42(2): 91–95.

Levin, R. 2014. *Dental practice trends: 8 permanent game changers*. Levin Group. Available at http://www.medicaiddental.org/files/Other%20Files/Roundtable_Presentations/2014Roundtable_DentalPracticeTrendsPP.pdf.

Reed, M.J., Corry, A.M., and Liu, Y.W. 2012. The role of women in dental education: monitoring the pipeline to leadership. *J Dent Educ* 76(11): 1427–1436.

United States Federal Trade Commission. 2012. Letter to the Honorable Stephen LaRoque.

Learning Exercises

1. For your current situation, whether you're a new graduate or experienced dentist, write down the biggest challenges you're facing in today's industry, from both clinical and nonclinical standpoints. For each challenge, identify what you believe the cause to be.

2. In terms of marketing, accounting, continuing education, technology, team building, and leadership, evaluate where your office currently stands with each category on a scale of 1–10 (1 being extremely lacking in these areas and 10 being extremely efficient). What actions could help you advance in each area?

3. Visit www.theadso.org and review the organization's vision, mission, values, and code of ethics.

4. From the DSO member list on the ADSO website, choose three DSOs, visit their websites, and evaluate their support models. What models are utilized? How do they differ from one another? What are their strengths? Weaknesses?

Part 6
Managing Staff: Human Resources/Compliance, Managing Dental Teams, and Staff Meetings

Chapter 22
Human Resources and Employment Compliance

Tim Twigg and Rebecca Boartfield

An Introduction to Employment Law

Many federal, state, and local laws govern your management of staff in a practice. Labor law impacts your decisions and actions from recruiting to compensating to evaluating to dismissing staff. While specific laws may apply based on the number of staff members in a given practice, a few federal laws are mentioned here simply to give you a sense of the legal climate in which you operate in a private practice or other organization:

Fair Labor Standards Act of 1938 establishes minimum wage standards for hourly workers that some states or cities may increase beyond the federal minimum. This Act also requires time and a half wages past a 40 hour work week.

Equal Pay Act of 1963 requires the same compensation for women and men with similar qualifications and responsibilities.

Civil Rights Act of 1964 and as amended by the *Equal Employment Opportunity Act* of 1972 protects individuals from employment discrimination based on sex/gender, race, color, religion, and national origin. Many states and cities have similar laws.

Age Discrimination in Employment Act of 1973 protects people aged 40–70 from employment discrimination.

The Pregnancy Discrimination Act of 1976 makes it unlawful to fire an employee based on pregnancy, childbirth, or related medical conditions.

As Zarkowski and Aksu (2008) summarize, "Federal and state laws have been written to protect employees from discriminatory practice, and serve as guidelines for employers in hiring and termination. Federal laws frequently require a minimum number of employees for a lawsuit to be filed. Most states have passed legislation similar to federal laws protecting civil rights and other employee benefits. State laws may only require the employment of one individual for a lawsuit to be filed. Employers should be aware of state employment law and civil rights protections afforded to employees.

Dental Practice Transition: A Practical Guide to Management, Second Edition.
Edited by David G. Dunning and Brian M. Lange.
© 2016 John Wiley & Sons, Inc. Published 2016 by John Wiley & Sons, Inc.
Companion Website: www.wiley.com/go/dunning/transition

Federal laws were passed, to protect specific classes of individuals. The Title VII of the Civil Rights Act of 1964, later amended in 1991, 42 U. S. C. S 2000*e*, *et. Seq.* prohibits discrimination in hiring and discharge and in employment, compensation, terms, conditions and privileges based on an individual's race, color, religion, sex or national origin. Title VII covers employers of 15 or more employees working at least 20 weeks of the year. Individual states also have state laws that protect the civil rights of their citizens. State law may be "stricter" than federal law, but can never conflict with the federal laws. For example, a state law aimed at protecting civil rights, in addition to prohibiting discrimination based on the qualities outlined in Title VII, may also include protection against discrimination based on height, weight or marital status, for example. Following passage of the Civil Rights Act, additional federal legislation occurred to protect classes of individuals."

An Introduction to Human Resources

Success with owning, running, and managing a dental practice requires many vital resources. These resources include financial resources, material resources, equipment resources, and of course "people" resources—otherwise known as *human resources* (HR). Human resources must be managed in view of compliance with employment laws such as those highlighted above.

While all of these resources are important, your human resources are critical and necessary because your systems, processes, and protocols are only as good as the people doing them. Without good people who stay with you long term, all of the best systems in the world won't ensure your success.

Every "real" company has an HR Department. Within these HR Departments, you will find processes that ensure the following:

1. Comprehensive job descriptions for each employee or position
2. Standardized recruiting and hiring protocols
3. Up-to-date policy manuals comprising applicable regulations
4. All of the necessary personnel forms to fulfill documentation needs and requirements
5. Processes for managing performance and employee engagement

When you're hired at places like Microsoft, Colgate, Walmart, Kraft, and Henry Schein Dental, you meet with HR on your first day of employment to complete a series of required processes. Think of HR as a system specifically set up to create success with your employees as well as comply with a myriad of regulations.

Like those companies, your dental office will need to have all of these same components in place. The number of people you employ may be lower, your annual revenue may be lower, but the requirements and the risks of not handling HR correctly are the same.

In fact, the risks may be greater because dentists don't take HR seriously. This could be because little or no time is spent on this topic in dental school, or because dentists erroneously believe they're too small to have to deal with it. As a result, most dental offices are *not* handling HR correctly and are vulnerable to serious liability. Today's reality is that dentists are at greater risk of a labor-related claim or lawsuit than a malpractice lawsuit.

The good news is when you have your HR bases covered, there is no more guess-work, no more flying by the seat of your pants, no more wishing and hoping. Most importantly, you are taking a giant step toward protecting what will most likely be (or already is) your most valuable asset—your practice.

Once you understand this need and the importance, the question becomes: "How do I accomplish sound HR practices at my office?" This chapter will provide you with the fundamentals of the three-principle HR components that are needed for creating a healthy and thriving dental practice.

In its most simple sense, HR is comprised of three principle components:

1. Foundational elements
2. Recruitment
3. Performance Management

Foundational Elements

For dental practices, there are four main areas of compliance that must be addressed: employment/human resources, recordkeeping/charting, OSHA, and HIPAA.

Employment/human resources are the trickiest because, unlike OSHA, HIPAA, and charting, you have spent little to no time learning about this area of your business. Sadly, most dentists are in the dark about this critical aspect of the business. Where do you begin? What do you need?

You start with these foundational elements:

1. A policy manual
2. Job descriptions
3. Personnel files

With these three elements solidly in place, you can build success with your all-important human resources.

Foundational Element: A Policy Manual

Policy manuals serve a variety of purposes that, if properly written, implemented, and used, can keep an employer out of legal trouble, or, at the very least, assist in prevailing if a charge is brought against an employer despite his/her best efforts.

When writing a policy manual, consider your audience. You don't want your manual to be too harsh, condescending, laced with typos, disorganized, or otherwise poorly done. Your policy manual is going to be one of the first impressions your employees have and will set the stage for your culture and climate. The experience of reading the manual should be a positive one.

Your manual should outline your expectations, communicate philosophies, explain employee benefits, and summarize practice policies. Be as concise and clear as possible. A confusing manual will be a hindrance not an asset.

In many cases, a policy manual fulfills an employer's legal obligation to provide written statements on certain matters to employees. For example, some states require employers to inform employees about what will happen to their unused paid leave upon termination.

Most importantly, the manual should address federal, state, and local regulations that are applicable to your practice, given the number of employees you have. The laws will vary on a federal, state, and local level—there is no "one-size-fits-all" law. You will need to know what these requirements are and include them. Here are some areas to consider:

- Overtime
- Pregnancy leave
- Family and medical leave
- Meal and rest breaks
- Military family leave
- Jury duty
- Voting leave
- Leave related to domestic violence
- Sexual harassment
- OSHA and HIPAA

It is not good enough to write a policy manual, stick it on a shelf, forget about it, and not revise it as laws change. In addition, it is prudent to modify the policies when changes are made based on business needs. A failure to keep the policies current will result in the employer following an obsolete policy that is not legally defensible.

Foundational Element: Job Descriptions

Job descriptions document the duties, qualifications, and physical requirements of a job. They help support why you felt one applicant was qualified and another was not, why you pay one employee more than you pay another, or why you terminated an employee for poor job performance.

If an employee or a government agency challenges a hiring or employment decision, one of the most important documents you will be expected to provide is a copy of the job description. This can be a key component to defending your employment actions.

When employees clearly understand what is expected, they have the necessary information to focus on the most important responsibilities and be more productive. One of the best ways to clearly and effectively communicate job expectations is with well-written job descriptions.

A good job description is comprised of the following key elements:

1. Title of the position
2. Exempt or non-exempt status
3. The name, or title, to whom the employee reports
4. A statement of the major purpose of the position
5. Minimum eligibility requirements for adequate performance
6. A description of the physical demands of the job and the type and amount of work to be performed
7. The essential duties
8. Any other information that would be of help in understanding the responsibilities of the job

Employers with 15 or more employees must comply with the Americans with Disabilities Act (ADA). If you have less than 15 employees, you are not relieved of compliance concerns as most states have disability laws that apply to smaller employers. By complying with ADA regulations, you ensure compliance with disability laws whether on a state or federal basis.

If a hiring or an employment decision is challenged, you may be required to show that the qualification standards used in the decision-making process are job-related and consistent with business necessity. In order to use a job description for this purpose, it must be prepared before advertising or interviewing for a job. A job description prepared after a claim is filed will not be considered as evidence.

Inability to perform nonessential or marginal functions of a job is generally not an acceptable reason to disqualify an individual with a disability when you're making employment-related decisions. It is, therefore, important to distinguish clearly what the essential functions of the job are on the job description.

According to the Equal Employment Opportunity Commission (EEOC), "Essential functions are the basic job duties that an employee must be able to perform, with or without reasonable accommodation. You should carefully examine each job to determine which functions or tasks are essential to performance. This is particularly important before taking an employment action such as recruiting, advertising, hiring, promoting, or firing."

When writing the essential functions on your job descriptions, consider the following:

1. Specify what employees actually do and the amounts of time spent on each function and task rather than a general description.
2. Describe the amount of work to be performed.
3. Keep sentence structure as simple as possible and omit words that don't contribute necessary information.
4. Avoid using the words "responsible for." An employee can be "responsible for" any number of duties and never do anything to accomplish them.
5. Begin each sentence with an active verb.
6. Include a percentage of time each essential function consumes as part of the whole job. Adding the percentage of time to each essential function involved helps clarify the level of importance that particular duty has as it relates to all other duties.

Well-written job descriptions are a valuable asset for employers, but only if they are kept up-to-date. They should be reviewed at least once a year and updated or rewritten as necessary and signed by the employee, with a copy given to the employee and a copy placed in the employees file.

Foundational Element: Personnel Files

Federal and state laws mandate recordkeeping requirements for employers. Everything from pre-hire to post-termination has some form of recordkeeping requirement to which employers should adhere. These records should not be kept all together in one place. Depending on the type of record, you may be placing the documents into one of three personnel files: the Regular File, the Confidential File, and the Form I-9 File.

The Regular File usually contains the following:

- Job application and resume
- Employment agreement
- Time and pay records
- W-4 Form
- Attendance and leave records
- Waiver and acknowledgement forms
- Direct deposit authorization
- Employee benefit and enrollment form
- Personnel change forms, such as changes in pay, title, and seniority
- Performance evaluations
- Property held by employee, keys, pagers, other practice property
- Continuing education records
- Disciplinary actions
- Promotion, demotion, transfer, layoff, leave, or termination

The Confidential File typically contains the following:

- Investigative records of grievances or complaints
- Workers' compensation documents
- Discrimination charges and related documents
- Medical information including the results of physical examinations
- Pre-employment and/or other drug-test results
- Work restrictions or accommodation requests and results
- Employment reference results, records of references provided to other employers after termination
- Wage garnishment information
- Credit card information
- Domestic violence information
- Documents that identify employees as being in a protected class
- Veterans' status

We recommend a separate file strictly for I-9 forms. If the U.S. Immigration and Customs Enforcement (ICE) agency conducts an audit of your I-9 forms, you do not want to give the ICE representative access to your personnel files. This would invite him/her to find other possible violations that could lead to potential fines.

The length of time required for keeping various records on employees varies with the type of information in the files. As a general rule of thumb, except for the Form I-9, keep all documents pertaining to employees throughout the employment relationship plus 4 years from the date of termination. If legal action has been taken or is pending, all relevant records must be retained until final disposition. For I-9 forms, upon termination, keep them 3 years after the date of employment begins or 1 year after the date when employment ends, whichever is longer.

Recruiting

Now that once you have the foundational elements in place, you can focus on getting the right people on your team. No management function is more critical than the ability to hire, train, motivate, and effectively manage qualified and competent people.

Good hiring practices and effective people skills have many common benefits. The most significant is a decrease in staff turnover and labor-related problems. Research suggests that direct replacement costs can reach as high as 50–60% of an employee's annual salary, with total costs associated with turnover ranging from 90 to 200% of annual salary (www.SHRM.org. Effective Practice Guidelines Series, A guide to Analyzing and Managing Employee Turnover). Imagine turning that cost into profit for your practice.

One of the most common hiring mistakes inexperienced dentists make is focusing on an applicant's skills and experience. While these are important, you shouldn't place too much significance on them. If someone's skills are not what you need, this can usually be taught or trained. As for experience, unfortunately, it does not always equate to proficiency at your unique practice.

Attitude and compatibility within the practice, on the other hand, cannot be taught or trained—it is either there or it is not. Thus, we recommend focusing first on attitude and compatibility, and then on skills and experience.

Another common mistake is limiting the methods used to evaluate applicants to just one or two aspects rather than taking advantage of the multiple modes of evaluation that are available. Here are ideas for evaluating applicants:

- Résumés/applications
- One-on-one interviews
- Group interviews with staff
- Reference checks
- Employment verifications
- Personality/job match assessments
- Skills assessments/working interviews
- Criminal/background checks

Your hiring success rate will increase with each added method you use to evaluate applicants.

Much like your applicant evaluation methods, it is a good idea to open up the sources you use for attracting and finding applicants. Look to some of the following resources for quality applicants:

- Current employee referrals
- Patients
- Suppliers/vendors
- Schools
- Employment agencies
- Professional associations
- State Employment Department
- Newspaper advertisement
- Internet job placement services
- Community networking

Once you have generated some good responses from your recruiting sources, you can begin to narrow down your applicant pool by doing some prescreening. To do this, develop qualifying questions that you will ask each candidate. The questions must be job related, but can range from work experience to behavioral situations. Typically, prescreening occurs over the phone. If the answers are unsatisfactory, then you have no obligation to move further with that applicant. For those applicants with whom you are impressed, invite them to move forward with an interview.

Require your applicants that move on in the process to complete an application, if they haven't already done so, before the interview. Unlike résumés, applications require the applicant to list specific information about previous employment, which can be verified more easily. The application should also require the applicant's signature attesting to the honesty of the information, authorize the information to be fact-checked, and acknowledge understanding that falsification of the application can be grounds for denying or terminating employment.

To prepare for the interview, develop a set of specific questions to ask. Avoid asking questions that will elicit a "yes" or "no" answer. Focus instead on behavioral-based questions that will elicit a more valuable and comprehensive response. A good rule to follow is that the applicant should talk about 70–80% of the time.

Make notes during and after the interview on a document other than the résumé or application. It is imperative to keep the notes focused on technical skills or experience, rather than potentially discriminatory issues. Close the interview by providing a brief overview of pertinent practice information and your philosophy. Inform the applicant of the next step in the process, but refrain from making any employment commitments.

As you narrow the candidates to two or three finalists, you may want each to complete a personality assessment for job match compatibility. Use the tool to assess perceived attributes, character strengths, and limitations relevant to the job in question. Care must be taken that the assessment does not discriminate, profile, or otherwise target certain groups or protected classes of prospective employees. Use only validated and approved assessments that are, ideally, dental profession-specific.

For your top 1 or 2 finalists, you may want to conduct a skills assessment or a working interview. Skills assessments and working interviews are not the same thing and should not be confused with one another. You may use either method, just ensure to follow the rules for each accordingly.

To conduct a skills assessment, limit time to 1 or 2 hours, do not replace a regular worker, do not have the applicant perform productive work, and have him/her sign a form confirming the voluntary and unpaid nature of the assessment. In this scenario, the person performing the skills assessment is *pretending* to perform a job duty; s/he is not actually executing it. For example, a hygienist can clean teeth on a model; a front desk person can create an insurance account for Mickey Mouse.

To conduct a working interview, none of the above is applicable. A working interview is just like employing someone for a few hours to a few days. They function just like regular workers, and there are no restrictions. They will, however, have to be paid just like normal staff members. A person cannot volunteer for an unpaid working interview. You will need to secure a completed I-9 form before commencing work as well as complete a W-4 form. In doing this, workers' compensation liability may be a factor if the person gets injured, and you may be a part of an unemployment insurance claim filed if the person is not hired.

Once you have your final candidate, the last step is checking references, verifying employment history, and/or performing background checks. Although you may manage this part of the process yourself, it is likely you will contract with a third-party agency. If you do hire an agency, ensure you know and follow all of the rules set forth by the Fair Credit Reporting Act (FCRA) or other applicable state laws. There are steps you must take to initiate these processes and reports you need to provide if the applicant is rejected as a result of the information provided.

By employing the selection process outlined above, you can assemble the members of your winning team.

Performance Management

Now, with your team in place, you must be committed to your team's success. This commitment means providing the tools, resources, training, support, and ongoing communication that will help them succeed. This leads us to the final HR component- performance management.

For several years, there has been an ongoing debate in the HR profession about the value of performance reviews. It has been the focus of Human Resources publications, as well as articles in the *Wall Street Journal* and *Businessweek*. It has been concluded that the standard, age-old annual performance review is no longer as effective and carries potential liability. Today a new, more relevant, meaningful, and productive approach is required. We are finding many employers having success with goal setting and ongoing feedback as their chosen method of performance management.

Managing performance with goal setting can be, at first, challenging because it is individualized for each employee. Nobody can give you the goals for your employees because only you know what you need from your employees to support your success.

If you're asking yourself "why goals?" the simple answer is: employee engagement. Employees who are motivated to make your business and their positions better will positively impact things like customer service, productivity, and morale.

In groundbreaking research, the Gallup group created the Q12 Survey. Gallup "conducted decades of research—writing, testing, and refining thousands of question items to find the ones that would best measure employee engagement. In 1996, Gallup finalized the 12 question items that consistently and powerfully link to business outcomes, including profitability, employee retention, productivity, safety records, and customer engagement."

The following are the twelve core elements that they uncovered as the best predictors of employee engagement and performance:

1. I know what is expected of me at work.
2. I have the materials and equipment I need to do my work right.
3. At work, I have the opportunity to do what I do best every day.
4. In the last 7 days, I have received recognition or praise for doing good work.
5. My supervisor, or someone at work, seems to care about me as a person.
6. There is someone at work who encourages my development.
7. At work, my opinions seem to count.
8. The mission or purpose of my company makes me feel my job is important.
9. My associates or fellow employees are committed to doing quality work.
10. I have a best friend at work.
11. In the last 6 months, someone at work has talked to me about my progress.
12. This last year, I have had opportunities at work to learn and grow.

As the manager/owner/employer, creating goals begins with you. You must know where you want your business to go in order to determine the best way to get there. You need to carefully analyze your business to determine what needs to be improved.

You want everyone, in their own way, working toward the achievement of the goals you established at the executive level. Things to keep in mind:

> ➤ The employee needs to be able to do the work; people can't achieve a goal that is not within their scope of influence or current capability.

➤ The employee must have the tools, resources, and access required to get the work done.

➤ Expectations must be well defined, and the employee must have sufficient time and bandwidth to meet milestones.

➤ Goals must be reasonable. The challenge of a stretch goal can be invigorating; an impossible target will certainly be frustrating and can be demoralizing.

➤ Managers must be prepared to offer guidance and coaching.

How goals are written can be critical to whether or not they will be achieved. A misunderstood goal will be ineffectual; an overly ambitious goal will hinder motivation. It's important that the goals be *S.M.A.R.T.* This common acronym stands for the following:

➤ *Specific:* Exact, accurate, clear, unambiguous, and without the use of generalities. You must specifically define what you expect the employee to do. Use action verbs when possible.

➤ *Measurable:* You will need to identify how success will be measured. What is the concrete criterion? This is usually stated in terms of quantity, quality, timeliness, or cost. This is how you will be able to *objectively* assess whether or not the employee is achieving the goals established.

➤ *Attainable:* Is the goal within the employee's capabilities? Is the goal part of the employee's overall authority? Goals need to be realistic—not out of reach and not extreme. If you can't answer this question: "How can the goal be accomplished?" the employee won't be able to either. Ensure that the employee has the resources and time, as well as access to necessary information (i.e., data, people) in order to be successful at reaching the goal.

➤ *Relevant:* The goals should matter to the employee and align with goals for the team, department/division, and organization. Be sure the employee understands how his/her individual goals contribute to the success and/or failure of the goals at higher levels. In this sense, you are giving the employee context for the work they do.

➤ *Time bound:* Specify a delivery date and/or schedule. When does the goal need to be completed? Goals should be grounded in a specific time frame or target date to create a sense of urgency and prevent day-to-day activities from getting in the way unnecessarily.

S.M.A.R.T. goals create shared understanding and expectations. The purpose is to help the employee, and the team, the department, and the organization succeed.
Pitfalls to avoid:

➤ Consider the employee's total set of goals. While each individual goal may be achievable, you may be assigning the employee more goals than s/he could reasonably be expected to successfully complete. Generally three to five should suffice.

➤ Don't create a situation in which safety, ethics, or morals will need to be compromised in order to achieve the goal. Be sure employees know you don't want short cuts (cheating), which can be dangerous, to become the manner in which a goal is accomplished.

➤ Don't create goals that are so narrowly defined that employees miss the bigger picture. You don't want employees to focus myopically on short-term gains and lose sight of the long-term effects on the organization.

➤ While goals should be time bound, don't make the time line inappropriately short. Too short of a time frame can result in long-term problems—short-term goals encourage short-term thinking.

➤ Think about whether or not the goal will influence risk-taking. Define acceptable levels of risk. You don't want your employees to take too much risk and put the organization in any kind of harm.

Once you've established goals, then you move on to the critical piece of monitoring employees' performance and providing important feedback, both positive and constructive. Goal setting will not work if the employee is not receiving feedback. How can anyone expect an employee to continue good work or stop bad work when s/he doesn't know what the employer wants? Feedback is fundamental and necessary in order to turn things around.

Before anyone can provide feedback, the employee's performance must be monitored to know what kind of feedback to give. Monitoring performance can be done in two different ways: quantifiable and behavioral. Here are a few examples of quantifiable methods:

- Sales/production/collection reports
- Deadlines met
- Error reports
- Budget forecasts

These methods specifically measure what an employee actually does day-to-day. They are objective—these things either happened or they didn't.

Here are some ways to capture behavioral performance:

- *Observation:* Probably this is the most effective method because it means you're actually observing your employees work. Nothing beats the power of direct observation.

- *Asking for an accounting:* This must be accompanied with regular one-on-one conversations with the employee in which you probe the employee to account for his/her performance, one way or another. Questions like: "Did you meet the expectation?" "What actions did you take to meet them?" Then you must listen, make some assessments, and perhaps ask some more questions in order to determine the best way to approach any feedback provided.

- Feedback from other sources like coworkers, supervisors, clients, patients, and so on.

It's important to remember that feedback means positive too. Sometimes employers get so wrapped up in what's going wrong, they lose sight of the fact that many things are going right, and employees should know both the good and the bad.

According to a recent article in the *Wall Street Journal*, there is a significant movement to encourage positive feedback in the workplace. The article states: "Fearing they'll crush employees' confidence and erode performance, employers are asking managers to ease up on harsh feedback. Accentuating the positive has become a new mantra at workplaces like VMware Inc., Wayfair Inc., and the Boston Consulting Group Inc., where bosses now dole out frequent praise, urge employees to celebrate small victories, and focus performance management around a particular worker's strengths—instead of dwelling on why he flubbed a client presentation."

With any feedback, it shouldn't be a one way street. In fact, the more you can structure the feedback as a dialogue, the better the outcome. The process of openly discussing positive and constructive feedback can be essential for building effective relationships, raising awareness, maximizing potential, and improving one's performance.

Regardless of whether the feedback being given is positive or constructive, there are a few principles to apply:

- *Timely*: Do not wait to provide feedback. Use the next available time that is practical to provide the feedback.
- *Specific*: Refrain from using generic phrases like "you did a great job." These are vague and won't give your employee the necessary insight to know what should be repeated and what should be avoided.
- *Objective:* This is particularly true of constructive feedback. It's about the behavior, not the person. Describe what happened, what you saw, how it impacted the client, the team, the business, and so on.
- *Continuous:* Giving both types of feedback should be a regular occurrence in the employee–employer relationship.

For constructive feedback in particular, focus on changeable behavior. In some cases, the person just won't be a fit and nothing can be done about it. What people say, how people go about their jobs, and how they interact with others can be managed and coached; other problems, particularly attitude, not-so-much. When you find yourself judging the person, not the behavior, you will know this relationship is probably not going to work.

One final note on feedback, in terms of goals that have been set, you should establish specific intervals at which point the employee's progress in accomplishing said goals will be measured and discussed. This will depend on the goal. Some goals will be reviewed sooner than others. Is it a goal to be obtained in 6 months? Is it a year? This will guide you in how quickly, and at what intervals, structured meetings should occur to discuss the employee's progress, or lack thereof.

With any performance management system, employers tend to get wrapped up too much in the past. Here are a few thoughts about why focusing on the future may be a more effective approach:

- We cannot change the past, but we can affect the future.
- Nobody wants to be "made wrong"—doing so creates defensiveness. Future-focused conversations get away from "let me tell you how wrong you've been" and move to "here is how I want you to do this task/job."
- People take it less personally. It removes the feeling of being personally attacked.
- Most people do not like getting negative/constructive feedback and most hate to give it. It can be a relief to all parties to not be in this situation.
- Future-focused feedback can contain the same constructive points, but done in a manner that doesn't further bash the employee with what went wrong that cannot be changed.
- We all know that when we are receiving negative/constructive feedback, we tend to tune out the speaker and start developing our responses in our head because we get defensive. Future-focused feedback allows the listener to be fully engaged.

Throughout this, it's important to not lose sight of ensuring appropriate documentation. That documentation can come in all different forms so long as you are tracking the employee's performance and the conversations you have had about it. This is particularly true for an employee who is not a high performer, who is not improving even with all the feedback, and is certainly not meeting established goals, which may very well mean you will have to terminate the employee's employment.

Disciplinary documentation should:

- State the reason for the counseling in specific, factual, scrupulously honest, concise terms.
- Outline the specific nature of the discipline.
- Describe the corrective action expected of the employee in specific, measurable terms.
- Warn of potential consequences if the employee fails to improve.
- Include signatures and dates from all parties involved.

Here are some examples of other forms of documentation:

- Any document containing the specific goals to be achieved
- Notes within a file on your computer
- Written statements from patients/clients/coworker/other
- Handwritten notes on a yellow pad

Remember that all of these notes and documentation, no matter the type, should be job related and objective. Do not pass judgment or document anything of a subjective nature.

Preventing Sexual Harassment

Zarkowski and Aksu (2008) succinctly describe the importance of preventing sexual harassment: "An important protection offered by the Civil Rights Act of 1964 is protection from sexual harassment. Two forms of sexual harassing behaviors are protected. *Quid Pro Quo* includes unwelcome sexual advances, requests for sexual favors, and other verbal or physical conduct of a nature or submission to them is basis for hiring, firing, or advancement. *Hostile environment* occurs when any type of unwelcome sexual behavior creates an offensive or hostile environment. The harassment does not have to result in tangible or economic job consequences. The dental office is an environment that is characterized by working relationships in which humor or inappropriate comments or behaviors, intended to be humorous, may result in allegations of creating a hostile environment. Examples of behaviors that could contribute to a hostile environment include the following:

- Unsolicited or unwelcome flirtations, advances, or proposals
- Ill-received jokes or offensive gestures
- Intrusive questions about an employee's personal life
- Suggestive facial expressions
- Abuse of familiarities or diminutives such as "cutey" or "my girl"
- Unnecessary, unwanted physical contact such as hugging or touching

- Suggestive comments about clothing
- Questions about sexual fantasies, sexual preferences, or sexual activities"

Tips on Dismissing Staff Members

Terminating a staff member's employment certainly is not an easy process. However, it may become necessary when a staff member has failed to meet expectation over time and documented efforts to improve performance have not been successful.

Attorney Michael Moore (*Dental Economics*, March 2010) recommends a somewhat "softer and gentler" approach to what has traditionally been called "progressive discipline"–not using the words "warning" or "discipline" during this process, suggesting these steps instead:

1. *Provide informal counseling.*
2. *Include a Decision Day* in which a staff member is paid but does not report for a work shift in order to reflect on personal goals and commitment to the practice.
3. *A Final Affirmative Agreement* in which the staff member agrees to commit to the practice and to correct performance issues within a specific time period and during which the staff member will not be terminated if the performance issue is being successfully addressed.
4. *Exit Evaluation* in which a staff member who separates (amicably or not) receives a letter encouraging her to report on a form anything negative about the practice.

While less aggressive, this four-step process is very similar to the process for dismissing staff presented at the end of Chapter, 23.

These practical tips will help you navigate the nuances of actually terminating a staff member:

1. Have a check written for all salary and benefits due (for example, unused vacation time, severance pay if you offer it).
2. Be firm and quick with you actions.
3. Do not get into a debate or argument with the staff member.
4. Typically, it is best to dismiss the staff member at the end of the week if you have temporary help available or a new hire available. If you don't have backup staff available, you may need to dismiss earlier in the week in order to hire a temporary or permanent replacement in a timely manner.
5. Do *not* allow the dismissed staff person to remain in the office after s/he is dismissed. Considerable damage could be done to a practice's reputation and team unity by an upset staff member knowing s/he is facing dismissal. See Chapter 16 for more information on employee embezzlement.

Final Note/Conclusion

To prevent problems related to human resources or lack of employment compliance, dentists need to (1) gain awareness, (2) have a commitment to do something about it, and (3) take action to address the inherent HR compliance risks to protect their practices.

You have the following options for tackling No.3: (a) do this yourself, (b) hire a labor law attorney, or (c) partner with and utilize the services of a firm that specializes in HR for dentists (see Chapter 21). Each has its pros and cons. Given what you have learned and the challenges associated with HR and employment compliance, partnering with HR professionals is the easiest, safest, and most cost-effective approach.

Regardless of the direction you choose, it is important to understand the importance, value, and need for addressing HR successfully.

References and Additional Resources

http://www.wsj.com/articles/everything-is-awesome-why-you-cant-tell-employees-theyre-doing-a-bad-job-1423613936.

http://www.wsj.com/articles/SB122426318874844933.

http://www.bentericksen.com/.

http://www.dol.gov/.

https://q12.gallup.com/public/en-us/Features.

Moore, Michael. 2010. Don't let your practice be held hostage. *Dent Econ* 100: 3.

Zarkowski, Pam and Aksu, Mert. 2008. Employment Law. Chapter 17. In: Dunning, David G. and Lange, Brian M. (Eds.), *Dental Practice Transition: A Practical Guide to Management*, Ames, IA: Wiley-Blackwell.

Learning Exercises

1. Skills assessments carry no liability for me because
   a. the individual is not an employee and I have not made a formal job offer,
   b. I keep the time under 2 hours, no productive work is performed, and I have a signed form verifying no wages and no promise of employment.
   c. I don't pay the prospective employee any money for the day they work, and
   d. I make the candidate a volunteer.
2. Today, the asset value of my practice is most in jeopardy due to
   a. economic recession,
   b. malpractice lawsuits,
   c. IRS audits, and
   d. labor-related judgments, penalties, and fines.
3. You are required to have an I-9 form for
   a. all employees,
   b. current employees only,
   c. employees hired after September 2001,
   d. minority employees only.
4. Employee performance management is best handled by
   a. focusing on past performance and citing past performance deficiencies,
   b. no less frequently than once a year from the date of hire,
   c. focusing on the future through individually established goals, and
   d. having a strict three-strike rule of progressive discipline

5. Well-written job descriptions are valuable because
    a. they communicate expectations, duties, qualifications, and physical requirements of a job;
    b. they ensure compliance with the ADA;
    c. they can be used to support employment decisions;
    d. all of the above

Answer key: 1. (b); 2. (d); 3. (a); 4. (c); 5. (d)

Chapter 23
Managing Dental Teams
Amy Kirsch

Managing dental teams effectively is one of the biggest challenges dentists face in their practices. As we all know, a motivated and well-managed team may improve productivity, profitability, and patient care. In this chapter, we discuss how to hire the right people, how to motivate them, and how to evaluate them effectively.

Before You Hire Anyone, What You Must Know

When hiring a quality employee, you must first know and be clear about who *you* are and what kind of team you need to surround yourself with to practice effectively. The most successful practices we work with are great students of their behavioral style and know how to use it in selecting and working with staff members.

In the early 1970s, the Carlson Learning Company described four major behavioral styles (DISC) that have guided many dental practices in their hiring practices and with team building meetings. They describe four general behavioral and personality styles to be aware of in your practice:

- Dominance
- Influence
- Steadiness
- Conscientiousness

Are you a "dominance" style? This is the visionary leader who loves challenge and change. You wear your heart on your sleeve and need followers who will implement your ideas for you. Having too many dominance styles in a practice is like having too many cooks in the kitchen.

If you are an "influence" style, you prefer working with people and motivating them. You have fun and love the people side of dentistry. However, if you hire a whole team of influencing individuals, you will have lots of fun but rarely run on schedule and may have issues with implementation and follow-through.

Dental Practice Transition: A Practical Guide to Management, Second Edition.
Edited by David G. Dunning and Brian M. Lange.
© 2016 John Wiley & Sons, Inc. Published 2016 by John Wiley & Sons, Inc.
Companion Website: www.wiley.com/go/dunning/transition

The "steadiness" style craves order, works and thinks about systems, loves harmony, and dislikes change and conflict. If you have too many steadiness styles on the team, you will be a low-key, happy group, but change will be difficult for you.

The "conscientiousness" style is the detail-oriented, analytical individual who loves research and working alone. If you have too many conscientiousness staff members on the team, you will have a very organized practice with lots of rules and regulations, but not enough people-oriented individuals with high customer service skills.

What is your behavioral style and what behavioral style would best complement you in the practice? Most of us are a combination of some of these. We need to be surrounded by others who have other strengths than we do. Many staff and doctors spend too much time trying to change other people's behavioral style, and it rarely happens. There is one factor that will not change: you are the dentist and the owner of the business. Your behavioral style will most likely remain the same for the duration of your career.

Therefore, hire staff based on their strengths and behavioral style, not just their skill set. Learning effective clinical and business systems is easy if you have a person with ability, a willingness to learn and a great training program. However, basic behavioral styles rarely change. Recruit and select staff members who complement you and your style.

An additional important point to consider when you hire someone is to trust your instincts. If there are red flags in the interview, you can almost count on wild forest fires when the person is hired. So often we have a gut feeling about an individual and ignore it, but after hiring hundreds of employees over the years, our instincts are almost always right.

How to Locate and Recruit the Best Staff for Your Practice

The best candidates for your position are not necessarily looking for a new job, so you will need to network to find the "right" person. The best place to start your networking is with your existing patients of record. Are any of your patients a good candidate for you? Perhaps one of their friends could be the team player you are looking for in your office. Let your patients know about the open position in your practice. Involve your staff in the hiring practice by offering them a "finder's fee" if they refer an applicant and you hire that person for the job. Most staff members are motivated to refer their friends to your practice and will be more vested in their long-term success and training.

Do not overlook the importance of placing a creative, descriptive, and exciting ad in the newspaper (if you are in a small community) and on the internet (Craigslist, Indeed. com, ziprecruiter.com). See sample ads below. You want to set your practice apart from the others on the internet and in the newspaper so you will attract the "cream of the crop."

When evaluating a candidate in today's competitive marketplace, quick response time and good interview skills are very important. The candidate should e-mail his or her résumé and be screened initially over the telephone by a competent staff member or the doctor to determine experience, job responsibilities, and salary needs. If the candidate appears to be qualified for the position, ask him or her to come in for a personal interview. If the candidate's résumé or application demonstrates good job experience and longevity, set up an interview with the doctor or Office Manager as soon as possible. Good applicants are hired quickly!

In the interview, ask interesting questions and listen more than you talk. Look for a person with a positive attitude and willingness to take on a challenge. Remember to trust your instincts! Ideally, the right candidate would be available for a working interview or skill assessment as soon as possible to evaluate his or her abilities and experience. The last part of the interview process would include a lunch meeting with the staff. After all, they will be intimately involved in the training and success of this individual, and you need their feedback and support in the hiring process.

Questions to avoid:

1. Marital status
2. Names and ages of spouses, children, dependents
3. Nationality, ancestry, lineage descent
4. If the applicant is pregnant or plans to have a family
5. Age
6. Race or color
7. Does he or she rent or own home
8. Religion
9. Dates of attendance or completion of school
10. Height or weight
11. Provisions for childcare
12. Who he or she resides with
13. General medical condition, state of health, or illness
14. Receipt of workers' compensation
15. Physical disabilities or handicaps
16. Organizations, clubs, societies, lodges
17. Military service, either foreign or national
18. Economic status
19. Refusal or cancellation of bonding
20. Name and address of relative to notify in case of emergency
21. How spouse/parents feel about person working
22. Sexual orientation

Sample Employment Ads

Growing, quality-oriented professional office desires enthusiastic, mature team member as Patient Coordinator. Outstanding work environment and benefits. Three days/week/Aurora. Please e-mail résumé to _____.

Full-time Practice Administrator for a small quality-oriented professional office. If you are a highly motivated people person with exceptional organizational skills and would like to be a member of our progressive team, please e-mail resume to_____.

Happy, high-quality, team-oriented dental office is seeking enthusiastic Financial Administrator to help our family of patients properly handle their accounts and schedule their appointments. Dental experience required. If this sounds like you, please e-mail your resume to_____.

Are you an enthusiastic, motivated dental person looking for a new opportunity? We have a leadership position for the right individual to take over the front desk responsibilities. Part-time or full-time. Please contact: _____.

An opportunity for a caring, enthusiastic person with a progressive professional office as Appointment Administrator. Please e-mail your resume to_____.

Appointment Administrator needed for a quality-oriented downtown professional office. If you have a high level of energy, excellent verbal skills, and people skills, please e-mail your resume to_____.

Downtown dental office requires full-time Patient Coordinator. If you are self-motivated, enthusiastic, and have good communication skills, please call Elaine _____ to become a member of our quality team. Benefits program offered.

Full-time position in a small professional office. Fantastic opportunity for an organized people person who is creative and detail oriented. To become a valued member of our fine team, please e-mail resume to _____.

Downtown area. Two-doctor restorative practice seeking mature-oriented individual with good verbal skills and an eagerness to learn.

Would you enjoy working in a cheerful, exciting, and professional atmosphere? Well, we're in need of an enthusiastic and caring person to join us in our quality-oriented practice. Experienced preferred, but not required.

Full-time position in professional office. Wonderful opportunity for an organized people person who is detail oriented. Excellent benefits. Englewood area. Dental experience preferred.

Would you like to be appreciated? Dental Hygienist needed for caring, progressive family practice. Great pay with benefits is offered for an enthusiastic individual with appropriate skills.

Our high-quality practice is looking for an energetic and organized Dental Assistant committed to excellence. 34 hours/wk. Coal Mine and Wadsworth. Experience required.

Our progressive dental team is seeking an experienced EDDA to help provide quality dental care. This full-time position comes with complete fringe benefits package and negotiable salary.

Progressive Cherry Creek general practice looking for that special Dental Assistant who loves working with people, enjoys multitasking, and is interested in personal growth and long-term commitment. Outstanding salary and benefits.

Young, progressive dental practice in a new facility seeking enthusiastic, self-motivated person to be full-time Dental Assistant. Experience preferred, but will train the right person.

Seeking an outgoing people-oriented team member who likes a challenge for position of EDDA in a caring office. If you are looking for this type of position with a good benefits package . . .

Telephone Screening

The following questions are examples of questions to ask in the telephone interview to determine if this person should move forward with a personal interview:

1. "What about our ad prompted you to respond?"
2. "Tell me about your dental experience."
3. "Generally speaking, what is most important to you about your current position?"
4. "Have you dealt with the public in previous positions, and how have you felt about it?"
5. "What do you like most about your current job?"
6. "The hours for the position are _____. How does that work for you?"
7. "Before we continue our discussion, let's make sure we are in the same ballpark on salary. What kind of salary are you looking for?"
8. "What would you say are the main responsibilities of _____?"

9. "What do you think are important characteristics of a good _____?"
10. "Ideally, what are you looking for in your next job?"

If the person "passes" the telephone screening/interview, schedule the potential applicant for a personal interview with the Office Manager or Doctor for approximately 30–45 minutes.

First Interview

Prepare for the interview by having an application for completion, a copy of the job description, and a DISC Profile. Determine what questions you will ask the applicant in advance and take great notes. Many doctors have a staff member sit in the interview for their feedback and impression. Questions to ask to determine a person's willingness, ability, values, and goals can include the following.

Questions About His or Her Most Recent Position

1. What circumstances led to your employment at _____?
2. What most influenced your decision to work there?
3. What are (were) your day-to-day responsibilities?
4. What are (were) the most important dimensions of your position?
5. What arc (were) the key responsibilities and/or objectives?
6. Describe the kind of client contact you have at _____.
7. Which of your responsibilities have you performed particularly well?
8. In what ways could your performance be improved?
9. What steps have you taken to improve in these areas?
10. What aspects of the position do you enjoy the most?
11. What aspects do you enjoy the least?
12. What do you consider to be a stressful situation in your current position?
13. Why are you seeking to make a career change at this time?
14. What types of people do you work best with within your current position?

Questions About His or Her Other Work Environments

1. Of the businesses you have worked for in the past, which did you like the most?
2. Which did you like the least?
3. Which positions/duties have you liked the most?
4. Which positions/duties have you liked the least?
5. Of the various environments in which you have worked, in which were you most productive?
6. Which of your past positions have best prepared you for this job?

Questions About His or Her Personal Effectiveness

1. How would you describe yourself?
2. What do you consider to be your greatest strengths?

3. In what areas could you improve?
4. What was the worst mistake you ever made in a position, and how did you handle it?
5. Where do you see yourself career-wise in 3–5 years?
6. How does the position we are discussing today pertain to these career aspirations?
7. If you could create an ideal job for yourself, what would that job look like?
8. Why are you attracted by this position we are discussing?
9. What attracts you to a career in dentistry?
10. Define for me what you think constitutes "patient service" in a dental office.

Second Interview/Skills Assessment and Lunch with Staff

The purpose of the second interview is to assess the competency or skill levels of the applicant on a different day in a different situation, and to communicate more about values and the job itself. Always check skill levels. Also, you may need to consult an attorney to ensure compliance with employment/selection law.

When checking for competence or skill levels, use three tools: Question philosophies about why specific skills are used or necessary for the position. Test whatever professional skills the applicant possesses. Role-play scenarios that the applicant is likely to encounter in the position.

Questions About Philosophies

1. What is the most important role of the _____?
2. Describe your infection control procedures.
3. Describe your sterilization techniques.
4. Describe your philosophy of periodontal care.
5. What is your philosophy of helping build the practice?
6. Give an example of how you can support the team.
7. What is your role in influencing patients to have (prediagnosed) dentistry?
8. How do you document financial arrangements?
9. What role do you perceive yourself having in staff meetings?
10. What role do you feel that appointment scheduling plays in the overall success of the practice?
11. Tell me what you would do to incorporate the philosophy statement into your day-to-day responsibilities here if you were hired. (You previously gave the applicant a copy of your philosophy statement on the first interview.)

Tests

Tests for Hygienist

Perform a quadrant or two of prophylaxis (on the doctor, or on a team member if doctor wants to observe technique). If performed on you or a team member, you must pay the applicant and file the appropriate I9 and W4 forms. Communication skills and empathy toward the patients can be observed.

Place/take/develop bite-wing x-rays on a staff member or doctor.

Tests for Dental Assistant

Place/take/develop bite-wing x-rays on a staff member or the doctor. Test generalized chair-side technique, test applicant's four-handed dentistry skills, have applicant set up operatory, disinfect operatory, and follow process through with sterilization of instruments and tray. However, the setting cannot be real or have anyone benefit from this work unless it is to be paid.

Tests for Financial Administrator/Appointment Administrator

Compose a thank you note for a referral and/or a welcome letter to a new patient on the computer to check for composition, spelling, punctuation, computer skills, and so forth.

Mathematically, figure financial arrangements on a fictitious case with proper documentation.

Ask them to problem solve a difficult insurance and/or EOB issue.

Role-Play Scenarios

Role-Play for Hygienist

The hygienist must tell an established patient that he or she sees signs of periodontal disease and that the patient may need to see a specialist.

The hygienist is aware that a patient has been delaying getting a crown for 2 years. Have him or her talk to the patient about going ahead with it.

The hygienist sees another staff member disregard an important practice policy. What would the candidate do about it?

Role-Play for Dental Assistant

When the doctor leaves the room the patient turns to you and says, "Do you think I really need that crown?" How would the assistant respond?

When the doctor is not in the room, the patient bursts into tears. What would the assistant do?

When the doctor leaves the room the patient says, "I think I need a second opinion." How would the assistant respond?

He or she sees another staff member disregard an important policy. What would the assistant do about it?

Role-Play for Financial Administrator

Present a patient with financial arrangements for a large case.

Handle an emotional patient who did not realize what the fee for a procedure would be.

Role-play a collection call (follow up on a financial arrangement) on an account over 30 days. Then, do the same thing for the account after it reaches 60 days.

The financial administrator sees another staff member disregard an important practice policy. What would the candidate do about it?

Role-Play for Appointment Administrator

Collect an over-the-counter fee.

Schedule an appointment.

Schedule an appointment for a pre blocked morning time when the patient "wants to come in after work."

The patient wants to call later to schedule his or her next appointment. How should the appointment administrator respond?

The appointment administrator sees another staff member disregard a practice policy. What would the candidate do about it?

Welcoming Your New Employee to Your Practice

Celebrate the decision to work with your outstanding team by sending the new employee a plant or flowers with a note welcoming him or her to the practice. Have the entire team sign the card. On the first day of work, make sure a staff member is assigned to the new employee and available to greet him or her and give a brief orientation. It should include where to park, where the lockers are, a tour of the office, lunch and break time suggestions, and an introduction to all the staff members.

Have a specific training program for the new employee for everyone to follow. The most successful team members are clear on their job responsibilities and what is expected of them. All staff members should also be aware of where the new employee is in the training process and what their role is in the training.

One last thought to remember: you are in control of setting the tone in the practice by hiring individuals who can follow through with your goals and vision. Hire well!

Job Descriptions

Clearly defined job descriptions and responsibilities are the backbone of the success of an employee and of the practice. A job description should outline the duties of the position as clearly as possible. The documented job description includes the standards and qualifications for the position. It serves as a guideline for hiring, interviewing, and future training. The job description also sets the groundwork for performance evaluations and managing the employee effectively. Table 23.1 provides sample job descriptions for these positions: financial administrator, appointment administrator, dental assistant, dental hygienist, and an infection control person. Qualifications are not listed in these example job descriptions.

Table 23.1 Position descriptions.

Financial Administrator Job Description
Overall responsibilities:
- Responsible for administering the day-to-day financial activities of the practice; accounts receivable; insurance; back up the appointment administrator

Maintain an accounts receivable system:
- Enter patient activity in computer
- Maintain accounts receivable activity
- Maintain a financial record for each patient
- Complete insurance claim forms as needed for each patient
- Prepare bank deposits
- Prepare statements for patients
- Follow up insurance claims
- Follow up delinquent accounts
- Arrange payment schedule with patients

Table 23.1 *(Continued)*

Insurance:
- Submit treatment plans for predetermination of benefits
- Prepare claim forms for patients with dental insurance
- Organize supporting materials for claim forms, such as radiographs or written narratives
- Electronically submit claim forms daily
- Assist in the resolution of problems with third-party payers

Billing:
- Send statements to patients each week, divided evenly by the alphabet
- Prepare and mail overdue account letters on the 15th of each month
- Call patients with overdue accounts
- Post checks received each day

Appointment Administrator Job Description

Overall responsibilities:
- Responsible for maintaining appearance and order of dental office, patient scheduling; patient management and correspondence

Office management:
- Open the office and turn on the lights at least 15 minutes before the first scheduled appointment of the day
- Ensure the reception room is neat and has a professional appearance
- Check the day's schedule for accuracy
- Facilitate the morning huddle

Scheduling:
- Establish and maintain a recall system
- Confirm patient appointments 2 days in advance by phone or e-mail
- Schedule according to the daily production goal
- Preblock the schedule according to procedures
- Maintain a paperless tickler file for patients with delayed and undone treatment

Patient management:
- Manage recall system each month with the hygienist(s)
- Ensure patient communication is timely with emails, text messaging, letters, and phone calls
- Welcome patients and greet all patients by name
- Accurately record patient dental, medical, and insurance information
- Accurately file patient information
- Collect money from patients at time of treatment
- Arrange patient records for the next day's appointments
- Assist in the treatment rooms as needed

Correspondence:
- Sort, organize, and distribute mail
- Prepare and send out welcome emails to new patients and referral thank you letters to patients
- Send out the weekly marketing note

Dental Assistant Job Description

Overall responsibilities:
- Responsible for assisting the dentist in the clinical treatment of patients

Clinical management:
- Check to ensure that units are ready, stocked, and clean at the beginning of each appointment
- Oversee cleanliness of treatment rooms
- Help in other areas of the office when necessary (answering phones, filing, assisting the hygienist, etc.)

Patient management:
- Go into the reception room and greet patients by name
- Seat patients in the treatment room and have proper setup for procedures
- Try not to leave the patient unattended in the chair

Table 23.1   (*Continued*)

- Anticipate and assist dentist's needs at all times
- Perform clinical procedures as delegated by the dentist
- Document the date of service, services rendered, all charges, and what procedure is to be completed at the next visit
- Give patient instruction and demonstrate where necessary, as directed by the dentist
- Update patient's health history and patient information semiannually
- Notify the appointment administrator if a patient should be called in the evening after a difficult appointment
- At all times show care and concern for patients
- Escort patients from the treatment room to the business area

Dental Hygienist Job Description

Overall objective:
- Responsible for providing hygiene treatment to patients

Equipment management:
- Before each appointment, check hygiene room for cleanliness
- Clean hygiene room at the end of the day; turn off equipment
- Maintain a supply inventory for hygiene treatment
- Review, select, and submit orders for patient education materials for the practice

Patient management:
- Gather and review patient charts for the day and the following day
- Work closely with the appointment administrator to keep the hygiene schedule full and productive
- Carefully review patient medical and dental history records and update as necessary
- Accurately chart each patient's periodontal and restorative health at each visit
- Provide thorough and gentle prophylaxis to patients
- Provide periodontal therapy as needed to designated patients
- Provide radiographs for patients as prescribed by dentist
- Provide topical fluoride applications for designated patients as prescribed by dentist
- Communicate with patients in an understandable and professional way
- Provide appropriate patient education to each patient and distribute the proper patient education material
- Preappoint 90% of the hygiene patients for their next hygiene appointment
- Strive to achieve your daily and monthly goals
- Perform other tasks assigned by dentist

Infection Control Job Description
- Properly discard all disposable items from each visit
- Assemble soiled instruments and place in sterilization area
- Clean treatment room surfaces with disinfectant solution
- Presoak soiled instruments in a disinfectant
- Process instruments in ultrasonic cleaner tank
- Rinse and soak treatment trays in disinfectant
- Sort and package instruments by tray for proper sterilization
- Load, activate, and vent the sterilization unit according to the manufacturer's directions
- Store instruments and trays in appropriate places

Buying a Practice with Existing Staff

One of the most challenging situations a dentist may find himself or herself in after purchasing a practice is establishing rapport with the "inherited" or existing staff. Many staff members are reluctant to have a new leader and are unsure of their future in the practice. To ensure a smooth transition for the doctor, staff, and patients, we recommend building rapport and opening the communication lines with the staff as soon as possible. For example, here are five key questions to ask the existing staff in a 15-minute initial interview:

1. Tell me about yourself.
2. What part of your job do you like the most?
3. What part do you like the least?
4. What do you currently like the most about how this office runs and what would you change?
5. What do you need from me (dentist) with regard to leadership and communication?

In this short interview, the dentist, as the new owner of the business, is looking for ways to motivate and meet the employee's needs. He or she is hoping to uncover the employee's "hot buttons," what motivates the employee, and what he or she likes and dislikes about the job. It also allows the dentist to establish whether he or she has the "right" person for the job and to make any changes in personnel. This type of interview also gives the staff members an opportunity to view the new dentist as a leader and begin to build trust.

Training Employees

The success of an employee often depends on the quality and quantity of the training program. Many skilled staff members have become frustrated and left a position when they were not able to perform their jobs effectively due to the lack of training. Every position in the practice needs to have a complete and accurate job description that becomes the basis for the training program.

After hiring the "right" person for the job, the dentist, office manager, or supervisor should meet with the employee to review his or her job description and responsibilities and specific training chart. The training chart (Table 23.2) is completed and reviewed with the employee. Depending upon the job and the new employee's skill level, many staff members may be involved in the new employee's training.

The goal of the training chart is to determine:

- Who will train
- When they will train
- How they will measure the training
- What kind of training

To ensure the training is effective, the trainer and the new employee need to have uninterrupted training time. Depending upon the nature of the training, they may need 15 minutes or over an hour. One of the worst mistakes many trainers make is training the new employees on too many tasks at one time and not allowing them to become proficient before moving on to the next task. Good trainers do the following:

- Set aside specific uninterrupted training time
- Describe the task to be learned
- Tell why this task is important

Table 23.2   Training chart.

Date: _____

Trainee: _____

Position: _____

	Tasks	Who Will Train	Type of Training*	Date of Training	Progress**
1					
2					
3					
4					
5					
6					
7					
8					
9					
10					
11					
12					
13					
14					
15					
16					
17					
18					
19					
20					

*Type of training	**Progress
A. One-on-one	Example responses:
B. Group training	Supervision needed
C. Outside source	No supervision needed
D. Peer training	Task mastered
E. Self-study	Can train others

- Show how the task is done
- Have the employee do the task with supervision

Obviously, it is important for the employee to take notes and ask questions during and after the training. The training chart is reviewed with the dentist weekly for an update of the training progress.

Employee Evaluations

Employees need and want feedback on how they are doing in their jobs. This promotes excellence and reduces conflict when they know what is expected of them. If employees do not know how they are doing, they may continue to make mistakes and feel confused about their responsibilities. Performance reviews are based on the responsibilities outlined in the job descriptions and help determine raises, probation, and termination of employment.

Each employee should receive a formal appraisal once a year on his or her date of hire or at another specified time. New employees should receive a formal performance review after 3 months of employment. Future reviews for the new employee may then be conducted on an as-needed basis.

The dentist or supervisor reviews the employee's job description and completes the evaluation form (Table 23.3). Note that the staff member also completes a self-evaluation. Then, the employee and the dentist/supervisor discuss the employee's strengths and weaknesses. Together they establish the objectives for the next time period. All individuals sign the evaluation form, and a copy is placed in the personnel file.

Table 23.3 Employee evaluation.

Performance Evaluation
(Filled out by doctor or office manager)

Date: _____

Employee name: _____

Position: _____

Characteristic and performance rating:
Rate each aspect of work performance on a scale of 1–5.
1: Exceeding the job requirements
3: Meets the job requirements
5: Unsatisfactory or unacceptable performance

Circle One Per category		Excellent			Unsatisfactory	Comments
Punctuality	1	2	3	4	5	____
Attendance	1	2	3	4	5	____
Attitude	1	2	3	4	5	____
Communication skills	1	2	3	4	5	____
Self-starter	1	2	3	4	5	____
Flexibility	1	2	3	4	5	
Quality of work	1	2	3	4	5	____
Speed	1	2	3	4	5	____
Telephone techniques	1	2	3	4	5	____
Computer skills	1	2	3	4	5	____
Charting	1	2	3	4	5	____
AR management	1	2	3	4	5	____
Insurance	1	2	3	4	5	____
Appointments	1	2	3	4	5	____
Radiography	1	2	3	4	5	____
Sterilization	1	2	3	4	5	____
Equipment care	1	2	3	4	5	____
Treatment procedures	1	2	3	4	5	____
Continuing education	1	2	3	4	5	____
Prophylaxis	1	2	3	4	5	____
Patient education	1	2	3	4	5	____
Preliminary diagnosis	1	2	3	4	5	____

Employee's Action Plan
Goal:

Table 23.3   (*Continued*)

Target date:

Goal:

Target date:

Goal:

Target date:

Signatures

Performance Evaluation Form
(Filled out by the employee)

Date: _____

Employee name: _____

Position: _____

Characteristic and performance rating:
Rate each aspect of work performance on a scale of 1–5.
1: Exceeding the job requirements
3: Meets the job requirements
5: Unsatisfactory or unacceptable performance

Circle One Per category		Excellent			Unsatisfactory	Comments
Punctuality	1	2	3	4	5	___
Attendance	1	2	3	4	5	___
Attitude	1	2	3	4	5	___
Communication skills	1	2	3	4	5	___
Self-starter	1	2	3	4	5	___
Flexibility	1	2	3	4	5	___
Quality of work	1	2	3	4	5	___
Speed	1	2	3	4	5	___
Telephone techniques	1	2	3	4	5	___
Computer skills	1	2	3	4	5	___
Charting	1	2	3	4	5	___
AR management	1	2	3	4	5	___
Insurance	1	2	3	4	5	___
Appointments	1	2	3	4	5	___
Radiography	1	2	3	4	5	___
Sterilization	1	2	3	4	5	___
Equipment care	1	2	3	4	5	___
Treatment procedures	1	2	3	4	5	___
Continuing education	1	2	3	4	5	___
Prophylaxis	1	2	3	4	5	___
Patient education	1	2	3	4	5	___
Preliminary diagnosis	1	2	3	4	5	___

Accomplishments
List areas of work in which you have performed especially well. Give examples.
Performance Improvement
Describe any performance area that needs improvement. (Think of specific tasks or behaviors.)

Raises

Raises in the practice should be based on two factors: merit of the employee and the health of the practice. Salary reviews should occur on a specific schedule each year. Salary reviews should not be tied to the employee's performance reviews, although performance reviews are a consideration in giving a salary increase.

Motivating and Appreciating Employees

Employees are any doctor's best asset and marketing tool. Motivated employees who know the difference they make are invaluable to the success of a practice. Dental practices that have high employee morale have many things in common:

- Shared values
- An environment of mutual respect
- Good communication between doctor and staff
- Teamwork
- No gossip or backstabbing
- A sense of ownership
- Challenging job
- Appreciation from the leader

Motivated staff enjoys a "family" atmosphere and a doctor who is committed to the long-term success of his or her team. Staff members like to have clear expectations and the freedom and autonomy to do their jobs. Many doctors feel the employee's salary and benefits should be enough appreciation for their team. In our combined 35 years of interviewing team members in dental practices throughout the United States, many employees crave and want the following from their employers:

- Be a good listener
- Say "please" and "thank you" often
- Give fair salaries and benefits
- Have spontaneous rewards for a job well done
- Remember birthdays and anniversaries in the practice
- Praise in public and criticize in private
- Give honest and direct feedback in a kind way
- Be a good role model

Many staff members have reported that they feel they are underappreciated by their doctors. Great leaders recognize the value of communicating their honest appreciation by sincerely complimenting the staff in front of patients. Patients love this, and so does your team. Other team recognition ideas include:

- Quarterly team outings (with a budget) planned by the different departments in the practice (bowling, shopping, manicures, baseball game, theater, laser tag).
- Spontaneous rewards are just as motivating as monetary rewards. Bringing staff a Starbucks latte to the morning huddle, giving them a $50 bill, or ordering a pizza for delivery to their home buys you a lot of motivation and positive attitude.

- Two round-trip tickets for the best "marketing" idea of the year.
- Having a masseuse come to your office and give staff a 15-minute shoulder and neck massage.
- Giving staff 5-, 10-, and 15-year loyalty gifts (watches, jewelry, bed-and-breakfast gift certificates).
- Schedule a staff meeting for 3 hours and surprise them with a shopping trip instead. Give them $200 and meet them for coffee at the end. Anything they do not spend they need to give back to you.

One of the most important keys to staff motivation is hiring motivated people. You cannot motivate a negative or unmotivated individual for very long. Keep your staff motivated by involving them in the practice decisions, providing regular feedback, and giving them challenging work.

Many practices have turned to a bonus incentive plan to help motivate and reward employees. If properly set up and administered, a bonus incentive plan can be a great motivator for staff. However, some bonus incentive plans are hard to track and may actually create a negative environment when the bonus is rarely achieved.

We have found the most effective bonus incentives programs are based on a 3-month rolling average of collections (not production!) and are achieved approximately 50–75% of the time. The bonus amount is determined by the percentage of staff salaries to collections and is distributed monthly. The individual amount is based on the number of days or hours worked.

Sample Bonus Incentive

1. Doctor commits to give staff a certain percentage of collections in the form of salary and/or bonus incentive. This percentage is based on the previous year's gross staff salaries in relation to collections. Usually ranges from 21 to 28%.
2. Bonus incentive is based on *collections*, not production.
3. Bonus incentive is based on a 3-month rolling average of adjusted collections.
4. Monthly gross salaries to be deducted from the predetermined percentage should include contract labor costs but not include spouse salary, staff benefits, or payroll taxes.
5. Formula and example:
   Step 1: 3-month adjusted collection average

Jan:	$68,000
Feb:	$64,000
Mar:	$66,000
Average:	$66,000

   Step 2: Monthly gross salary: $18,363 (Based on May profit and loss statement. This will change each month based on the gross payroll and contract labor that is paid in that given month.)
   Step 3: $66,000 × 28% (example) = $18,480
   Step 4: $18,480 − $18,363 = $117
   Step 5: $117 to be split among employees (based on hours or days worked)

6. Examples at 28%:
    $67,000 × 28% = $18,760 − $18,363 = $397
    $68,000 × 28% = $19,040 − $18,363 = $677
    $69,000 × 28% = $19,320 − $18,363 = $957

How to Handle Challenging Staff Members: Focus on the Behavior, Not the Person

Most dentists want to perform dentistry and do not want to deal with staff performance concerns and conflict issues. Unfortunately, as a business owner, you will at some time in your career experience these challenging situations. After many years of handling team conflict and having successful outcomes, here are some tips that we have found helpful:

C: Communicate within 24 hours
O: Out of area
N: Neutral
F: Facts
L: Listen
I: Investment
C: Conclusion
T: Trust the movement

C—Communicate within 24 hours: Address the situation as soon as possible, but when your emotions are in control. It is best to do this before the end of the day so that you will not take this problem home with you.

O—Out of area: When a situation is noticed or brought to your attention, make sure that you address it behind closed doors.

N—Neutral: It is your responsibility to remain neutral and nonjudgmental, especially when there is more than one individual involved. Remember, there are three sides to every story: yours, theirs, and the truth.

F—Facts: Stick to the facts. It is important to discuss the specific concerns related to this situation. At times, previous situations will be mentioned that may have no relevance to the resolution of this matter. The more factual you can keep the matter, the better.

L—Listen: In order to gather the facts, you must first listen. Remember that you have two ears and one mouth for a reason.

I—Investment: Your employees are an investment. Your primary goal is to resolve and move forward with any conflict situation. It is much harder and more costly to replace an existing employee than to hire and train a new one. However, if the problem continues, it is more costly to keep this individual.

C—Conclusion: As the dentist and owner, it is best to challenge the employee to think about the possible solution. Whether you are addressing a concern with an employee or an employee is coming to you with a concern, it is best for the individual to come up with a possible solution. Your goal is to have employees work out situations on their own. In the event they do come to you, they may have already solved the problem. When you need to address an employee, ask what *he or she* can do to improve the situation. This often leads to ownership and a higher level of accountability.

Lastly, document these situations in the employee's personnel file. Verbal situations could turn into written forms of communication down the road, which could lead to possible termination. One can never document too much.

T—Trust the movement: This is an old saying, but it remains true to this day. Trust what people do, not what they say. Actions speak louder than words. This age-old cliché will keep your business thriving and will help create a great place for all of you to work.

Disciplinary Process Leading to Staff Dismissal

As an employer, one of the more stressful tasks is managing an employee who is not performing at the level required in his or her job. It is important to have a disciplinary process in place to reduce the likelihood of wrongful discharge litigation and also to allow the employee an opportunity to improve performance. There are some standard steps in the progressive disciplinary process:

1. A verbal warning with written verification placed in the employee's personnel file
2. A written warning detailing the exact problem and what the employee is expected to do
3. Possible suspension without pay
4. Termination

All of these steps should be well documented and signed by the dentist and the employee. A copy of all written documents is placed in the personnel files. Each dentist should be aware of state and federal guidelines prior to dismissing any employee.

Managing dental teams can be stressful at times, but the time spent in developing a high- performing team is well worth the rewards you will receive as a business owner. Taking time to hire "right" and taking time to train a competent dental team will result in a team that treats each other with respect and kindness while putting the patient first. Having a solid team who shares common values and skills is crucial to practice success and patient retention.

References and Additional Resources

Moawad, Karen and Bender, Lynne Ross. 1993. *Managing Dental Office Personnel: A Management Tool for Structuring and Administering Personnel Policies in the Dental Practice*. Tulsa, OK: Penwell Books.

www.ada.org. American Dental Association (ADA) (especially, *Basic Training II and III, Employee Office Manual, Fast-Track Training: The Basics for Dental Staff*, and *Smart Hiring: A Guide for the New Dentist*).

www.dol.gov. U.S. Department of Labor (DOL).

www.eeoc.gov. Equal Employment Opportunity Commission (EEOC).

www.pathways-to-performance.com. Pathways to Performance, Inc.

Learning Exercises

Discover Your Behavioral Style

1. Answer the following questions and circle the answer to decode your behavioral pattern.

    Are you active/outgoing (DI) or more reserved (SC)?

    If you circled "active/outgoing," are you a relater with others (I) or a director of others? (D)

    Are you more concerned with persuading or impressing others (ID) or getting the results you want (DI)?

    If you circled "more reserved," are you more concerned with how you are to complete a task (S) or the quality of the task (C)?

    Are you more accepting of others (SC) or assessing of others (CS)?

2. Do an internet search on "behavioral styles" and compare your answers to what you discover on the web. The only limitation to this exercise is the accuracy of the observer him- or herself—a limitation that can be easily overcome by additional information from others who work with you.

Conflict Case Studies

Case Study No. 1

An employee barges into your office and breaks into tears. She proceeds to tell you about another employee who has been mean to her. How do you gain control of the situation, become a fact finder, and ultimately have the employees resolve the situation themselves?

Case Study No. 2

Sally, your dental assistant, is not following OSHA protocol. When and how do you approach her? What conflict solution should you use?

Case Study No. 3

Margie, your long-term dental hygienist, is upset about her schedule and wants to add another 20 minutes to each appointment. What conflict strategy should you follow?

Case Study No. 4

Last month, your accounts receivable was very high, especially in the over 90 days category. In your last meeting with Virginia, your office manager, she assured you the money is in the mail and she is confident the AR will be under control next month. In reviewing this month's AR report, the AR over 90 days has crept even higher. What is your plan of action with Virginia? What conflict principle do you want to use?

Chapter 24
Staff Meetings
David Neumeister

Staff Meetings = Empowered Team = Delighted Patients

Every dental office has a unique current that runs through it, like a river. It has a temperature and a movement that can be felt as you first wade into the flow. A river's current is the energy force that guides every drop of water, just as the office spirit of camaraderie creates an aura for the actions of every single staff member. The energy field in the office also determines the satisfaction level and the sense of security for every patient. The force of supportive enthusiasm is ignited by the dentist and fueled by every staff member at every moment of patient contact.

The environs of a dental office are often not welcoming, not calming. Your office can be uniquely inviting for staff and patients but it takes intentional thinking. Success takes time. A healthy office energy flow cannot be forced onto a group of people by a benevolent dentist. Neither can it be manufactured by everyone taking a course or reading a book. Once the energy flow is moving, it takes vision and a passionate determination to alter. It develops its own momentum as it moves through the day with its own weight and purpose. New patterns and behaviors take a long time to be nurtured and become a smooth part of the flow.

Your patients can feel the unique current when they walk through your front door. They sense the pace and energy in the reception room, in the hygienist's chair, when you come in to provide the clinical exam, and when they take out their checkbook to pay for their care. They respond to the diagnosis and recommendations in your office according to a subconscious sense of trust, quality, and energy in the office. Patients can feel tension: they can be intuitively aware of hidden agendas, and they will express their reaction by delaying treatment, saying "no," or even taking their records to another office. Some of their judgment is based on your new equipment and your clinical expertise, but their excitement to act now is based on a sixth sense of comfort and peace that comes from the feeling of ownership and security exhibited by the team of people that had an impact on them. It is critically important that you grow and motivate the team you have selected. That is why you need spirited, purposeful, staff-driven meetings.

Practice success is not just about fixing teeth. Teeth do not have emotions, people do. Teeth are easy.

Dental Practice Transition: A Practical Guide to Management, Second Edition.
Edited by David G. Dunning and Brian M. Lange.
© 2016 John Wiley & Sons, Inc. Published 2016 by John Wiley & Sons, Inc.
Companion Website: www.wiley.com/go/dunning/transition

How do you create a healthy, patient-focused aura in a dental office? It begins with the dentist defining personal success very clearly and moves on to building a team of dedicated, motivated professionals who carry that energy and commitment into everything you do as a dental professional. Every successful dental team needs to learn, grow, bond, share, and support your mission as a dentist.

Whether you see three patients a day or thirty, whether you have four or twenty-four individuals working in the same building, you need staff meetings. In fact, the busier you are, the more patients you see, the greater is your need to regularly stop, sit down, look into the eyes of your work friends, and learn how to define mission, collaborate, and build the daily energy necessary for consistent success.

You can attempt to teach or will this motivation onto your staff. You can buy some allegiance with bonuses or force dedication, for a time, with sheer willpower. But, if you are to raise the ceiling on patients wanting extraordinary quality services and if you are to grow your monthly production, you have only two choices: you can either work faster or you can empower your team.

You do not develop a team just because the king rules the kingdom. If a commitment to serve the patient is not lived by your team members, you do not have a team. Unless they understand the vision, believe in the dedication required, and are willing to hold each other accountable for defined outcomes, you do not have a team. Staff meetings are foundational to the success of a team. Remember, effective staff meetings are absolutely essential both to the success of the team and your dental practice.

Dental team: A group of people with different background skills and abilities working together toward a common goal for which they hold themselves accountable, and for which they are held accountable as a group.

It is not instinctive for a young dentist to regularly set aside productive chair time in order to gather everyone together to share and learn. In many average dental offices, staff meetings are not held at all or are regularly scheduled and postponed in favor of something more important. In some cases, staff meetings are grudgingly held and barely tolerated by the dentist or the staff in the practice. "I do not have the time for staff meetings," "I have never experienced one really valuable staff meeting in my life," "I have enough trouble getting the work done now, why would I want to call a meeting and waste valuable time?"

Dentists often believe success is a matter of knowing the technical material, learning the business skills, and surrounding themselves with an honest, diligent staff. It is true that you need technical and business expertise. Equally valid is the necessity for a talented, devoted support team, but it does not stop there. To be successful, day after day, year after year, you need to continuously motivate, train, reward, and challenge your team to understand and value your devotion to your patient's oral health and your team-shared vision of quality service.

The difference between average and excellent in any organization is the difference between common knowledge and daily application at every moment of public contact. Being successful every day absolutely requires focused, productive, and regular gatherings of your work group.

You will do more to improve your happiness and success as a professional by regular, focused team meetings than you will by taking a full week of the best dental education course in the country! Let me tell you why that is true.

You know your stuff. You graduated from a good dental school and have passed your boards. You have your license in hand, and now you have a dental practice. You have a setting to work your gifts in the public arena and actually get paid for it. All the patients in your community do not realize yet how good you are, but that will happen soon enough. You assume the key to your success as a dentist is literally in your hands.

But success is *not* in your two hands. Contentment at night when you are in bed waiting to fall asleep is not about your technical skills. Being able to do the dentistry is just the beginning. Contentment is found in knowing the patient with an old loose bridge who called today can fit in the schedule tomorrow morning without upsetting your other patients or your dental assistant. Contentment is found when the local school principal is first told she needs four quadrants of scaling and root planning and she does not get angry and ask why no one ever told her she had periodontal disease before today. Contentment is found when you leave the operatory and the patient quietly asks your assistant why root canals cost so much and your assistant has practiced an answer that builds confidence and security in the patient's decision to have this service provided today. That is the contentment that allows you to fall asleep with a smile on your face as you look forward to your professional decision to work every day to help people keep their teeth for a lifetime of health.

How do you get a group of unique, gifted, and dedicated people to rise above their differences?

How do you motivate these individuals to work as a team? How do you encourage them to value service to the patient the way you do?

How do you build a sense of responsibility within a group of people who each came from different life experiences, with different personalities and different personal needs?

What types of meetings are necessary for a successful office? These criteria are recommended:

- Start each day and establish congruency of focus.
- Share personal successes and celebrate victories.
- Share basic business information of the office.
- Bring new staff members into the family and experience your office philosophy.
- Learn of changes in dental techniques, materials, and office systems on a regular schedule.

This can all be productively accomplished with just two meetings: a morning huddle before the start of each day and a team meeting once a month for a few hours. The total time required might vary from 3 to 5 hours a month, which is carefully devoted to allowing each person to understand, connect, and contribute to his or her own success and the success of the dental office.

Successful meetings: How would you know if you had one?

1. The participants would predictably look forward to coming.
2. The time would be productive and accomplish growth and improvement in office systems.
3. Everyone would feel like they, personally, made a difference in the process of making a decision.
4. The team would want to think and act more effectively as a result of participating in the meeting.

If we use these points as criteria for success, imagine what has to be in place to accomplish our goals. First, we have to agree on what makes a group of people a team.

There are many settings where a group of people get together and act but no one would confuse the group with a team. You have visited established restaurants where it feels like the staff members do not talk to each other. Questions are repeated and you are left alone at the table for long periods. You sense that no one is in charge, and you have either been ignored or, if served, concluded that they really do not care if you come back for a second visit.

Sometimes it seems as if the wait staffs in some restaurants do not even like each other. Very quickly the service falters and next your perception of the quality of the food diminishes and you wonder why you came here in the first place. It does not take long to decide you are not coming back. Have you ever experienced a dental office like this?

Conversely, you have also been in restaurants where everything is seamless. The greeter tells you who your waitperson will be and he or she arrives quickly. Everyone seems devoted to making sure you have whatever you need. They actually look for ways to be responsive to your questions and desires. They can tailor the menu to meet your dietary needs, and they smile as they ask if there is anything else they can do to be helpful. And, no surprise, the food is terrific also.

What makes the difference? How does a group of people, each with a different background and experience, become an integrated unit that is capable of meeting the needs of a single customer, a couple on a date, a family with children, or a large group celebrating a wedding anniversary? Each visitor has a unique expectation and a unique perception of that particular restaurant. A successful restaurant finds that people return again and again because the experience was predictably warm and responsive. The food was well prepared, but food alone would not make this a return experience. Quality food is important, but quality food is not enough.

Quality dentistry is important, very important, but it is not enough to make a successful dental practice.

Order WITHOUT Control

Definition of success for the team: the entire staff enjoys, participates, takes away lessons, and improves service to the patient and to each other. Definition of success for the dentist: you develop rapport, educate, challenge, affirm, and grow a team of people to expand your ability to help patients make better choices about oral health.

You have an orderly pattern to your office systems without having to control or dictate the daily patient encounters in the delivery of oral health services in your office. You involve your entire staff in the process of patient service. Their confidence and authority to act comes from shared goals and common expectations for success. You can focus on direct patient care while your team demonstrates the attentiveness and service you would want if you were a patient in a dental office.

Team meetings must be:

Regular but team-driven
Focused but flexible
Fun but productive

In order to become regular, team meetings need to be scheduled at a definite time with no opportunity to change the date or shorten the length of the meeting. The staff should know this time is as indispensable as lunch and the direct deposit paycheck at the end of the month. Everyone, including part-time team members, should make a dedicated effort to be present for the entire meeting, every time. Staff members are paid for the full time of the meeting, and any food or incidental costs are paid for by the dentist.

Morning Huddle: 15 Minutes Before the Start of Each Day

Just as the daily schedule provides the itinerary for the day, morning huddle is the GPS device to get you there efficiently. Huddle is held 15 minutes before the start of each day. The goal of the huddle is to smoothly connect the daily expectations of each person in the office. It is an opportunity to share information that is usually known only by one team member but for which whole-team awareness is important to establish congruency in delivery of service. Figure 24.1 portrays the activity of a morning huddle. The dentist needs to know there is a difficult patient who needs anesthesia coming into hygiene at midmorning, and the assistant needs to know that the front office staff will call the one o'clock patient to be sure she has taken the required prophylactic antibiotic that was forgotten last time. The person handling financial arrangements wants the hygienist to have the mother of both children this afternoon stop at the desk to make the insurance co-payment. The dentist may want the receptionist to ask the guardian to stay in the office at 4 o'clock to approve the necessary care for a special needs child.

This daily exchange of unique information makes the day flow harmoniously for everyone. It is part of how the patient begins to perceive the office energy currents that intuitively inform them that this office is well managed. Patients reflect the confidence, warmth, and assurance they witness within the office.

Each person must come to morning huddle prepared. Some staff members may come to the office 20 minutes early that morning to prepare, and some may stay a little late on the day before. If you have a hygienist who starts at 9:00 a.m. every day, s/he would need to prepare the afternoon before and give the information to someone else to report for her/him. If each person expects to participate three or four times at different points in the fixed agenda, a great deal can be accomplished in just 15 minutes or less.

The business office comes with information about overnight schedule changes, patients having financial arrangements to make, or payments due today. They may also have information about special insurance requirements for a patient or have knowledge about the family of a new patient coming in today. They may know of a patient who must be seen exactly on time this morning because of a previous scheduling problem. The hygienist will know who needs x-rays, who has pending dental treatment as yet unscheduled, which patients need dental exams, and who in today's schedule might need a treatment plan/plan of care, or a new comprehensive exam. The dental assistant will know which patients need special precautions, what set-ups will be needed for each patient, and which rooms will be used. The dentist is responsible for knowing which patients may need special care and which ones may have recently completed treatment by a specialist. The dentist must also help the scheduling coordinator know which time in the day is appropriate to see an emergency patient if someone should call and need to be seen today.

Every team member is also encouraged to bring news of special happenings with any practice patient. Who, on today's schedule, has recently been in the newspaper, had an anniversary, been in the hospital, or graduated from school. Huddle is also the time when anyone can offer news about any patient of record who has had a significant milestone such as a wedding or birth of a baby. These patients might get a

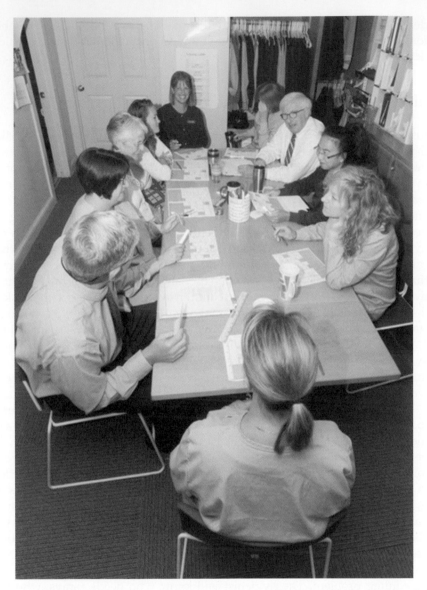

Figure 24.1. Dental office morning huddle with a comprehensive agenda is held at 7:45 a.m. each morning. Everyone comes prepared to share key information for the day.

congratulatory card, with sentiments from multiple team members. Huddle is the time when a specific person would put a congratulatory card on the staff table so that it can be signed during the day and mailed that evening.

Huddle is one more way you can create the expectation that each individual is responsible for the success of every other team member. Each person has an opportunity to be the one who satisfies the expectations of the patients visiting your office today. The quality of this meeting sets the tone and pace for the day. This allows patients to routinely leave the office glowing with praise for the congruency and professionalism of your office.

Table 24.1 Morning huddle agenda.

- Start by 7:45 a.m., end by 7:55 a.m.
- Announcements for the entire office
- Schedule changes for today
- Business
  - Patients who may need help opening the front door
  - Patients who need to make or confirm financial arrangements
  - Hand off patients
  - New patients
  - Next preblock time for hygienist and dentist
- Hygiene
  - Patients who need medical history updates at the front desk
  - Patients with outstanding treatment
  - Patients who need an FMX, treatment plan, or conversion exam
  - Patients who need a dentist check
- Assistants
  - Patients who require extra time or have special needs today
  - Patients who require follow-up from yesterday
  - Emergency time today
- Gift ideas for patients
- Equipment or supply needs
- Thought for the day

When everyone comes to this huddle prepared, you can begin to develop today's current of energy with a motivated, healthy team of individuals each possessing a desire to contribute to the whole. There must be a routine list of business office, hygiene, assistant, and dentist responsibilities that is used each day. If you do not start with common information and shared expectations, you will not feel linked throughout the day when the inevitable emergency call comes in or a patient arrives 20 minutes late. Morning huddle starts promptly 15 minutes before the start of the day and can be completed in 10–12 minutes.

Table 24.1 provides details for a huddle agenda.

Importantly, the companion website for this book has a digital recording—Morning Huddle at Dental Health—lasting approximately 7 minutes to help you to more fully understand these important meetings. As the old saying goes, "seeing is believing".

Monthly Team Meeting

The entire office gathers monthly on a firm date and at a known time, no excuses. These meetings should eventually be off-site so that there will be no interruptions and so it is obvious to the team that you are making an independent commitment to time and space for focused discussion and personal connections to enhance your daily work. There is a safe narrative that will lead to an orderly, patient-focused, and emotionally satisfying gathering that every person will look forward to every single month.

Early in a dentist's career staff meetings are called only when there is a crisis. They are seen as a time to fix what is wrong. The topics are often critical issues that require urgent action, and there is little discussion about long-range issues that impact your practice

Table 24.2 Monthly dental team meeting.

Location: _____

Moderator: _____

Record keeper: _____

Evaluator: _____

Start time: _____, end by _____

Meeting Agenda

Rewarding experiences—personal and professional

Action list

Reports

  Hygiene

  Dentist

  Supplies

  Gift account

Housekeeping list

Education topic

Evaluation

harmony. When dentists have greater experience, there is more planning and more time allowed for issues at a staff meeting. Still, staff meetings often remain a negative, complaint time controlled by whoever has the biggest problem or the loudest voice. This is not an experience anyone is willing to have a second time.

Six parts to predictably successful monthly team meeting:

1. Rewarding experiences
2. Action list
3. Reports: hygiene, dentist, supplies, gift account
4. Housekeeping list
5. Education topic
6. Evaluation of monthly team meeting

Table 24.2 provides the basic organizational structure for a monthly team meeting.

Rewarding Experiences

During the rewarding experiences portion of the meeting, everyone will share at least one personal and at least one professional experience that have occurred in the last month.

This time is devoted to a leisurely sharing of experiences by each person in the room. After one person starts, the sharing moves calmly clockwise around the circle giving each person an opportunity to tell his or her story. This allows a friendly, relaxed, and unhurried opportunity for people to share who they are, both personally and professionally. They can first tell the group what brings them satisfaction and reward outside of the office environment. Some dental colleagues find it not only easy but necessary to share home experiences. Some team members would have shared these personal highlights even if it meant bringing a photo or a personal memory to work during a busy day. Other team members will be less open about their lives outside of work, and that is fine. This process is not about revealing confidences. However, everyone *must* have a couple things that have happened each month that brought them special satisfaction. If one team member hesitates to offer an experience, offer her or him an opportunity to wait until the last person in the circle has had a chance to share and then come back to the less talkative team member.

No one is allowed to skip over sharing personal rewarding experiences. It is important to connect with each person as an individual and know a little about what makes them unique.

As the leader of the team you can support your quieter team members—and there will always be some reluctant individuals—by following up privately and asking more questions about their interests and strongly encouraging them to do more sharing at the next meeting.

Each person should express one or two personal rewarding experiences that have occurred in the last month. This could be an award a child achieved in scouts, an activity successfully accomplished at church, or a vacation experience including some photos of this special trip. This allows both the effusive and the less secure person a predictable time to tell the group a little more about who he or she is and what subtleties that person contributes to your team. This is part of connecting as humans on a social and emotional level so that work life has the potential to become a support network. It is easier to work effectively with coworkers who know and understand your family life, your hobbies, and the life experiences that make you a unique individual. These social connections enhance professional responsibilities and build a depth of empathy for the day when someone is sick or the sterilization area overflows. Those days will happen.

This rewarding experience time also allows opportunity for sharing a couple of experiences that have been professionally rewarding to each team member during the last month. Celebrate why you enjoy coming to the office each day. Tell one another what is working well for your patients. These experiences should involve named patients and other staff members. It is meant to cheer the successful patients and to affirm the behaviors and actions of fellow team members.

This rewarding experience time also provides a vehicle by which the business office and the clinician's treatment can elaborate on the interconnectedness of everything that occurs in a good office. The hygienist can thank the scheduling coordinator for moving patients on the day her daughter got sick and she had to leave on short notice. The assistant can thank the hygienist for encouraging a patient to complete her whitening experience before she had the bicuspids crowned, allowing the shade to match more perfectly. The dentist can affirm the person who takes new patient phone calls because of all the detailed information she collects on the phone, facilitating a better first visit experience.

The subtle message infusing this rewarding experience time is that we are all human beings with a home, with a circle of friends, and with unique life experiences. We also happen to share similar values in this dental office with an opportunity to make a difference in the lives of our patients and in the lives of our fellow teammates. The emphasis during this first item on the staff meeting agenda is on leisurely sharing.

Action List

During this part of the meeting, employees will follow up on activities from past meetings. A scribe or note taker should be assigned for tracking and posting the action list, housekeeping list (below), and other key points from the monthly staff meeting.

The second item on every meeting agenda is the action list. Through this section you demonstrate that decisions that are made by the team at a staff meeting are either put

Table 24.3   Action list.

Post on Monday Following Staff Meeting

Action	Who Is Doing It	Due Date or Completion Date
_____	_____	_____
_____	_____	_____
_____	_____	_____
_____	_____	_____
_____	_____	_____
_____	_____	_____
_____	_____	_____
_____	_____	_____

into action immediately or require more research and are returned to a future meeting for a more complete discussion.

Table 24.3 is an example outline of an action list.

An example of topics on this list might be the specific technical definition of an Current Dental Terminology (CDT) code for periodontal maintenance visits. Someone might volunteer to research that definition and report back at the next team meeting. That item, requiring follow-up reading, would be placed on the action list. Another example of an action list topic might be the dates and cost of the regional continuing education meeting scheduled next summer. An individual might be asked to get all the information, post the list of speakers and dates in the staff room, and then place the topic on next month's action list for a decision about members of the team who might want to attend.

Perhaps someone in the business office receives questions about implants and asks if he or she could learn more about this service. The group might then decide to invite a local oral surgeon to come to a lunch meeting in your office and discuss advancements in implant treatment modalities. The team members could determine which surgeon they want to learn from, and someone could be asked to make a contact for a lunch session.

The companion website for this book includes a sample action list.

You might even find more referrals from that oral surgeon after he or she discovers the quality of your office and your staff. If a decision is made by the group, that item would go on the action list for reporting at the next team meeting.

One objective of this list is to affirm to everyone that suggestions that are supported by the group are followed up and completed. A second objective is to make sure good ideas are not lost. Within days of your team meeting, this list should be posted in the back office so that it is visible to every staff member during the month between gatherings of the team.

Reports: Hygiene, Dentist, Supplies, Gift Account

What reports are important, what data do you track, and who does the tracking? First, the dentist must establish the vision for success in patient care, hygiene services, financial payments, and all other office systems. This creates the outcomes to be measured and discussed by your team. In this way you encourage a shared vision for exactly what constitutes "order without control" in your office. Once the vision is understood and valued by the team, it is the dentist's responsibility to have a staff member in charge of tracking every essential, team-selected outcome. Agree, in advance, to the desired target for success in each of these business areas and determine who in the office is primarily responsible for tracking and achieving the desired outcome. If any of these numbers are significantly outside the desired target range, the person in the office known to be primarily responsible for that outcome should be prepared to discuss possible solutions and help set in place an action plan for improvement. The dentist may sometimes check the data during the month, and the dentist will certainly build support for achieving success; however, the dentist is not presenting the report and is not the first one to comment on the report. This staff meeting is a team-driven model, not a dentist command model.

After months of tracking and evaluating office procedures, it becomes easier for the staff member in charge to report on the successes and the weaknesses of your chosen outcomes. An example is as follows: If your objective is to have office supplies at 6% of production and you have made one person responsible for ordering supplies, that person can budget purchases to stay in the selected range. If the monthly results are unusually high, the responsible person can explain what purchases were necessary and if or how the total will be decreased in the coming months. Eventually the most rewarding role for a good leader-dentist is to act as cheerleader for the empowered team, whose members act as if they are responsible for the success of the dental office.

There is a delicate but necessary balance between your real need to focus on specific results to be fully successful in the business of dentistry and still allow the individual team members to take responsibility for their own actions and results.

This part of the meeting is devoted to sharing selected office information with everyone. A team supports actions and decisions more fully if its members understand the "why" behind a decision. People do not argue with their own data. Practice management software programs also allow you to readily generate reports for and review/analysis.

Hygiene report: During the report section of the meeting there would be a summary of the activities on the hygiene side of the practice. This report is essential whether you have one part-time or a mixture of part-time and full-time hygienists. These data are useful for the team today and are useful for you as your practice grows and you track changes in the flow of patients and staff over the life of your career. This report might include the number of patient visits, number of sealants, number of quadrants of scaling and root planning, number of periodontal maintenance visits, dollars per hour produced, and number of broken appointments as a percentage of total hours available in the last month.

Dentist report: There would also be a report of the dentist's new patient numbers, production success, future pre blocks scheduled, insurance billing, and accounts receivable tracking.

The necessity of strong dental leadership cannot be overemphasized. Determine your indices for success, monitor the level of achievement, celebrate your good numbers, and determine, as a team, how to improve your weak numbers. The targets you choose to track will slowly evolve as your practice experience grows. You may start out tracking production and collection numbers and move on to separate the dentist numbers from the hygienist numbers. You may track accounts receivable over 90 days and then realize that a better number to track is percentage of daily production collected at the front desk each day. There are no perfect data points for your office. As your collaborative abilities increase, so will your awareness of the subtle pieces of information that influence your desired outcomes. The critical element is that you, as a group, decide what measures success for your dental office and that you, as a team, determine how to achieve your chosen definition of an effective dental practice.

Supplies report: Another report that should be a regular part of the shared information at your staff meeting is the supplies report. It should be given by the individual on the team who is responsible for ordering, purchasing, and tracking supply costs. The target for supply expense might be 6% of your office monthly production. Your actual cost for supplies is compared to the target, and a report is given by the person who orders supplies for your team. The supply expert would report monthly success and year-to-date success. You could even report hygiene supply cost, goal versus actual, as well as dentist supply cost, goal versus actual, to give you a better idea where your expense was in variance. The objective is for the entire office team to feel ownership in the process to stay under a specific overhead target each month and to share that information in a way that allows input for improvement.

Gift account report: The gift account is a reporting of small gifts that have been given to patients since the last meeting. One person is in charge of sending cards and pre-purchased gift certificates to patients who, for example, celebrated an anniversary, who received an award, or who were admitted to the hospital with an injury. Any staff member at any time can suggest that a gift be sent. One person in the office is designated as gift officer to have cards and certificates on hand and to be the person to send messages whenever appropriate. Any one staff member could sometimes sign the card, or multiple staff members might sign the card, as appropriate. There is no need to notify the dentist when it is decided to recognize an individual. The gift officer has an allowable monthly maximum to work from, and within that parameter, he or she is free to send gifts anytime during the month. Announcement of the recipient's name and the gift is made at the gift account section of the agenda. For some in the room, this is the first time they may realize that recognition was given.

The objective of the gift account is to provide every staff person an opportunity to recognize some of the special people who have entrusted their care to your team. Each person in your office should feel a personal responsibility for remembering and rewarding your patients. Staff recognition antennae should be on alert all the time. Imagine the buzz in the community when flowers and a card from two or three staff members arrive at the hospital for the new baby. Or just imagine the number of friends who might learn of the gift certificate to a local bookstore that is received with a signed personal card from your office when a student in your care was inducted into the National Honor Society.

The companion website for this book includes samples of these reports: monthly supply expenses, front office, and hygiene department.

Housekeeping List

In this part of the meeting, discuss any nonurgent ideas or questions that came up since the last team meeting.

A blank sheet "housekeeping list" is posted in the staff area at the beginning of the month. It has space outlined for the topic of interest, the name of the person who wants to raise the issue, and the approximate time required to allow group discussion. Every staff person is encouraged, during the month, to put any original idea he or she has or any question that arises on the list. Anything placed on the housekeeping list does not require urgent action and would generally benefit from some consensus building

Table 24.4 Housekeeping list.

Item to Discuss	Who	How Much Time
_____	_____	_____
_____	_____	_____
_____	_____	_____
_____	_____	_____
_____	_____	_____
_____	_____	_____
_____	_____	_____
_____	_____	_____

Post immediately after last staff meeting.

before an action is taken. If the air-conditioning is not working, for example, that needs attention immediately and would not be added to the housekeeping list. If, however, you are wondering about having a cleaning service come in three times a week instead of the current two times, that question should be placed on the housekeeping list. It is a question that could be answered spontaneously by the dentist on the day your assistant had a concern about something on the carpet. Or, it could just be forgotten or ignored by a team member. However, if this question is placed on the housekeeping list by the individual who recognized the problem, at any time during the month, it will lead to a staff meeting discussion and understanding of all the issues surrounding office cleanliness. An office conversation will acknowledge the desire of the team member to have a very attractive office. It will also allow every team member to appreciate the consequences of cleaning his or her own work area, the cost of current vendors, and public perception of cleanliness in your office. Table 24.4 is an example outline for a housekeeping list.

By putting this and similar topics on the housekeeping list, posted on the staff room wall, it encourages every team member to think, every day, about ways to improve the office. Their input and advice and questions are encouraged. This is part of empowering your team to take responsibility for the success of the practice.

Using a housekeeping list takes a staff question out of the realm of the dentist or office manager being a one-person, autocratic, problem solver. The staff member may wish someone could just go out and buy different magazines for the office, but this is a good time to pause and ask for the issue to go on the housekeeping list for the next month. Then the whole group can have a discussion about patient reading habits and marketing to specific patient interests, and after this, you may give a staff member a budget to be responsible for all patient reading material. This is a situation when the best action could be to give an immediate answer. Alternatively, depending on the issue, you could help others get involved in the solution. It also allows the staff member and the dentist time to think about an issue and obtain more background information before the full team discusses the concern. Most important, this type of sharing is part of allowing everyone to be part of the learning and decision-making process.

Decisions that are owned by the team are more likely to be valued and implemented as a team. Individual team members do not argue with a decision that was developed as a group. Putting a question that is not urgent on the housekeeping list for full discussion will, by itself, lead to dramatically diminished back office chatter about who makes decisions and how they are made.

There are definite concerns that ultimately fall to the dentist alone to make the decision. This housekeeping list activity does not transfer all leadership responsibility to the group. If there is a patient care decision to make regarding the choice of dental laboratory, or if the cost of some suggestion is prohibitive or the timing is inappropriate, it will be up to the dentist to make the decision. A housekeeping list during staff meetings is not one step toward absentee leadership. This is the highest form of leadership, creating a real-life experience of shared responsibility toward a shared team vision of an ideal oral health environment.

The staff and the office will have benefited even in situations where the dentist encouraged full discussion and the group's choice cannot be immediately accomplished. Examples might include adding another front desk staff member, purchasing a new piece of equipment, or remodeling of the building. First, they benefit by feeling that they are a valued part of a team working in all ways to make the office better. Second, they will have a fuller understanding of all the factors contributing to the perceived problem. Remember the cleanliness problem that was raised earlier? It could even be that each person does more end-of-day cleanup in their respective area, thereby eliminating entirely the need for a third day of cleaning. Third, they will witness the leader–the dentist–seriously listening and valuing and affirming the input of a group of dedicated and empowered team members.

Empowerment is not a matter of giving your staff power. They already had power in the talents and skills they possessed when you invited them to join your practice. Your role as leader is to grow that ability and release that power in a focused way. *Leadership is the ability to create an environment where it is easy for people to succeed and feel better about themselves in the process. Remember, our goal is order without control.*

Other items you might find on the housekeeping list could include such things as the scheduling of the floating holiday around the 4th of July each year. Having a housekeeping list, discussion lets the team decide which adjoining day to take, either the day before the 4th or the day after. Other examples of housekeeping list subjects might be a question about the appropriate background music or air temperature for the office. There may be a concern about the repeated denial of insurance claims by one specific insurer, or a change in insurance definitions in the CDT Manual.

There will be five to fifteen items on this list each month. Most items will be discussed, consensus developed, and action taken that day. A couple of items will require the moderator to ask for volunteers to act as a short-term task force to obtain more information or write up some possible solutions. In this case the item will be added to the action list schedule for a specific future meeting. Regardless of outcome, you have established that ideas for success are encouraged, heard, debated, and decided upon, and an action taken.

When a dental assistant asks you why you use a specific brand of whitening material, you might simply tell her your reason. There are times this would be most appropriate. You might also suggest that she put it on the housekeeping list and let the whole office reflect on the myriad choices of whitening materials. You might find that there are newer products that another staff member knows about that are even more effective.

Bringing this topic to a full staff meeting discussion demonstrates that you value the opinion of every member of your team on this subject. Front desk staff, assistants, and hygienists should all learn about the best whitening materials for your patients.

Everyone–even the business office staff, who is also asked about whitening materials–will have a better understanding of the range of materials available and the benefits of the products you endorse. Most important, you also make real your commitment to empowering everyone to become an expert. A team is only as strong as its weakest link.

Housekeeping is not only a way to involve your team in problem solving; it is additionally a way to educate your entire office on the narrative behind some actions that may be taken for granted. This is particularly true for newer team members. Very importantly, it is also a way to model a behavior you want your whole team to emulate. If you demonstrate the respect that comes from truly listening to the emotion behind the words and concerns of your team members, they will give their fellow teammates the same respect. If you ask sincere questions, you will be more certain you have all the information necessary before a decision is made. Then you respect the will of the group and, finally, are certain the chosen action is implemented. The individual team member will expand his or her sense of ownership and commitment to the office. This establishes the foundation that allows each person to feel personally responsible for what happens each day in your office. If the results of that patient visit or that teammate encounter were not healthy, you want that business office person, that assistant, or that hygienist to take responsibility for initiating an action to achieve a different result.

If you, the dentist and leader, demonstrate integrity to the process of really being present and listening to your employees, they will learn how to do this with your patients. They will be more willing to do this with each other, and they will come to model this behavior outside the office as well. They just may become better spouses, better community members, and better citizens because they work in your office.

This is difficult to accept for most dentists: sometimes when a problem arises the best solution is not to provide answers. Instead, the preferred action is to ask questions to help the individual discover a solution based on the questions you asked, leading him or her to think about the problem differently. Having staff meetings like this will make some decisions take longer to achieve, but the long-term implementation will be much better. Team decisions are thick decisions that infuse actions and decisions of every person every day. This creates the energy and comfort that your patients feel at every moment of contact.

The companion website for this book includes a sample housekeeping list.

Education Topic

The education topic is a unique learning opportunity each month that can be done internally or externally. Staff members are engaged in an education topic at a team meeting depicted in Figure 24.2.

Have fun with this portion of the meeting. This item should be scheduled last on your agenda, but the topic should be planned and scheduled for every meeting. This is a critical section that is often omitted from dental team meetings. Every team gathering is an opportunity for internal systems growth or external subject learning.

Internal systems growth: Internal systems ideas for the education topic section might be new dental materials, causes and treatments for bruxing, when to do implants, your new patient experience, verbal skills, dental office emergency procedures, OSHA training, insurance coding and tracking, or production goals and equipment maintenance. You also need to occasionally revisit and fine-tune all the assumptions and

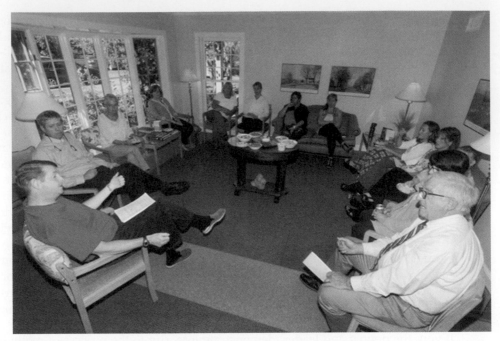

Figure 24.2. Monthly half-day staff meeting with the entire team and a guest speaker—in this case a local pharmacist explaining new pharmaceutical regulations.

actions about what is required to be a successful dental office. Your team meeting is also an opportunity to educate your staff and yourself about the changes and challenges of a modern dental practice. You want to make your office a full-time learning organization.

Use the educational topic portion of the meeting to introduce or expand new ideas and services to the team. You could provide the educational session yourselves by doing a thorough review of whitening techniques or the effects of and treatments for temporomandibular joint disease.

External subject learning: The education topic section often involves bringing in an outside speaker to add depth to your knowledge and add breadth to the staff. Invite, in turn, each of the specialists you refer to and ask them to come and explain why they got into dentistry or what they particularly enjoy doing in their specialty field. Some of your team may not even have met these people, and they will benefit intellectually and also have a more convincing answer when the patient asks what it is like to have wisdom teeth removed by this surgeon. Imagine the goodwill created when orthodontists can come to your office and explain why they enjoy repositioning teeth. They could bring successful case models and photos to help your team understand treatment options and referral time frames. This opportunity is especially appreciated when new specialists move to the area. They are anxious to meet all the referring dentists and to connect with the staff. This introduction time will be remembered by the specialist and by your staff many years into the future. Every few years it is helpful to have a guest return for a second or third visit, as treatment protocols change or new health risks become more of a topic of public discourse. It also creates quite a buzz among your staff members when they can tell their colleagues that they heard, at their office, a lecture by the local periodontist or oral surgeon a few weeks ago.

There are many other community members who have important background information that would expand your ability to help your patients. Many of these topic experts would relish the opportunity to see your office and visit with your staff. They just might also refer their clients and friends to your office because you take the time to be very thorough in educating your whole staff.

Imagine the benefit to your patients and your staff if the diabetes counselor from the community hospital could come and tell you about what he or she advises patients regarding oral health and the oral-systemic implications of diabetes.

Creativity and a willingness to take a risk are the only limitations to the number of informative and successful learning opportunities available to your team. How about inviting a hospice trainer to come talk about listening to a patient who might have recently lost a loved one? Other good hour-long topics would include a pharmacist, a counselor for eating disorders, a tobacco cessation expert, or a drug and alcohol counselor.

In this era of ubiquitous information sources with a blizzard of confusing claims and recommendations, how can you possibly read enough, learn enough to be informed? And then, how do you keep your staff informed? One way you can do this is by having 1 hour of every team meeting devoted to office education.

Why would you provide an hour every month for an education topic with the entire office team?

1. It ensures that your patients receive more complete healthcare. This develops a level of empathy and awareness that patients can see and feel. This will be a unique experience for many of your patients, who are accustomed to being rushed through the model of healthcare that says "time is money."

2. It grows the skills and confidence of every team member. Your senior certified dental assistant and your newest front desk trainee will benefit from these education opportunities. Each person will learn firsthand new background to procedures, new words to explain, and new ways to be helpful to every patient seen. Your patients will benefit, team interaction will be enhanced, and each employee will take home a new awareness that provides an enhanced level of personal satisfaction.

3. It allows you to put more responsibility for treatment descriptions and patient trust building on your highly informed and motivated team members. When the person who answers the new patient phone call knows the consequence of a diabetic with periodontal disease, he or she speaks with a confidence that could make a positive impression on the patient. When the hygienist knows the laboratory sequence involved in making an all-ceramic crown, he or she has a much more convincing answer to the patient who wonders why a simple crown costs so much. When your assistant has met the surgeon and talked with and seen photos of multiple implant cases, he or she has not only the words but also the sensitivity to help the anxious college student who has just suffered a serious fall and lost a front tooth.

You can also use this education time to maximize the benefits of attending a continuing education course as a team. What if you asked each person, in advance of a full-day course away from the office, to come to the next meeting prepared to list three new things learned during the day and two things to do differently as a result of what has been learned? Imagine how much more engaged your staff would be if they had to report at next month's meeting. Imagine the outcome if someone takes notes and posts the "two things I will do differently" list on the staff bulletin board so that anyone can go by and check the results of the commitment a few weeks later.

You could use the education time to write an office mission statement, draft No. 1, and then 2 months later you could go back and fine-tune your chosen outcomes. At a future meeting, during the education topic section you could then set up criteria for measuring progress toward your mission. Each person might be asked to identify things he or she could personally accomplish that would have the greatest impact on the newly defined dental office mission. Post these impact statements so that each person is self-linked to actions that help achieve a higher level of participation.

Your imagination is the only limitation to the growth that is possible during this regular section of team learning.

Evaluation of Monthly Meeting

This section of the meeting involves a discussion of criteria for success each month. Evaluate every team meeting to help bring the group to consensus on the chosen outcomes for every meeting.

You could identify the "how would you know?" criteria for a really perfect team meeting. List the specifics of "ideal" in advance so that everyone knows what success looks like. Possible criteria could include the following:

Start on time, 8:00 a.m. or 1:15 p.m.
Did everyone participate?
Were all subjects covered to the satisfaction of everyone?
Did everyone learn new things?
Was it fun?
Have everyone rate their responses on a scale of 1–5, with 5 being terrific and 1 being terrible.

Length and Frequency of Team Meetings

When do you have these meetings, how often are they held, and how long does all this take? Once you get over the fear of losing control of a group conversation and you decide the risk/reward balances in favor of having these meetings, these are natural questions.

Table 24.5 presents a sample staff meeting schedule.

Start simply by having these meetings in the office, at the start of your day, 1 day a month. Begin by setting aside 2 full hours when you are fresh in the morning and let everyone build comfort with the process. After 6 months of growth, go to 3 hours and maybe eventually take a half day every month to build your team. Developing confidence and trust in a process of openness and sharing is more important than any one result. Early success is just getting everyone to speak up and being clear about building group decision dynamics. Early in the learning there are no wrong answers, and the only fault is a lack of involvement by individual team members.

The companion website for this book includes a sample team meeting evaluation.

Table 24.5 Staff meeting schedule.

Permanently Posted in Staff Room

Month	Host	Notes	Moderator	Evaluator	Guests
January	Shirley				
February	Heidi	Shirley			
March	Jackie	Heidi	Shirley		
April	Tom	Jackie	Heidi	Shirley	
May		Tom	Jackie	Heidi	
June			Tom	Jackie	
July				Tom	
August					
September					
October					
November					
December					

Successful team meetings are a lifelong journey whose destination expands as you travel.

Moderator for the Staff Meeting

For the first few meetings, have some senior staff members moderate the meeting. The agenda provides order to the process, so the moderator only has to keep the discussion moving, close topics when consensus is reached, and end at the appointed hour. The moderator is not the expert with the answers but, rather, a facilitator of conversations to build a harmony of result. The moderator does not call for votes or rule on opinions. The objective is openness of ideas and group consensus. "Are we agreed that Susan and Bill are going to post the sterile area schedule by Friday and everyone will select their day to be responsible so the system can start on the first of the month?" This is the role of the moderator.

One other significant obligation of the monthly moderator is to draw in the quieter team members. When the subject of discussion naturally involves a person who is known for his or her reticence, it is an expected part of the process that the shy person will speak up. It is also the responsibility of the moderator to draw them into the conversation. "Martha, you work with this every day, what do you feel about the discussion we are having?"

Eventually, every single person in the office should be the moderator. If there are six people in the office, then each person will be moderator of the office staff meeting two times each year. Even the new dental assistant, just a few months in your office, is placed in the schedule so that he or she can confidently step right in and facilitate the meeting.

Getting Started: What to Do If You Do Not Already Have Monthly Staff Meetings

1. Select a regular day of the week each month for a 2-hour meeting, like the third Wednesday of the month at 8:00 a.m. Do not change this date or time; do demonstrate your absolute commitment to meeting and growing regularly. A

few months later, expand the time set aside to 3 hours, and perhaps eat at 11:00 a.m. that day and work from noon until the end of the day's schedule.

2. For your first monthly staff meetings, start simply. Establish a rotating schedule for just two people, perhaps moderator and scribe (note-taker), for the balance of the year. To make an easier transition to regular focused staff meetings, you might have only two or three sections instead of the full six. Perhaps start with an educational topic, reports, and rewarding experiences. I urge you to always include the rewarding experiences section and be leisurely about this section, allowing individuals to share themselves. You might have only office rewarding experiences for a few months to focus on successful patient experiences. It is easy to ask your staff to share success stories that involve three or four team members, and it encourages a focus on what is working well in your office. You can always expand the rewarding experiences section as time permits. I suggest you always do the rewarding experiences section first. It sets the tone for the balance of every single meeting. It elevates enthusiasm and reinforces the importance of a team working together for the rest of every meeting. Always start with rewarding experiences, whether you allow 2 hours or a full day for your gathering. Some easy education topics for your first meetings might include some of your referring specialists. They enjoy sharing some interesting cases, and everyone learns more about personalities and referral patterns.

3. As your success grows and the team learns that staff meetings are not just filled with the dentist complaining about the most recent crisis, you can expand the agenda and the time allowed for meeting. You could add the meeting evaluation responsibility and add a housekeeping list so that more ideas could be generated between meetings.

4. Ask for suggestions of topics that staff would like to learn more about during future staff meetings. Give them some ownership of what new learning will occur. You may have a couple of subjects like whitening and implants that you feel the need to explore early in the process. The education focus will attract considerable positive interest, while the idea of closing the office, buying bagels, and paying your team to share ideas for improvement will probably raise some early uncertainty for everyone.

Dentists naturally favor consistency over creativity, they often gain order by taking control. Staff meetings are a growth opportunity that begs for a fresh spirit of energy and challenge. Most dentists are highly perfectionist personality types. Dentists also are fearful of starting anything new unless they know exactly how the process will turn out. As a rule, dentists would rather not attempt something new than risk the possibility of making a mistake. This is not about allowing yourself to do something you may regret. It is about beginning a journey for all of you. Staff meetings create a horizontal environment where each person feels responsible for the success of the whole. Staff meetings create a higher ceiling for your practice. This is an evolving process and a personal journey that has its own reward.

If you dare to dream of smiling each day as you drive to work; if you think patients can be grateful and send appreciative notes when they find an emotional match in your office; if you can imagine a team of people whose members are individually motivated to do well and who are comfortable encouraging each other to do well, you desperately need staff meetings. Your entire team will benefit on a daily basis when they join in the shift to greater personal success and practice success as you grow people through motivating staff meetings.

If you have ever experienced the inner peace that comes from a healthy, positive current of energy as you blend your talents with the gifts of your workmates, you know the value of an authentic team. If you can surround yourself with gifted people and establish an orderly process for the journey together, you will enjoy your dental profession to the fullest. You made your own good fortune, and you made theirs too.

Other Ideas for Staff Education Topics

- Learn about behavioral styles and personality styles by finding someone to give a self-scored inventory to your whole office. Post the results so that everyone on the team can see how unique communication styles complement others to make a complete team. The options that grow out of this include learning how to use behavioral styles to help patients and learning how to use this information when you hire new team members.
- Ask each staff member to come to the next meeting with "the most difficult question you get asked." Put all the questions in a box and have a staff member draw a question out of the box and offer a good response. Then ask the whole team to brainstorm other possible answers and write out for the meeting notes some better answers to the question. Continue this until all the questions have group-developed comfortable responses. This may require two meetings to complete, but your verbal skills will improve dramatically. At the same time, the group is learning practice values and dental terminology.
- Invite a communications professor from a nearby college, a family health therapist, the infection control expert from your hospital, a stress management counselor, the local rescue service, the fire safety expert, the owner or hostess of a fine dining establishment, or a marketing expert for some other service business.
- Identify what you do well in patient relations by asking everyone to come with a list of their five or ten favorite patients and have each person tell the group why the patients they chose are special. What are the common themes of these patients, and how can you build on these positive feelings? What can you do to attract more of this type of person to your office?
- Give each person $50 and ask him or her to use it to have a real quality customer service experience before the next staff meeting. At the next meeting, allow each person to describe what exactly made the event go well or not so well. Keep a list of the qualities and feelings necessary to have an emotionally satisfying experience. Then you can brainstorm how your individual team members can do more of this quality service in your office. Stop and ask each person to write down three things he or she can personally do to improve the quality of the patient visit. Post the list and then, next month, ask each person to report on how it is going. What do your employees see that tells them it is making a difference in the patient perception of quality in your office?
- Invite an independent financial planner to discuss life insurance needs and retirement planning to your staff.
- Ask your staff for ideas and be creative. This is fun for everyone and part of the energy that makes your office a special place to enjoy each day.

Several other chapters in this book complement this chapter, especially Chapters 2 and 3 on financial statements and practice financial analysis and Chapters 22 and 23 on human resources and staffing.

Book Companion Website

The book companion website at www.wiley.com/go/dunning/transition includes additional material for this chapter that is not included in the printed version of the book. Please see 'About the Companion Website' at the start of the book for details on how to access the website.

References and Additional Resources

Blanchard, Ken, Carlos, John P., and Randolph, Alan. 1996. *Empowerment Takes More Than a Minute*. San Francisco: Berrett-Koehler.

Blanchard, Ken, Cuff, Kathy, and Halsey, Victoria. 2014. *Legendary Service; The Key Is to Care*. New York: McGraw Hill Education.

Brown, Brene. 2012. *Daring Greatly*. New York: Penguin Random House.

Chambers, David and Abrams, Ronald. 1992. *Dental Communication*. Sonoma, CA: Ohana Group.

DISC Personal Profile System. 2001. Minneapolis: Inscape Publishing.

Frazer, R.L. and Associates. Emotional Intelligence Workshop, Personal Coaching Workshop. www.frazeronline.com.

Haines, Stephen G. 1995. *Successful Strategic Planning*. Menlo Park, CA: Crisp Publications.

Keirsey, David. 1998. *Please Understand Me II*. Del Mar, CA: Prometheus Nemesis Book Company.

Lancaster, Lynne C. and Stillman, David. 2002. *When Generations Collide*. New York: HarperCollins.

Lencioni, Patrick. 2002. *The Five Dysfunctions of a Team*. San Francisco: Jossey-Bass.

Rath, Tom. 2007. *Strengths Finder 2.0* New York: Gallup Press.

Learning Exercises

1. Imagine that you have purchased a dental practice in which staff meetings were rarely held. How would you begin the process of adding a morning huddle? What are the reasons you would give to make your staff look forward to setting aside this time? In the beginning what would your agenda include?

2. Now imagine you want to add a regular monthly staff meeting to discuss broader topics. What are easy topics you could include in your first few meetings? What would you do to be certain that the staff understood the importance you place on everyone helping to improve your office?

3. Picture your staff after a year of monthly meetings. You can see they value the learning that occurs and all would agree there is a greater sense of community in your office. The problem you experience is that some staff members dominate the meeting and others are reluctant to speak up. What things could you do to draw in the quieter people? What things could you do to increase the sense of enthusiasm and anticipation for your regular meetings?

4. What are some of the possible topics you could have on the agenda that would increase the staff knowledge about developments in dental materials or new technology?

5. How do you plan a staff meeting so that everyone can be present from the start and there are few interruptions?

Part 7
Money Management: Insuring a Practice; and Personal Finance, Investments and Retirement Options

Chapter 25
Insuring a Dental Practice

James E. Spitsen

Insuring a Dental Practice

1. We are not going to get into a deep discussion of risk management and the principles of the risk management process in this chapter. That being said, we are going to give a brief overview of the topic so that you will able to see where insurance falls. It is likely that you have practiced some aspects of risk management in your daily lives and you were completely unaware of it at the time.

    Risk management is the identification and analysis of risk exposures in your business or personal life. The process includes evaluation of those exposures in order to arrive at a plan as to how you are going to deal with the risks you have identified.

    Let's look at an example. A young general dentist new to practice stated that he/she was very uncomfortable performing impacted third molar extractions and wondered if he/she had to do them in order to have a successful practice. The dentist preferred to refer those to an oral surgeon. Referring procedures you are uncomfortable with to a specialist is an excellent risk management tool. In fact, it is called Risk Avoidance.

    When you have *identified the risks* that concern you, whether financial or professional, you can arrive at how you are going to handle the risks you have identified, such as the one discussed above.

    There are several ways to handle risk. We briefly discussed *Risk Avoidance*, which is a conscious decision not to do something in order to avoid a potential negative outcome. You avoid a potential negative outcome of a bony third molar extraction by referring the procedure to an oral surgeon whose job it is to accept that risk.

    Risk Acceptance is the decision to accept a potential risk as necessary to your ability to do business. As a dentist, everything you do for a patient presents some level of potential risk. You can't practice dentistry or any other profession really without taking on some risk.

    Risk Transfer is where insurance falls in the risk management process. If you own or purchasing a building, then there is the risk that it could burn down. If it did, it is unlikely that you would have the personal funds to rebuild. So, you pay a premium to an insurance company and for a fraction of the cost to replace the building the insurance company takes on the risk of replacing it at the time of loss.

Dental Practice Transition: A Practical Guide to Management, Second Edition.
Edited by David G. Dunning and Brian M. Lange.
© 2016 John Wiley & Sons, Inc. Published 2016 by John Wiley & Sons, Inc.
Companion Website: www.wiley.com/go/dunning/transition

The insurance company accepts these risks with the understanding that some of the buildings will in fact burn but most will not, so the law of averages should work in their favor.

You can also transfer risk by contract. If you lease space, it is almost certain that your landlord will require you to carry certain limits to cover your potential liability should a loss occur. That landlord will also require you to name him/her as an additional insured on your policy. By doing this, the landlord is transferring his/her risk of leasing the premises to you, back to you.

If you make a decision to accept a risk and decide not to transfer the risk to someone else either through contract or insurance, you have *retained that risk*. Some might call this *self-insurance*. Let's go back to that building you own. Everyone has the option to purchase flood and earthquake coverage from either their insurance provider or the Federal Government. However, the fact is that if your building isn't in a flood zone or an area prone to earthquakes, you usually do not purchase insurance to cover that risk. With that decision, you have retained the risk of potential loss to your property due to flood and earthquake. Taking a high deductible on an insurance policy is a form of risk retention as well.

So, insurance is one of the many risk management vehicles you will utilize but it is not the only vehicle you have available. Insurance exists because you cannot avoid all of the potential risks of being in business and you cannot afford to self-insure potential risks on your own.

A good risk management plan is one where you have identified the risks you face, make a decision as to how you will handle those risks, put your risk management plan in to place and then monitor it and make changes as needed. Your insurance agent or broker should be tasked with assisting you in this process since you are the dentist and they are the insurance professional.

There you have it! The *Risk Management Process* in a nutshell. You didn't go to dental school to study this, but it is imperative that as a business person you have a grasp on this process as well as an idea of where to go for the expertise you need to guide you through the process.

2. In every state in America you will find two or three insurance agents that specialize in insuring dentists. Your state association will know who these agents are and so will your colleagues who have been in practice for any length of time. You should find out who these agents are, interview them, and work with the one with whom you feel the most comfortable and who has the knowledge you need to protect your business. There are nuances to insuring a dental practice, so it is wise to work with an insurance professional who knows more about it than you do.

    In addition, there are insurance companies that specialize in insuring dental practices. It will always be in your best interest to choose an insurance company that has designed and implemented an insurance program for a dental practice. As we get into specialized coverage areas later, you will see why this is important. An insurance company that specializes in dentists will also provide their clients with risk management expertise to help their insureds reduce their exposure to loss, which helps everyone in the end.

3. Now we are going to get in to the nitty-gritty of insurance. Basically, we are going to look at insurance that personally protects you the dentist; insurance that protects what is yours and finally we are going to look at insurance that protects you from others. When speaking of "you the dentist" we are including you as an individual and you as a legal corporation. If you organize your practice as a

corporate entity, make sure you always name the corporate entity on all of your insurance policies.

We are going to look at them in that order. So, professional liability insurance, which you want to look at first, will actually be one of the last types of insurance discussed.

When we talk about insuring *you the dentist*, what are we talking about exactly? We are going to discuss those lines of insurance that protect your health, your revenue stream, and your life. These are the more personal lines of insurance that protect *you*.

Health Insurance

If you are under age 26 and have generous parents, you may still be covered under their family health insurance plan. If this is the case, make sure you thank them profusely as they are doing you a great service. Once you hit age 26 however, the government says you are on your own.

The *Affordable Care Act* is currently the law of the land and rules all health insurance in America. The Affordable Care Act, (ACA) was implemented on January 1, 2014 after having originally been signed in to law in 2010. As a future small business person, this is very important to you.

As of January 1, 2014, everyone was required to have health insurance and there are penalties for those who choose not to get it. If you earn under a certain amount per year, you may qualify for health insurance premium subsidies from the government. However, as a dentist, you won't qualify, your hygienists won't qualify, and most likely your chairside assistants won't qualify either.

The good news for the small employer is that you no longer have to go in to a high risk state run health plan or form a small group plan just to get health insurance if you have had an adverse health history. Effective with the ACA, no one can be denied coverage.

In the past, it was not uncommon for the spouse of a dentist to work a job that provided group health insurance because the dentist was not able to qualify for an individual health policy due to preexisting medical issues. That is no longer necessary with implementation of the ACA.

Since you will likely be a small employer with fewer than fifty employees, you will not have to offer group health insurance to your employees under the ACA. This doesn't mean you cannot make health insurance part of a benefit package for employees, rather it just means there is no penalty for not offering it.

Let's get back to health insurance for you, now that you know you must have it. Exactly what type of plan is best for you? The correct answer is, "that depends." It depends on what your health status is, it depends on your level of health care utilization, and it depends on your financial wherewithal. There will be three basic types of plans to choose from; *high deductible HSA qualified plans*; *deductible plans with co-insurance*, and *deductible plans with co-insurance and co-pays*.

High Deductible HSA Qualified Health Plans

High wage earners are drawn to higher deductible plans in order to keep their monthly premiums down. Certain high deductible health insurance plans qualify for *Health*

Savings Accounts (HSA). However, if you are a high wage earner with significant health issues, a high deductible plan may not be in your best interest.

HSA Qualified High Deductible Health Insurance Plans must have minimum deductibles as set each year by the federal government. Some plans will also have co-insurance after the deductible though it is usually best to purchase a plan with 100% co-insurance, which means that after your deductible is satisfied, the health plan picks up 100% of covered costs.

With a HSA, you are able to fund a high deductible through the use of a savings account that provides special benefits. First, you can fund the account with pretax dollars or deduct the account if you funded it with post-tax dollars. Either way, the money and the earnings on the money in the HSA are tax free if you use the funds for qualified medical expenses. If you use the money for nonqualified purchases, you pay your normal tax rate on the money and also a tax penalty.

After age 65, you can use the money saved in an HSA for anything you desire. If you continue to use the funds to cover qualified health expenses, the money used is tax free. If you decide to take some of the money and purchase a boat, you pay your normal tax rate on the funds drawn out but there is no additional tax penalty. Make sure you consult with your accountant and/or tax advisor if you decide to use the funds in a Health Savings Account for a nonqualified health expense.

So, what are qualified and nonqualified medical expenses as they relate to HSA? Your best source for information on this topic is found in publications 969 and 502 from the Department of the Treasury Internal Revenue Service. You can find both of these online using the IRS website www.irs.gov.[1]

Deductible Plans with Coinsurance

If you venture out from high deductible health plans into lower deductible plans, there are many issues to consider. The deductible options are greater, from lower deductibles of around $750–5,000 or perhaps even higher. There are high deductible plans that don't qualify for Health Savings Accounts due to a myriad of reasons but usually due to the inclusion of prescription benefits payable before the deductible. With the passage of the ACA you will see more co-insurance levels than were normally seen in the past.

If you have a deductible insurance plan with co-insurance, it means that even after you pay your deductible, you will still pay a percentage of covered expenses based on the co-insurance level in your policy and the out of pocket maximum.

For example, let's say you have an individual health insurance plan with a $2,500 deductible and 80% co-insurance that will apply up to the "out of pocket maximum." You are single, so this plan covers just you. Your "out of pocket maximum" is $6,500.00. While skydiving you break your leg in two places. The result is medical expenses totaling $50,000.00. Your deductible will apply to the first $2,500 of medical expenses. After the deductible you have a balance of $47,500 in medical expenses. Since you have 80% co-insurance, the health insurance company is going to pay 80% of the remaining bills until you have paid out a total of $6,500 out of your own pocket, which includes your deductible. If you didn't have the "out of pocket maximum," you would pay the $2,500 deductible as well as 20% of the remaining $47,500 for a total of $12,000.00.

---

[1] www.irs.gov

It is important that you watch the co-insurance percentages in your health insurance quotes closely as well as the out of pocket maximum. Under the ACA you will have your choice of plans in the categories of Bronze, Silver, Gold, and Platinum. A Bronze plan may have co-insurance of 60%, which means you could pay 40% after your deductible up to the out of pocket maximum. The premium may look appealing but a serious injury or health event could cause personal financial hardship.

In a Platinum plan, the co-insurance may be 90%, which means you would pay 10% after your deductible up to your out of pocket maximum. The monthly premium will be considerably higher than a Bronze plan. But if you have a health condition, or the monthly premium is easier to budget for than a potentially large hospital bill, then a Platinum plan may make more sense.

Deductible Plans with Co-Pays and Co-Insurance

This type of plan is identical to the plan above, except that the company has co-pays for certain health expenses such as office visits, emergency room visits, and so on. The co-pay limits or "fixes" initial out of pocket expense, but if your office visit results in more tests or an actual hospitalization, then you will have deductible and co-insurance expense.

The Affordable Care Act has not been a stagnant law since it was first approved in 2010 and there is no reason to believe it will quiet down in the near future. It has and will remain a politically charged juggernaut for years to come. Because of this, it is important that you rely on someone that specializes in health insurance to help you find the plan that is best for you based on not only your health but also financial wherewithal and your appetite for assuming risk.

Almost all health insurance plans require that you utilize a physician that is a member of your health insurance company preferred provider organization, (PPO). For a physician to be a member of a PPO, he/she usually has to sign a contract that will limit or "cap" his/her reimbursement amount for office visits and medical procedures. You will have the same issue with many of the dental insurance plans you work with as a practicing dentist.

There has never been more change in the health insurance industry than there has been since the implementation of the Affordable Care Act. Make sure the insurance professional you utilize to help you establish this coverage specializes in health insurance. Shopping for this coverage via internet on your own is not advisable as you may see a monthly premium you like but the deductible, co-insurance, and co-pays may lead to more out of pocket expense than you would have had if you hadn't paid so much attention to the price. Use an insurance professional!

Dental and Vision Insurance

We won't discuss these two lines of insurance in great detail as you will likely not need to carry either. Both of these types of insurance have limited benefits. Dental insurance usually covers two diagnostic/preventive office visits each year per covered person. It may have a lifetime limit of $1,000 on orthodontia and some other limited coverage as well. Since you are a dentist, it is unlikely you will need this coverage. However, you will likely accept dental insurance from your patients and that is discussed in Chapter 13.

Vision insurance is equally limited. A vision plan will have a co-pay for an annual exam and limited coverage for frames, lenses, contacts, and so on. Some plans provide reduced costs or discounts for procedures such as Lasik.

Disability Insurance

Disability Insurance is likely the first business-related insurance product you are offered. Disability insurance provides money to you should you become disabled due to a covered illness or injury. Disability covers your personal living expenses. Most disability policies allow you to purchase up to either 70 or 80% of your normal gross earnings. You cannot insure 100% of your normal gross earnings as you would have paid taxes on your normal gross wages. You can't bring home more income on disability than you did while working. If you did, this would be a *moral dilemma* as you have no real incentive to return to work.

As a third or fourth year dental student, you will begin to hear from many insurance professionals trying to sell you disability insurance. However, as a dental student do you need disability insurance coverage? You have no income, in fact it is likely you have nothing but debt and probably a negative net worth. So, why should you look at disability insurance while you are still in school?

The short answer is "yes," you should look at disability insurance when you reach your last year of dental school. The main reason is that you have now invested a lot of money in your chosen career! So, if you become disabled while you are still in dental school, you want to preserve some financial ability to live. Another reason is to preserve future insurability as well as the ability to increase your limits at a later date.

If you were born after January 1, 1960, your full normal retirement age is 67.[2] It is important that you purchase a disability policy that will pay benefits to your normal retirement age and one that pays regardless of any other benefits you receive.

There are two basic forms of disability insurance policies; individual disability policies and association or group employer disability policies. Within these types, there are several different provisions that set them apart. Let's talk about the two policy forms first.

An individual policy is just that. It is a policy sold to you based on *your* current occupation, earnings, and health. The rates you are charged are based on those factors as well as the amount of insurance you wish to purchase.

An association or employer group disability policy is much like a group health policy. Group disability policies are usually designed for a particular group, whether it is an employer group or an association. Group disability premiums are usually more competitive than an individual policy premium but there are usually some trade-offs for the lower rate.

As a dentist, you want to look for a disability policy that was designed for dentists. You want to make sure it covers your occupation either as a general dentist or other dental specialist. This type of policy is called an *own occupation* policy. Before you purchase any disability policy you will want to know the definition of *occupation*. If it is *any occupation*, it means the policy doesn't usually pay if you can perform any job functions that correlate to your level of skill and education.

[2] Chapter 25

For example, after 10 years in practice as a general dentist, you develop arthritis in your hands and are no longer able to practice. However, you are able and qualified to teach at your alma mater. If you are covered by a disability policy with an *any occupation* definition, then you may not receive any disability benefits. Under a properly defined *own occupation* policy, since you cannot practice as a general dentist, the disability policy would pay your benefits.

Within the "own occupation" definition, you also have to make sure there are no limits on time. Some "own occupation" policies will pay for a true own occupation disability for 5 years and after that the policy definition changes to "any occupation." This of course helps the insurance companies keep the monthly premium lower, but also can seriously affect your disability benefits.

Individual disability policies are usually guaranteed renewable, or noncancelable and guaranteed renewable. So, what do these two terms mean?

A guaranteed renewable disability policy is one in which as long as you pay your premium, the insurance company cannot cancel your policy and they cannot change your terms. However, they can raise your premium.

A noncancelable and guaranteed renewable disability policy cannot be canceled if you pay your premiums, the terms of the policy cannot change and the premium cannot be increased.

As a dentist, unless you go to work in corporate dentistry or for a very large office and you are not a member of the American Dental Association, you will encounter group disability policies offered through either the American Dental Association[3] or your state dental association.[4] It is likely that an association group disability policy is neither noncancelable nor guaranteed renewable, so why should you look at an association group disability policy?

Disability insurance through an association usually costs less than individual disability policies. They may also have a definition of *own occupation* that is much stronger for you as a dentist than for an off-the-shelf individual disability policy. In addition, an association disability policy may have some additional coverage built-in that is designed for dentists, such as loss of use of hands benefit.

If you leave the association however, you may become ineligible to keep their disability policy. Also, since the association disability policy is built on a group disability platform, the premiums can be increased over time. Ask your association or their insurance professional about the history of the insurance plan, for example, has it ever been canceled? Have the premiums ever been increased on current policyholders?

Now comes the hard part, which policy is better? The answer is not easy. The short answer is that obviously there is a place for both of these policies.

For a brand new dentist, cash flow is usually not the greatest. Since you can actually purchase disability insurance as a fourth year dental student, cash flow can be even worse! Early in your career an association or group disability policy may make sense because you can get more bang for your insurance buck. Later when you have started to earn more, you will need more disability coverage. This may be a great time to layer an individual policy with your current group plan.

Should you decide to go with an individual disability policy as a fourth year dental student, make sure you meet with a trusted insurance adviser who has your best interests in mind. Check the marketplace for individual policies. Compare the

---

[3] You can find out more about the ADA-sponsored group insurance plans at www.ada.org.
[4] Insuring a Dental Practice.

coverage, especially the definitions of your occupation. Have your insurance adviser provide the insurance company ratings for each of the insurance companies they are recommending.

There are also other provisions to discuss regarding disability: the cost of living allowance (COLA) and guaranteed purchase options to name two. Review these options with your adviser and have them explain them to you fully. Also make sure you discuss with your insurance adviser, as well as your accountant, both the amount of disability coverage you need and how you will pay for it. You do not want to structure your disability so that the benefits paid to you are taxable.

Whether you are looking at an individual disability policy or an association-sponsored or group plan, you need to find out if the policy "offsets" for any other benefit you may earn. If you become totally disabled, you may qualify for Social Security Disability Benefits. If so, some disability policies will reduce the amount of the benefit they pay to you so that the total of their benefit plus the Social Security benefit equals the amount of disability you purchased. There are disability policies that do not offset for other benefits received. You should look for those policies.

When you begin practice and borrow money to purchase equipment or sign lease papers to get equipment, it is not uncommon for the financial institution or leasing company to require that you carry enough disability insurance to cover the loan or lease payments. You should always try to avoid assigning your personal disability policy to a lender or leasing agent. If a disability occurred, they would get the primary payment and you would get the leftovers.

Instead, there are disability products designed to meet the needs of lending institutions and leasing companies. They are called *"Reducing Term Disability Policies."* These policies meet the needs of the lender or leasing entity without tying up your personal disability benefits. The policies are written to cover your payments for the term of the loan or lease as long as you are disabled.

Business Overhead Expense

Somewhat related to disability insurance is *business overhead expense* (BOE). BOE coverage pays your continuing business expenses such as rent, leased equipment payments, payroll, and interest on loans. If you are disabled from an illness or injury, you don't want to be placed in the position to have to use your personal disability insurance benefits to try and keep your office viable. BOE coverage takes that burden off your shoulders.

BOE coverage is usually a short term policy payable for up to 2 years maximum. If you are unable to return to work after 2 years, your practice is gone as your patients have found other dentists. The premium is usually very reasonable since the policy pays only for 2 years.

If you practice alone, you would purchase enough BOE coverage to cover everything. If there are two dentists in a practice, you would each insure your share of the covered expenses.

Many people confuse Business Overhead Expense insurance with the Business Interruption insurance found in a property insurance policy. The big difference between the two is that BOE pays if *you* are unable to work due to illness or injury. Business Interruption insurance pays if your *premises* is unavailable to use due to a covered loss such as fire or storm damage. We will discuss Business Interruption in detail later; so we won't go in to the actual coverage here. The important fact to remember is that they are two very different types of insurance. Business Interruption is usually automatically included in your property policy but you have to apply and qualify for BOE coverage separately.

Life Insurance

For some reason, life insurance is the insurance that everyone loves to hate, but if you are ever a beneficiary of a life insurance policy, you will see just how much good can come from having a life insurance policy in place. Years ago there was a commercial on television and the announcer stated, "Life insurance isn't for you, it's for the ones you leave behind." Well, that is partially true. Life insurance *is* for those you leave behind but it can also be a useful tool for you as you do tax, estate, and business succession planning.

The two questions most asked about life insurance are, "How much life insurance do I need?" and "What is the cheapest life insurance policy I can buy?" The short answer to the first question is, "I don't know" and the answer to the second question is usually, "Term or Group Term."

As a fourth year dental student you may or may not need much life insurance at all. If you are single and without much debt, you may need enough life insurance to take care of your final expenses only. If you are married with two children and your spouse is dependent on you and the potential income you will make as a practicing dentist, you may need a significant amount of life insurance.

When you graduate and begin to practice, you may borrow money to purchase equipment. Many times the lender will require you to have life insurance in place that is assigned to the lender to cover the value of the loan. Some lenders even require you to assign your disability insurance as mentioned earlier.

If you become a partner in a dental practice, it is not uncommon that as part of the contract you agree to purchase your partner's portion of the practice from the estate should the partner die. This is common in "Buy/Sell Agreements'." Coming up with that money could be troublesome. But, if you have life insurance in place to cover that exposure, the life insurance could completely fund the purchase of the practice.

So, how much life insurance do you need? The answer is; "more than you probably think you do!" Sitting down with your life insurance professional or adviser will go a long way to help you come up with a dollar value with which you are comfortable investing.

There are many variations of life insurance but we are going to discuss two of them: *term life* and *whole life*. Just as with individual disability insurance and group disability insurance, there is room for both in your portfolio.

Term insurance is the most cost-effective vehicle for delivering higher death benefits at low cost. Whole life policies are more expensive as they are considered, "permanent insurance." They build cash value and are around for as long as you pay your premium or until you have "paid up" the policy.

Term policies are only in place for the term of years selected, usually from 10 to 20 years. They are a great policy as long as you die within that time period. If not, the premiums paid in are gone and there is no death benefit or cash value. The premiums are usually very reasonable since the likelihood is that you will outlive the period of years selected.

Whole life policies are not limited by a time period and as long as you pay your premium the policy is in force. Some whole life policies are considered "paid up" after a certain number of years or payments. Some policies you may pay on until you reach age 100. A whole life policy can be designed in many different configurations to meet your needs.

Whole life policies do build up cash values that you can actually tap into in the future if you need the money. You can also draw out of the cash values similar to a retirement plan.

Let's look at some premium differences between whole life and term life:

We will begin with the rates for a 24-year old male. Let's call him Jim. Jim is looking for a $500,000.00 term policy. The longest term policies most companies offer is a 20-year level term. This means that the premium stays the same for the first 20 years, but in that 21st year, watch out!

Jim has no health issues so he gets the best rates the insurance company has to offer. Based on your health and lifestyle your policy could be rated in classes that usually range from "smoker" to "super preferred."

A 20-year level term policy for Jim carries an estimated annual premium of $245.00. That is a lot of potential payout for a $245.00 annual investment. Remember though that a term policy builds no cash value and if you are still alive at the end of the 20-year period, you have nothing. The premium in the 21st year will jump to over $2,000.00 annually, so you may let the policy expire at the end of 20 years, especially if you are still in good health.

In contrast, that same $500,000 death benefit in a whole life policy could cost anywhere from around $3,000 per year up to close to $10,000 per year depending on the plan you choose and of course your current health and lifestyle choices.

If the policy is for a female, the rates will be slightly lower since females usually out live males, their rates are lower. In this same scenario a female would have term rates around $210 and whole life premium rates from around $2,800.00 up to around $8,300.00 depending on the plan chosen.

There are several differences between the term plan and the whole life plan. First, as stated earlier, the term plan premium will increase dramatically after the level term period ends. Term plans build no cash value so if you are lucky enough to live to the end of the level term premium period, that premium is gone forever.

The whole life premium on the other hand has been building cash value. If you invested $2,800 per year in premiums in a whole life policy, you could expect a cash value at the end of 20 years to be quite significant. Most likely the policy would be worth more than the total of paid premiums over those 20 years.

But I know what you are thinking; you can come up with $210.00 or $245.00 much more easily than $2,800 or $3,000 early in your career and that is likely very true. You are young and invincible so you will opt for the term policy and roll the dice that you will remain healthy so that when the one term policy becomes too expensive, you can apply for another low-cost term policy to take you out further.

But what if you don't stay healthy? What if something happens in that 20-year period that renders you uninsurable? Heart issues, cancer, Parkinson's, and even diabetes are medical conditions that could either severely limit your ability to purchase life insurance or rule you out completely. Your level term premium has ended, the annual premium now has skyrocketed but you have no other life insurance in place or available. That is the gamble you take when you rely on term life insurance only.

If you do begin with only term life insurance, there is a safety valve available in some policies. The safety valve is the ability to convert the term life policy any time during the level premium period to a whole life product. If you purchase a term policy make sure the policy is convertible to a whole life product. That way you have at least some ability to keep some permanent insurance in place if you become uninsurable later on.

It is always amazing that the insurance professional who will convince you to purchase an individual disability policy due to its increased safety and security over a group- or association-based disability policy will turn around and recommend a term life insurance policy over a whole life policy. As it was stated earlier regarding the two types of disability insurance, there is room for both term- and whole life insurance-based policies in your personal protection portfolio.

Life insurance companies offer all kinds of bells and whistles to go along with their basic death benefit. Some of the more common that you can choose from include the following:

1. *Waiver of premium:* If you become totally disabled, your premiums are waived for the period of your disability.
2. *Guaranteed purchase option:* Purchase of this rider guarantees that you will have the opportunity to increase your death benefit by a certain amount during the policy period without having to provide any evidence of your current insurability.
3. *Accelerated benefit rider:* A certain portion of your death benefit could become payable to you due to a diagnosis of a chronic or terminal illness.
4. *Family term rider:* This type of rider lets you add some coverage for dependent children, usually up to a certain maximum. This coverage can be quite beneficial for three reasons; the cost is usually very competitive, you likely wouldn't have any other individual policy on your children, and third, many companies allow you to convert the rider to a permanent policy for the child once the child is no longer dependent, usually at age 21.

There are many other riders available on life insurance policies. Your job as the purchaser of the product is to take a look at the cost of these riders to see if you feel they are cost-effective for the additional coverage that is provided. If your insurance professional shows you a premium with all or some of these riders already "built in" to the premium, have them break them out so you can see what they cost.

Life insurance can be used in many ways in addition to just protection for those you love. You can use life insurance policies to fund the buyout requirements in a partnership buy/sell agreement. Life insurance is commonly used to cover estate tax liability so that more of an estate can pass to the heirs instead of the government. Since life insurance proceeds are tax free, it is a great way to avoid tax liability.

A dedicated life insurance professional can help you make the decisions best for your individual circumstances when it comes to how much life insurance to purchase and the type of plan that fits you the best.

We have now discussed the major insurance types that protect you including health, disability, and life insurance. Now we will move on to protecting that which belongs to you.

Protecting What Belongs to You

In this section we will discuss insuring all that you physically need to practice dentistry. If you graduate dental school and become an associate, you may not have to worry about this for a while. If you graduate and buy in to a practice right away or decide to start a practice from scratch, you will quickly learn just how much of a financial investment is required for you to practice your craft. Dentistry is one of the most expensive professions when it relates to equipment and supplies needed just to open your doors. In this section we will discuss insuring your building and business personal property from risks of loss.

Purchasing insurance to cover the loss of your office and dental equipment is fruitless if you don't stay on top of what it would take to replace your office should a loss occur and how much it would take to put you back in the position you were prior to the covered loss. It also doesn't help if you don't keep your insurance professional informed when you make large purchases or major changes to your building or dental office property.

In the world of insuring a dental practice it is good to know that many insurance companies have designed "package policies" that build in the most needed coverages into a policy that only requires a few personal additions or deletions to meet your individual practice needs. These packages can cover your building if you own it (or are required by contract to insure it), your contents, your loss of income due to a covered cause of loss, even some losses that affect your physical practice but didn't occur at your office, just to name a few.

There are some other coverages in package policies that can offer protection from some of your potential liability from third parties but we will discuss those later.

Insuring your Building

Building Coverage: Building insurance premiums are based on the construction materials used in the structure, the square footage, distance to fire stations, rivers, flood plains, upkeep, and so on. If the dental practice is the only tenant of the building, then this is ideal. If the practice is located in a strip mall or office building, the other tenants of the building will weigh in the decision of the insurance company as to how much to charge or whether they want to offer coverage at all.

When it comes to insuring buildings and contents you want to insure them for their *replacement cost*. If you purchased a panoramic x-ray in 2015 for $30,000 and it is lost in a fire in 2025, the cost of that pan may have increased to $37,500.00. You will want the policy to pay the replacement value at the time of the loss. Likewise, if construction costs in 2015 are $150.00 per square foot for a building like yours, but in 2025 they are $225.00 getting $150.00 won't help you replace your building.

Your insurance professional can help you arrive at the cost to replace your building. Don't be fooled by thinking you should insure the building for the amount you paid for it, unless you just built it. The insurance company typically is looking for the replacement cost for that building if it were burned to the ground. Though you don't insure the land value or the foundation since both usually survive in any loss, the replacement cost of your building could be very different than the cost to purchase the building.

Insuring your Business Personal Property

As with your building, replacement cost at the *time of loss* is your goal when insuring your business personal property (BPP). Between your insurance professional and the dental office supplier you have chosen to work with, you can stay current on the insurance amounts or limits you would need should a loss occur. Utilize the professionals that are available to you and value their opinions. Your insurance professional is your partner, not an adversary just trying to get you to spend all your hard earned money on insurance premiums.

Within your BPP you could have electrical equipment that needs specialized coverage. From a digital telephone system to computers to digital x-ray and even a CAD CAM system with a mill, you can have electrical exposures that can severely affect your equipment and those exposures may not be on your insured premises. It is important to make sure you separate your electronic equipment values and insure them within the insurance package but do so with an electronic data equipment form or endorsement.

Electronic data processing equipment (EDP) is very important as it provides additional coverage due to off premises causes of loss such as a power surge caused by damage to an electrical transformer located a half mile from your insured premises.

If you own your building or if you are leasing it but are required by your lease to provide all insurance, you can also add the values of your heating and ventilation and air-conditioning to this coverage. This can be very important especially if your air handling units are located on the roof of your building and subject to the increased chance of lightning strikes.

Business Interruption

Business interruption coverage protects your revenue stream if your business is closed due to a covered *property loss*. Just as disability and business overhead expense protect your revenue from an accident, illness, or injury, *business interruption* takes care of that exposure due to property losses. Many dentists have looked at business interruption coverage thinking they have disability insurance. Don't make that mistake. They are very different types of insurance.

Policies designed for dentist offices will provide business interruption coverage in two basic forms, both of which are usually included in the policy. Dentist specific policies will allow you to purchase a daily limit of coverage for a certain number of days. For example, you could purchase a limit of $5,000 per day for 30 days. What this does is remove the requirement to prove the amount of your loss for those 30 days. You just have to prove that you were closed due to a covered loss in order to collect the benefit. This can be a real time saver versus proving your actual loss.

The second type of business interruption insurance coverage that is either built-in to the policy or available to you is *Actual Loss Sustained Business Interruption*. With this type of coverage, you have to prove your loss using tools such as tax returns, patient schedules, receivables, bank statements, and so on. You may have to enlist the assistance of an accountant. Actual loss sustained business interruption coverage usually pays up to 1 year as any practice should be back in business before a year is over. The coverage can also pay partial benefits once you are back in business as your patient load builds backup after the loss.

Policy Deductibles and Co-Insurance

Let's briefly discuss the role of policy deductibles and co-insurance. You may refer to this as having some "skin in the game."

A *deductible* is a monetary amount that is your responsibility to pay should a property loss occur. If your property policy has a $500.00 deductible, it means the insurance company will subtract that amount from the total value of a loss and pay you the difference.

For example, your dentist office suffers a covered loss due to water damage from a water line that bursts in an operatory. The practice suffers a $2,500.00 loss and they have a $500.00 deductible.

Covered loss:	$2,500.00
Deductible:	−$500.00
Amount payable:	$2,000.00

Deductibles help keep you from turning in every small claim that may provide a payout from an insurance company. Deductibles can be low or high depending on your comfort level or insurance company requirement. Higher deductibles help reduce the overall premium for the property insurance policy. With a dental office property policy it may not make sense to purchase a high deductible because the price difference may not make taking the higher deductible worthwhile. Ask your insurance professional for a couple of insurance options at different deductible levels so you can see which level makes the most sense to you from a cost savings and overall comfort level.

Co-insurance on a property policy is a potential penalty that awaits you should you decide not to insure your building and/or contents at replacement cost. If you purchased a building for $250,000 but it would cost $500,000 to replace it if it burned to the ground, you could have a real problem.

The co-insurance penalty could apply in this situation. The penalty would state that you recover only the portion of the loss relative to the percentage of the amount of coverage you *did* have versus the amount you *should* have had. We call this "did over should" in the insurance world. You *did* have $250,000 worth of coverage. You *should* have had $500,000 worth of coverage. You had half the amount of coverage you should have had, so if your covered loss was $200,000 you would collect half of that amount, or $100,000.

You do not want this to happen and there are two ways to make sure it doesn't. The first and best way is to make sure you have your building and contents values up to date on their replacement values. Your insurance professional and your dental office supply company can assist you in keeping your values current.

The second way, and everyone should do this, is to make sure that your insurance professional deletes the co-insurance penalty clause from your policy. This is also called "to waive co-insurance" in the package policy. This will get rid of the co-insurance penalty but if you are still underinsured, it only allows the policy to pay up to the limit purchased, you still have an uninsured portion you will have to deal with personally.

Ancillary Policy Coverages

Package policies for dentists include many other ancillary coverages that are thrown in by the various insurance companies. Coverage for signs not attached to the insured building, trees and shrubs, property of others, money and securities, fine arts, and so on. You should get a list of the extra policy coverages that the insurance company is including in the package. Insurance companies that specialize in insurance plans for dentists will add coverage for office specific exposures such as some coverage for gold and silver even though it is unlikely you have much gold and silver on premises any longer.

Flood and Earthquake

Flood and Earthquake insurance is usually excluded in all insurance policies these days. If you want the coverage, you have to request for it. You usually purchase these coverages only if you are located in an area subject to flood or earthquake occurrences.

Most flood coverage is provided through a government program called the National Flood Insurance Program, or NFIP for short. The program is sold through local insurance agents but the program is run actually by FEMA (Federal Emergency Management Agency). If your practice is located in a flood zone as defined by FEMA, you may be required by your lender to carry flood insurance. Your local municipal codes may also require you to carry flood insurance if you are located in a flood zone.

The best advice is to make sure you don't purchase or build a practice in a flood zone. You can check the flood risk of any location by visiting www.floodsmart.gov[5] and checking the flood risk profile for that location. The higher the risk, the higher the flood insurance premium you will pay.

One final thought on flood insurance. You can't wait until a flood is threatening your property to apply for the coverage. There will be a 30-day wait from the time you apply until the time the coverage becomes active. If there wasn't a waiting period, everyone would wait until a flood was threatening their property before applying for coverage.

Earthquake insurance is a bit different from flood insurance. You can usually purchase earthquake coverage from the insurance company that insures your practice. That is of course unless you live in earthquake prone areas such as California. In earthquake prone areas you may have to purchase earthquake insurance from a governmental or quasi-governmental agency.

The deductible levels for both flood and earthquake coverage are usually much higher than your normal package policy deductible. Flood and earthquake coverage overall premium costs are relative to the exposure or risk the location presents. The higher the potential hazard, the higher the premium will be.

Protecting You the Dentist from Others

There are a few types of insurance that we could have discussed in the previous section because they are usually insured through the package policy we discussed in that section. However, the insurance is really protecting you from the actions of others so they really fit in this section the best.

In your dental practice office package insurance policy you will find coverage for *Employee Dishonesty*. The limit is low, around $25,000 but can be increased for an additional premium. Employee dishonesty protects you the dentist if an employee steals money, supplies, or services from your practice.

[5] National Flood Insurance Program website.

Employee dishonesty claims are not as rare as you would think they are or should be. You were trained to perform dentistry, not to run an office. However, the less "hands on" you are in the business side of dentistry, the more likely it is that an employee dishonesty claim could occur. When you delegate deposits, check writing, business account reconciliation, and so on to one or two people and you take a "hands-off" position, you open yourself up to a claim.

Don't ever think that having a relative, close friend, or even your spouse in this position would remove the threat of employee dishonesty. It can and has happened in situations where all these were involved. There are as many stories of how employees steal from employers as there are stars in the sky.

So, how can you control this exposure, even when you can't eliminate it? The answer is to take a "hands on" approach. Some suggestions are as follows:

- Sign all checks. Never delegate this. Seeing all expenditures helps.
- Never let the same person who makes the bank deposits reconcile the accounts or handle the checks.
- Since there are fewer and fewer paper checks written, get in to your bank accounts or financial management software and look around. Know your vendors so you will notice if there are payments made to entities you are not familiar with.
- Everyone in your office that handles money, whether it is coming into the office or going out from the office, must take at least one full week off per year for vacation so that someone else can do his/her job. While the person is on vacation the substitute may notice if something doesn't look right. If the employee refuses to take a full week off or continually cancels a vacation, a red flag should go up immediately in your mind that a full audit may be needed.
- The less controls you choose to utilize, the higher the employee dishonesty insurance limit you should purchase.

Hopefully, you realize this is an important insurance coverage and make sure you have adequate limits and adequate controls. The subject of embezzlement is discussed in Chapter 16.

Workers Compensation

You are probably wondering why workers compensation insurance is listed under insurance products that protect you the dentist. In fact, most dentists opt out of covering themselves for workers compensation, which is your option under the policy. You usually purchase workers compensation coverage only to cover your employees. In most states, you are required to purchase the coverage.

To understand why worker compensation is in this section, let's have a brief history lesson. During the industrial age, manufacturing in America skyrocketed. There was no OSHA to ensure working conditions for employees were safe. If an employee was injured on the job, his/her employer may or may not have taken care of him/her. If the employer chose not to take care of the injured employee, the only recourse was for the employee to sue the employer for negligence.

Well, it didn't take too long for the government to learn that most employers back then chose not to take care of their employees. Negligence claims were difficult to win and expensive. So, in order to provide for the employee, workers compensation insurance was born. But there were trade-offs. The employer had to purchase the coverage to protect the employee, *but the employee had to waive his/her rights to sue the employer for negligence as his/her part of the deal.*

So, workers compensation protects the employees should they be injured on the job, but it also protects the employer from every employee suing them for negligence when they are injured on the job.

Workers compensation insurance is the closest thing to socialized insurance that we have in America just for the following reasons:

1. The coverage is mandatory.
2. Both the employer and the employee have to waive some rights in order for it to succeed.

It is considered a "no fault" type of plan in that if the employee is injured on the job, whether it is the employer or the employee at fault, coverage will apply.

As stated earlier, most states require an employer to purchase the coverage. Some states make you purchase workers compensation coverage from a state facility. These are called "Monopolistic" States. The current monopolistic states are Wyoming, Washington, North Dakota, and Ohio. The remainder states allow you to purchase the coverage in the open market. Some states, such as Missouri, make you purchase the coverage only if you have a certain number of employees. Most states make you purchase the coverage even if you have one employee.

There are four basic types of benefits payable under a workers compensation policy: medical expenses, lost wages, permanent disability, and death benefits. In addition, there are some benefits for retraining employees if they can't return to their old job. But for the most part, in a dental office you are looking at medical expenses and lost wages.

Dental office work can result in a myriad of injuries to employees: needle sticks, bites, carpal tunnel, and low back injuries seem to be the most common. Usually, none of these types of losses, except perhaps back injuries, ever lead to total disability.

If an employee presents him/herself to you and states, he/she want to file a workers compensation claim, or if you witness or become aware of an employee injury while he/she is at work, you are obligated to file a workers compensation claim. Not only is this the law, it is also the right thing to do. It also protects you as the dentist since it begins the running of the statute of limitations and it bars the employee from filing a suit against you for negligence. That doesn't mean the employee can't work with an attorney if he/she is injured. What it means is that the attorney will be working with the employee to ensure that the medical bills are all paid, the correct amount of temporary disability benefits are paid, and that the employee is compensated for any permanent total or permanent partial disability they may suffer as a result of the injury.

Employers Liability

There is another coverage provided under a Workers Compensation policy and that is called "Employers Liability Coverage." Employers liability is sometimes referred to as Part 2 coverage under a Workers Compensation policy. It is designed to cover types of loss not covered by the Workers Compensation coverage in the policy. This could include claims of gross negligence as well as claims by spouses for loss of consortium. Unlike Workers Compensation coverage, you must prove negligence in order to collect under the Employers Liability Coverage. It is a seldom used coverage and it is unlikely you will ever see it used in a dental practice. Employers' liability will show up on your Workers Compensation Policy showing three limits: bodily injury by accident; bodily injury by disease each employee; and bodily injury by disease policy limit. The base policy limits are low but you can increase them if you like.[6]

Workers Compensation Policy Audits

Workers Compensation is the only policy you will likely ever work with that is auditable by the insurance company or state program. The initial premium is based on your estimate of the annual wages of those employees covered by the policy. Let's say those wages equal $200,000, not including your wages, assuming you opted out of coverage. The insurance company applies a rate to the estimated premium, adds an amount called an "expense constant," and arrives at a premium.

If at the end of that policy period the actual wages paid to your employees was $225,000, you would owe premium on the additional $25,000. If on the other hand your actual payroll was $175,000, you would have a refund of a portion of the paid premium coming back to you as you over paid on the actual payroll. You never want to grossly overestimate your payroll. If you do have premium dollars coming back to you at the end of the year, the insurance company isn't paying you any interest on their use of your money for the year they held on to it. However, if you grossly underestimate your payroll, not only will you owe more at the end of the policy year, but the insurance company will also likely automatically increase the payroll on your renewal policy if you hadn't already increased the payrolls at your renewal.

General Liability Insurance

General Liability Insurance in a dental office mostly provides premises liability coverage. But what is premises liability you ask? Well, let me tell you a story about premises liability. When I was a small child I accompanied my mother as she took my grandfather to the doctor. I was around 6 years old. In those days, it was not uncommon to wait for a long period of time to see the doctor and a 6-year old can get impatient. I pulled a chair over to a drinking fountain, climbed on the chair, and proceeded to get a drink. Well, the chair slipped out from underneath me and I fell, hitting my lip on the fountain and splitting it open and causing me to let loose with cries of pain, fear, and anguish. Guess what? We got in to see the doctor immediately after that occurred! Back then, we would never have thought of accusing the doctor of being negligent and that the negligence caused my injury. No, the doctor stopped the bleeding, put a piece of tape on my lip and sent me on my way. Who knows, he may have even charged my Mom for the visit!

Today that same incident could lead to allegations of negligence, permanent facial scarring, as well as pain and suffering. That is premises liability and your General Liability policy covers that exposure.

How about a story from a dental office you ask? Gladly. A young chairside assistant comes out in to the reception area to call the next patient, Mrs. Jones. Mrs. Jones is

---

[6] Visit www.irmi.com to find out more about Employers liability Insurance.

elderly, unsure on her feet and has a dislike for dentists, so she is quite anxious. The assistant helps Mrs. Jones up out of her chair and holds her arm as they walk down the hall toward the operatory. On the way, Mrs. Jones stumbles and falls, breaking her hip. Later, her family alleges that their poor Mom tripped on a piece of frayed carpet in the hall. Mrs. Jones sues you for negligence. It is your General Liability policy that protects you from claims like this.

Within General Liability coverage there are two other coverages that are worth mentioning. The first is "first aid" coverage. Sometimes it is referred to as "premises medical payments" coverage. First aid coverage helps you nip potential claims in the bud by offering to pay for medical expenses as long as there is no allegation of negligence or the desire to be compensated for "pain and suffering." This is an excellent coverage that has stopped many claims in their tracks.

The second and more important coverage is "Nonowned and Hired Automobile" coverage. This is an undersold coverage, some agents even exclude it to keep the package premium down. But it should never be excluded.

But you don't have any autos in your dental practice you say. Nonowned and hired auto coverage isn't for autos owned by the dentist, it protects you the dentist in another way. If you send your office manager to the post office and he/she drives his/her own vehicle, do you think you have any potential liability if your employee causes an accident? The answer is "yes." Even though your employee's personal auto insurance would be primary, once the other party found out that they were on a business errand for you, the floodgates can open. You can almost guarantee that your employees do not purchase high automobile liability limits on their own and it is unlikely you have ever asked them what their limits are.

There is also the aspect of the "hired" auto side of the coverage that covers your use of temporary substitute autos but the real protection comes from the "nonowned" side. Always purchase nonowned and hired auto coverage and at a limit equal to your general liability limit.

General liability also includes many other subareas of coverage that may have lower or similar limits to the main general liability policy limit. If you lease your office space from a third party, there is coverage for damage to premises rented to you. The policy will also have coverage for personal and advertising injury as well as products and completed operations coverage.

The general liability policy will exclude coverage for your professional liability. As a professional, the insurance company wants you to purchase a separate policy to cover that exposure. A Professional policy that is designed specifically for you will be discussed in the next section.

When you lease out your office premises or take out a loan for equipment your lender will likely ask you to produce proof of insurance coverage. The lease agreement will indicate the level of insurance coverage they require you to purchase and they will require you to name them as a loss payee or as an additional insured. This is common and your insurance professional can get this for you quickly.

Always send the full lease to your insurance professional for his/her review, not just the insurance section of the lease. There can be wording and requirements stated in other parts of the lease that the agent will need to review. Of course, you should always, always have an attorney review all contracts you are about to sign and do it before you sign it. Some landlords will put crazy provisions in lease agreements that assign liability to you that your insurance policy will not cover. It is your job and the job of your insurance professional and attorney to root out those provisions and have them removed.

We have seen provisions in a dental office lease that required the dentist to indemnify, hold harmless, and provide general liability coverage for the landlord, not just for incidents that occurred on the dentists' insured premises, but also for all incidents that occurred in the entire office building complex and parking lot. It is provisions like this that need to be removed.

Umbrella Policies

An *Umbrella policy* extends additional limits over the top of your general liability coverage, your nonowned and hired auto coverage and the employers' liability coverage under your workers compensation policy. An Umbrella provides an extra layer of protection. However, Umbrella policies almost never provide excess coverage over your professional liability policy. These policies are designed as an adjunct to a general liability policy. If your dental practice owns automobiles, the umbrella provides excess coverage over the auto policy as well. As your assets grow, the addition of an Umbrella policy can add more protection. If you purchase an Umbrella policy to add more protection as your assets grow, make sure you have adequately raised your professional liability limits and you have more exposure there than from a general liability exposure.

Professional Liability Insurance

Here we are! Whether we call it professional liability, dental malpractice, medical malpractice, or errors and omissions coverage, we are talking about the same insurance coverage. This coverage protects you the dentist, as well as your staff, from allegations of injury due to negligence. Whether it is pulling the wrong tooth, performing a root canal on the wrong tooth, injuring a nerve, prolonged numbness, aspiration of a crown or drill bit, or whatever else can be aspirated, your protection for the actual practice of dentistry comes from your professional liability policy.

In the "good old days" we would sell professional liability insurance to our clients and most of them would never have cause to use it. It was always there as a safety net but claims were few and far between. These days we don't speak to our clients in terms of, "if you ever have a claim," but more often, "when you have a claim." The society we live in today is different than it was 30 years ago. The likelihood of you having a professional liability claim is much more likely now than it was then.

The average Dentist Professional Liability policy is written with a limit of $1,000,000 per occurrence and a $3,000,000 policy aggregate and no deductible. This means that the policy will pay up to $1,000,000 for any one claim but the policy won't pay more than $3,000,000 in one policy year for all claims combined. Defense costs are usually paid in addition to the per occurrence limit.

Most professional liability policies also have a small sublimit of liability coverage for "first aid." If your patient swallows his/her crown, the first aid limit will cover the costs of the x-rays and physician visits necessary to follow the crown through the patient's system. If allegations of negligence arise, the first aid payments stop and the claim handling process begins.

Claims Made and Reported Policy Forms

The average policy is written on a "Claims Made and Reported" basis. Some insurance companies also offer to write Dental Professional Liability insurance coverage on an "Occurrence" basis. Your insurance professional can help you decide which is best for you but we will discuss each briefly.

Claims Made insurance coverage was designed by insurance companies during the 1970s after some court cases concluded that each new occurrence policy provided a fresh set of limits each year for a claim. This was called "stacking policy limits." A claim would be turned in and the insurance company thought that their maximum exposure was $1,000,000, which was the policy limit when the claim occurred. Some inventive attorneys and courts concluded that some subsequent policies could also be applied putting a whole lot more money on the table.

Claims Made policies closed that loophole. These policies are written so that they cover only claims that are reported during the policy period. Once that policy expires, no claim can be reported against it. In order to cover your past acts, a claims made policy contains a prior acts date, also called a retroactive date, that works to apply your new policy all the way back to the original date of your first professional liability policy.

For example, you pass your boards and your license is issued on June 1, 2015. You had accepted an associate position to begin the date your license is issued. On your application you would want the policy to begin on June 1, 2015. This will also be your prior acts date for future policies. In 2016, when this policy expires, the new policy will have policy dates of June 1, 2016 to 2017 but the prior acts date will be June 1, 2015. The new policy now covers you back to 2015 because the prior claims made policy has expired and no claims can be reported against it. If you had reported a claim during that first policy year, the policy would cover the claim no matter how long it took to close it, but once the policy expires, no new claims can be reported against it.

Occurrence Policy Forms

Occurrence policies are different in that the policy that was in effect at the time an alleged negligent act occurs is the one that will always respond. So, if you are notified on June 1, 2017 of a claim from an act that occurred in 2015, it would be the policy that was in effect in 2015 that would respond. An easy way to remember this is that *Occurrence* policies look back for coverage and *Claims Made* policies look forward for coverage.

There are pros and cons for both policy formats. Claims Made policies are more cost-effective than occurrence policies. However, with an occurrence policy you don't have to worry about keeping your prior acts date on each new policy or risk having to purchase a tail endorsement if you don't qualify for a free tail.

When you retire, you don't have to worry about purchasing "tail" coverage with an occurrence policy like you do with a "claims made" policy.

Tail coverage is what protects you when you stop purchasing claims made coverage. If you have been with your professional liability insurance carrier for many years, the insurance company will usually provide your tail coverage for free when you retire. This free tail coverage is usually provided only after you have been with the insurance company for a certain number of years and you may have to meet minimum age requirements. For example, the policies may state that you have to been insured with them for 5 years and have attained a certain age, usually age 50.

If you become disabled, the "tail" is also provided at no charge.

There are few circumstances where you may want to purchase a "tail" endorsement before retiring. If for example, you decided to go back to school for specialty training and didn't plan to practice or moonlight as a general dentist while in school you will have to decide whether you want to purchase the "tail" or roll the dice and take your chances. Understand though that tail coverage can be expensive.

Occurrence policies cost more because you are basically "prepaying" for your retirement tail in each policy.

If you carried low limits when you first started as a new dentist but 10 years later decide to increase your limits, the occurrence policy would not increase your past limits of liability, but only those limits going forward after you raise them. With a Claims Made policy, if you increase your limit of liability 10 years later, many companies apply that higher limit all the way back to your policy prior acts date. Some companies do not do that and they utilize what is called a "split liability retro date endorsement." This endorsement basically keeps the limits low for past acts and only increases the limits going forward. You may want to avoid this type of scenario if possible.

If you are ever presented with an allegation of negligence by a patient, or maybe it is even just a comment made by the patient when a procedure doesn't go the way the patient thought it should have, you should discuss this with your insurance professional immediately. It may be prudent to put your insurance provider on notice of a potential claim. If nothing ever comes out of the incident nothing is lost. If an actual claim does arise you have the comfort of knowing it was reported in a timely manner to the insurance company. Problems can arise when you do not communicate these incidents to your insurance provider. Remember that they are your partner in helping protect you, your reputation and your assets.

Employment Practices Liability Insurance

Employment Practices Liability Insurance protects you the dentist should one of your current or former employees accuse you of actions such as wrongful termination or sexual harassment, just to name two. Do not confuse this with the Employers Liability Insurance Coverage discussed in the Workers Compensation section. They are completely different.

Your package insurance policy, if it is purchased from a company that specializes in insuring dentists and other professionals, will almost always have some coverage to defend you should an employment practices liability issue arise. Many companies will offer you the opportunity to purchase higher limits for an additional premium. The higher limits will also contain some indemnity limits in addition to defense limits.

Employment practices liability insurance was the hot new insurance coverage just a few years ago. Wrongful termination, sexual harassment, failure to promote, hostile work conditions, and promoting a female over a male or a male over a female claims were all the rage. The insurance companies jumped right in to offer some coverage to help alleviate the potential financial burden of an employment practices claim. Who knew that in just a few years employment practices liability insurance would take a back seat to our last insurance product we will discuss, cyber liability.

Cyber Liability Insurance

Cyber liability insurance is one of the fastest growing areas of insurance ever. It wasn't that long ago that the closest thing to cyber liability insurance you could purchase was identity theft coverage and that only protected you personally. Cyber liability insurance for a business has almost become a mandatory coverage to purchase. Modern dental practices are so digital that your business and patient information will always be at risk.

As stated, regarding so many of the other lines of insurance discussed, many package policies for dentist offices have a very limited amount of cyber liability protection built-in to them. Most of these "giveaway" coverages are inadequate to protect you from a full blown loss of your patient data whether due to a system hack or simply a lost laptop computer that held copies of all your patient records.

The insurance industry responded quickly and with not only insurance policies to help with your potential financial loss, but also with plans, programs, and templates to help their insureds meet their requirements under the HIPAA/HITECH Security Act.[7]

In September of 2013, the final rules under HIPAA/HITECH went into effect that laid out your responsibilities should your patients protected health or personal information become compromised due to a failure of your system. Your responsibilities can be costly and burdensome. Patient notification and credit monitoring for patients are two potential responsibilities that can prove to be costly.

You also have to be able to show you have programs in place to reduce the chance of a data breach occurring.

Even at a time when you read or hear of security breach after security breach, the cost for a practicing dentist to purchase a well-rounded cyber liability policy has actually gone down and the coverage parameters as well as the back room services, such as public relations and patient notification assistance, have grown. Why is that you ask? The answer is a simple matter of economics. First, more professionals are purchasing Cyber Liability Insurance coverage, which brings down the cost for everyone. Second, dental offices are putting in more controls to protect their systems from potential hacks.

Even so, the coverage is important for dentists to purchase. Never underestimate the power of a former employee scorn or that lost laptop mentioned earlier.

A good risk management plan to minimize your cyber liability exposures coupled with a good cyber liability insurance policy is a great combination that will help you sleep more soundly at night knowing you have done all that you can to keep the bad guys out of your patients protected health and personal information.

Identity Theft Plans

An identity theft plan for the most part isn't actually insurance. When you purchase an identity theft plan you are purchasing a set of services that will assist you should your personal identity be compromised. A personal identity theft plan protects you much like a cyber liability plan protects your business.

Your personal identity can be compromised in any number of ways. You could lose your wallet or purse. Someone could get your Social Security Number and date of birth and begin applying for credit cards and loans. Your checking and savings account numbers could be compromised.

[7] Find more information on the HIPAA/HITECH Security Act at www.hhs.gov.

Identity theft plans help provide the leg work to get the after effects of identity theft undone. These plans work with your credit card companies, credit bureaus, banks, the IRS, and so on to help you sort out what is right and wrong, make corrections, and correct your credit scores and accounts. They can quickly lock down your credit so that no one can apply for credit or loans using your name, Social Security Number, and date of birth.

Identity theft plans are cost-effective and help protect you from those who try to profit from your success.

Summary

That is an overview of insuring a dental practice in a nutshell. A very, very large nutshell! Here are a few takeaways from all the information that you have just digested:

- Risk management is a process to be planned and thought through; insurance is just one aspect of an overall risk management program.
- You aren't the first dentist to need specialized insurance for your profession. However, if you aren't careful, you could pick an insurance professional who is working with his/her first dentist! Don't let this happen.
- Likewise, choose an insurance company that has a specialized program for dentists. Any insurance company can insure your building and contents. But if they have policies designed for a dentist, they will include coverage that a regular insurance policy won't contain.
- You don't have to reinvent the wheel. Utilize the expertise of your local and state dental association as well as practicing dentists in your area for their suggestions.
- Keep your insurance professional in the loop when making changes to your practice. The purchase of a cone beam CT would warrant a call to your insurance professional before it is delivered. Having the insurance professional find out about the purchase a year later or worse, after a loss occurs is not how you want to run your practice.
- You can become insurance poor paying premiums to cover all your potential exposures. Work with your insurance professional to design the overall insurance program that meets your personal, contractual, and financial needs.
- You have to be involved in the business aspect of dentistry in order to protect your assets. Utilize your professional team to assist you including your insurance professional, attorney, and accountant. Never sign a lease or contract without having your team review the documents before you sign.
- Keep informed because insurance is fluid and constantly adapting to new exposures and providing solutions. Meet with your insurance professional regularly to stay on top of what is happening both in the dental industry and insurance marketplace. Ten years ago we wouldn't have had a section on Cyber Liability and Employment Practices Liability would have barely been mentioned. Today they are two of your larger exposures.
- A well-executed risk management program and insurance plan provides what we in the industry call "sleep insurance." You want to be comfortable that you have your exposures identified and planned out so that the plan allows you to sleep well at night.

References and Additional Resources

American Dental Association Member Benefits. ADA Group Insurance Plans. Available at www. ada.org/en/member-center/member-benefits/insurance-resources

Employers Liability Coverage. Insurance Risk Management Institute. Available at www.irmi.com/ online/insurance-glossary/terms.aspx#E

Head and Horn, 1988. Essentials of the Risk Management Process, ARM 54. The Institutes. Risk Management Principles and Practices. Available at www.theinstitutes.org

Health Savings Accounts and Other Tax-Favored Health Plans. Publication 969 Internal Revenue Service. Available at www.irs.gov/pub/irs-pdf/p969.pdf

Health Insurance Portability and Accountability Act (HIPAA). Privacy, Security and Breach Notification Rules. U.S. Department of Health and Human Services. Available at www.hhs.gov.

Health Information Technology for Economic and Clinical Health (HITECH) Act. www.healthit.gov.

National Flood Insurance Program, Federal Emergency Management Association. www. floodsmart.gov.www.fema.gov.

Retirement Planner: Benefits by Year of Birth. Social Security Administration. Available at www. socialsecurity.gov/planners/retire/agereduction.html

Learning Exercises

1. It is the beginning of your D4 year and time to get a plan together as to what you will do after your boards are passed and your license is issued. After a short search you are approached with the offer to purchase an existing practice. While contemplating all that goes into business ownership, you realize that it is important to include a risk management plan part of your decision process.

   a. What are the four main elements of a good risk management plan?

   b. Since you can't avoid all risk and still practice dentistry, what are three ways to deal with some of the risks that you will face?

   c. Name some professional resources you could bring into your decision-making process and what their role might be to assist you.

2. In the middle of your D4 year you begin to get inundated with offers to purchase disability insurance. Even though you have no income and if fact, have nothing but debt, disability insurance companies clamor to provide you with offers for coverage.

   a. Do you even need disability insurance at this point in your career when you currently do not generate any revenue? If so, why?

   b. Compare and contrast the major differences between an individual disability policy and an association group disability policy?

   c. While signing a lease for new equipment for your dental practice, the leasing company wants you to assign your disability policy to them just in case you become disabled. Why do they want you to do this? Is it a good idea? What is an alternative to assigning your personal disability to cover a business expense?

3. You have been in practice now for 9 months. One of your favorite patients is in the chair getting ready for you to place his/her brand new crown. As you move the crown into position, the patient shifts to the right, slightly bumping the crown and in the blink of an eye and a slight swallow, the crown is gone . . . at least for now!

    a. Who do you inform of this incident and how quickly?

    b. What insurance coverage is immediately available to assist in making sure your favorite patient is taken care of and under what circumstance would the insurance company stop paying the patient under that coverage?

4. Your patient Frank is also a local insurance agent. He has been after you for a long time to "provide you with a quote" to insure your dental practice. He intimates that he pays you a lot of money for the dental work you provide to his family and it would sure be nice to have you as a client.

    a. What are some key questions you could ask Frank regarding insuring a dental practice?

    b. Why is it important to work with professionals specializing in dental practices?

Chapter 26
Personal Finance, Investments, and Retirement Options

William "Dana" Webb and Brian Lange

Finance

Developing a Philosophy About Money

From many years of helping people build and maintain wealth, it has become apparent that most people do not have a philosophy about money. When asked about their philosophy, they usually develop a blank stare. The truth is that most people have never given it a thought. For this reason, it is important to first discuss the philosophy of money.

When you hold a dollar bill in your hand, you have three choices:

1. You can spend it. Most Americans know how to do this. With one of the lowest savings rates in the world, taking time to explain to Americans how to spend money is not time well spent. We will assume the reader has an understanding of this concept.
2. You can lend it. This is what most Americans do when thinking they are building wealth. The truth is no one you know has ever built or maintained wealth lending money. The term "lending" may be new to some readers. Let me give you examples. If you purchase a U.S. government bond or note, you are lending your money to the federal government. If you purchase a corporate bond, you are lending your money to that corporation. If you purchase a municipal bond, you are lending your money to that city. If you put money in a certificate of deposit or money market, you are lending your money to that financial institution. In other words, bonds, notes, CDs, money markets, fixed annuities, and so forth are lending instruments. You are lending your money and in return receive interest. Let us repeat: no one builds or maintains wealth lending money. But if you do the third thing, you will build and maintain your wealth even in retirement.
3. You can own things with it. Wealthy people own things. Think about it. Do you think Bill Gates is wealthy because he knows how to lend money? He owns a company. Do you think Warren Buffett is wealthy because he lends money well? He owns several companies. How about Donald Trump? He owns real estate.

Dental Practice Transition: A Practical Guide to Management, Second Edition.
Edited by David G. Dunning and Brian M. Lange.
© 2016 John Wiley & Sons, Inc. Published 2016 by John Wiley & Sons, Inc.
Companion Website: www.wiley.com/go/dunning/transition

Throughout the pages of history, owners build and maintain wealth. While it is true that what is best to own changes from time to time, it has always been owners who build financial security. You can build wealth owning real estate, your own business, stocks, or collectibles, just to name a few. What to own is up to you, but you must be an owner to build or maintain wealth.

One more thought. You should carry this philosophy with you the rest of your life. Most Americans think they should view their money differently during their retirement years. Remember: your money does not know how old you are. With interest rates at historic lows and people living longer, you must continue this philosophy into retirement to prevent outliving your money.

Being Committed to Your Financial Goals

It has been said that most people "want" to be rich, but those who build wealth are "committed" to being rich. In other words, those who build wealth are willing to sacrifice more than most people to attain their goals. Wealth builders understand that if they want a different outcome in their lives, they need to change the way they think, act, and react. Most people want a different outcome in their lives, but they do *not* want to change the way they think, act, and react. To build wealth most people need to make some fundamental changes in their character.

Be ready to spend more time focused on your wealth-building program. This is why it is very important for your spouse to share your goals. Many wealth-building trains have been derailed by a spouse not willing to allow the needed time away from the family to pursue this dream. It is so much easier with an understanding spouse, or better yet, one who can work alongside you to help you reach your goals.

Be ready to do without. You will not be able to keep up with your neighbor. They will be spending their money on the appearances of wealth, probably with too much debt. Wealth builders live way beneath their means. For example, most people think wealthy people drive expensive automobiles. The average age of a vehicle owned by a millionaire is 11 years old. In other words, those who build wealth rarely have an emotional need to keep up with the Joneses.

Be ready to use "good" debt when appropriate. Too many people do not understand debt. They either think all debt is bad or they have too much "bad" debt and not enough "good" debt. Good debt is debt against something that will probably go up in value over time. This would include mortgage and education debt. Bad debt is debt against things that go down in value almost as soon as you purchase them. This would be vehicle debt and credit card debt. Have as much good debt as you can handle, but eliminate bad debt from your life for good.

Finally, more often than not, building wealth is a by-product, not a main focus. Most wealthy people will tell you they were so busy doing what they loved, that the wealth was a side benefit. That is why so few wealthy people retire. They could retire financially, but they do not want to stop doing what they love. Find a vocation that you love and be the very best at it. Never stop learning. If you will read one book a year concerning your vocation, you will be light years ahead of most of your competition.

Saving Money versus Saving Buying Power

One of the biggest myths when it comes to building wealth is that if you save money, you will build wealth. For most people this is impossible. If you want to build or maintain wealth you must save buying power, not money.

When Ford introduced the Mustang in 1964, the price was about $2,000. Today it is over $35,000. Most think the cost of the car has increased. NO!!! The dollar today is weaker than the dollar of 1964, so it takes more dollars today to buy the same thing. Read the previous sentence again. Generation after generation teaches their offspring to "put your money in the piggy bank and save it for a rainy day." They teach their children to save money, an item that goes down in value every year. The child grows up, cannot figure out how to build wealth, and the parents scratch their heads. How can anyone build wealth saving something that goes down in value every year?

The problem is even worse for those who are retired. They have held the wrong definition of the word "safety" their entire lives. They believe safety is holding on to the dollars they have. Change your definition of safety now. Do not wait another day. Safety is not the preservation of principal, safety is the preservation of buying power.

Suppose one retired in 1964 and had $100,000. If he believed safety meant holding on to the principal, he might have invested in a long-term bond paying 5%. He received $5,000 per year, and when the bond matured, he received $5,000 plus the $100,000 back. He thought he was safe because he still had his principal. But he was not. When he received his first $5,000 in 1964, when the Mustang was $2,000, he could have purchased two and a half Mustangs. When he received his $5,000 in 2015, the Mustang was $35,000 and he could have purchased less than one-sixth of a Mustang. *Conclusion:* If his definition of safety was to hold on to the principal, he was successful. However, what good did it do him? The standard of living continued to drop year after year as his purchasing power was eroded.

So, what mistake did this retired person make? He placed his money in a lending instrument and lost his buying power. Had he owned something with this money, his $100,000 would have had a better chance to have a rate of return high enough so that he would still have been enough to purchase the Mustang in 2004. In other words, to build or maintain wealth, we must be owners, not lenders, throughout our lifetime. But to do that we first need to create a budget and live within it.

Building Wealth

Making Decisions from the Revenue Side, Not the Expense Side

There are basically two parts to every financial business model. Some people in the company are in charge of bringing in revenue. Others have the job of controlling expenses. Both are important. However, when a major decision is made, it must be made from the revenue side. Too many businesses today make it from the expense side.

For years legendary CEOs (chief executive officers) would add new streams of revenue to their corporations to increase the value. This was done by creating new products or services to sell or by buying smaller companies and continuing to sell their products or services. Both increased corporate revenues.

Today, CEOs seem to be more CFO (chief financial officer) minded. They try to increase the value of a company by cutting expenses, not by increasing revenue. In the short term, this can work; in the long term it is usually a bad decision. Take the case of a widget company that moved jobs overseas to cut labor costs. The company even built a factory overseas to produce widgets between 8 a.m. and 5 p.m. But what really happened? The factory overseas produced the agreed-upon widgets between 8 a.m. and 5 p.m., closed down for 1 minute, then reopened again at 5:01 p.m. to continue to manufacture widgets for the bootleg market until 7:59 a.m. the next morning. How much can that company really save now that they have to cut prices on their own widgets to compete with the bootleg market widgets, which are produced 16 hours out of every 24-hour period? In other words, every day, twice as many illegal widgets are produced with the same quality as the legitimate ones.

I tell that story because I find most families and new business owners also make decisions from the expense side. When hurricanes swept through the Gulf Coast area, forcing gasoline prices higher, we could tell wealth builders from those who would never build wealth just by listening to their conversations. Most people were talking about how they were cutting expenses in other areas of their budget to pay for the increase in gasoline prices. In other words, they were making decisions from the expense side of the ledger. Wealth builders were talking about how they would need to increase their income to pay for the rise in gas prices. Hourly people asked to work overtime. Sales people focused on making a couple of extra sales per month. Retired people would talk about getting more aggressive with a portion of their investments. In other words, these people were focusing on increasing income, not cutting expenses.

People who build or maintain wealth make decisions from the revenue side. Successful businesses are built from the revenue side. Therefore, you must also think this way when building your dental practice while still managing overhead.

Investment Choices

Now that you understand you must be an owner to build or maintain wealth, what should you own? There are many things you can own; however, our advice would be to narrow the list to the following:

1. Own your dental practice. That may be tough to do at first, but make that one of your goals. This would be the business that you own.
2. Own the building in which your dental practice is located. This will be a longer-term goal for most dentists and would be the commercial real estate in your portfolio. If you purchase or build a building with more square footage than you need, you can rent out the remaining square footage and have another stream of income.
3. Own what you invest in your retirement plan. This will give you a chance to own mutual funds. Make sure the mutual funds you own have all stocks in them with no bonds. Remember, bonds are a lending instrument. Your stocks, which represent ownership, will help you build more wealth over the long term.
4. Only after you have accomplished the first three items should you begin to own other things. At this point, you may want to own single-family homes or apartment buildings to rent. You may wish to own individual stocks or another business that your spouse would operate. You will have many choices, but choose the investments that best fit your personality and character traits. For example, do not try to be a landlord if you lack the time or temperament to do it.

It should be pointed out that the comments above are directed toward your business life. Do not forget your personal life. You should be an owner there too, and your first purchase should be a house. Most people should structure the purchase of this house with an 80% first mortgage, a 10% second mortgage, and 10% down. This should be your only personal debt. Always pay cash for your other purchases, including automobiles. Too many young people start their adult lives with vehicle debt and credit card debt because they saw their parents do the same thing. Wealth builders have neither. This does not mean they avoid using a credit card. This means they pay the entire bill when it arrives and never let interest accumulate.

One final word of caution on this topic. We cannot tell you how many times newly retired people have told us they were so busy making money during their career that they failed to build wealth. We know you have studied hard to be a dentist, but never confuse making money with building wealth. If making money takes all of your focus, then hire a competent financial advisor to help you stay focused on your wealth-building plan. Doing this will be a good investment.

Understanding the Basics of Financial Planning

There are a number of concepts and terms you need to become familiar with even if you do not plan on doing any investing. At the very least, you should be able to understand what your investment counselors are recommending. Investment Dictionary (http://www.investmentterms.net/) defines/explains any and all investment that you might have questions about. You should also know how to go about selecting your investment manager. A guide to how to choose the best investment manager can be found at (http://www.scholtzandco.com/individual-investors/how-to-choose-the-best-investment-manager/).

This robust website sponsored by the American Institute of Certified Public Accounts also provides a wealth of information about personal finance and investing: http://www.360financialliteracy.org/Topics/Investor-Education

Below is a glossary of some of the common investment terms with which to become familiar. This is by no means an exhaustive list.

Glossary of Some Basic Terms Related to Investments

Bond: A bond is a debt investment in which an investor loans money to an entity (typically corporate or governmental) that borrows the funds for a defined period of time at a variable or fixed interest rate. Bonds are used by companies, municipalities, states, and sovereign governments to raise money and finance a variety of projects and activities. Owners of bonds are debt holders, or creditors, of the issuer (www.investopedia.com).

Derivative: At its most basic, a financial derivative is a contract between two parties that specifies conditions under which payments are made between two parties. Derivatives are "derived" from underlying assets such as stocks, contracts, swaps, or even, as we now know, measurable events such as weather. Conditions that determine when payments are made often include the price of the underlying asset and the date at which the underlying asset achieves that price (www.simple.com/blog/what-are-deriviates-really).

Diversification: A risk management technique that mixes a wide variety of investments within a portfolio. The rationale behind this technique contends that a portfolio of different kinds of investments will, on average, yield higher returns and pose a lower risk than any individual investment found within the portfolio (http://www.investopedia.com).

Dividend: A payment made by a corporation to its shareholders, usually as a distribution of profits. When a corporation earns a profit or surplus, it can reinvest it in the business (called retained earnings), and pay a fraction of this reinvestment as a dividend to shareholders (www.wikipedia.org).

Dow Jones Industrial Average: The best known U.S. index of stocks. A price-weighted average of 30 actively traded blue-chip stocks, primarily industries including stocks that trade on the New York Stock Exchange. The Dow, as it is called, is a barometer of how shares of the largest U.S. companies are performing. There are hundreds of investment indexes around the world for stocks, bonds, currencies, and commodities (www.nasdaq.com).

Global Fund: A mutual fund that includes at least 25% foreign securities in its portfolio. The value of the fund depends on the health of foreign economies and exchange rate movements. A global fund permits an investor to diversify internationally (http://financial-dictionary.thefreedictionary.com).

Growth Fund: Mutual fund (unit trust) that invests in the bonds and stocks (shares) of any promising entity of any nation, but maintains a significant percentage (typically 25 to 50%) of its assets in highly reliable . . . securities (www.businessdictionary.com).

Hedge Fund: A fund, usually used by wealthy individuals and institutions, which is allowed to use aggressive strategies that are unavailable to mutual funds . . . Hedge funds are exempt from many of the rules and regulations of government other mutual funds, which allows them to accomplish aggressive investing goals (www.investorwords.com).

Income Fund: Mutual fund . . . or any other type of fund that seek to generate an income stream for shareholders by investing in securities that offer dividends or interest payments. The funds can hold bonds, preferred stock, common stock or even real estate investment trusts (REITs) (www.investinganswers.com).

Index Fund: An index fund (also index tracker) is an investment fund (usually a mutual fund or exchange-traded fund) that aims to replicate the movements of an index of a specific financial market, or a set of rules of ownership that are held constant, regardless of market conditions (www.wikipedia.org).

International Fund: Usually refers to an investment or mutual fund composed of international bonds and foreign company stocks (www.investinganswers.com).

Market Capitalization: Large Cap, Mid Cap, and Small Cap Stocks: Market capitalization, commonly known as market cap, is calculated by multiplying a company's outstanding shares by the company's stock price per share. A company's stock price by itself does not tell you much about the total value or size of a company; a company whose stock price is $60 is not necessarily worth more than a company whose stock price is $25. For example, a company with a stock price of $60 and 100 million shares outstanding (a market cap of $6 billion) is actually smaller in size than a company with a stock price of $25 and 500 million shares outstanding (a market cap of $12.5 billion) (www.mutualfundstore.com).

Mutual Fund: An investment security type that enables investors to pool their money together into one professionally managed investment. Mutual funds can invest in stocks, bonds, cash, and/or other assets. These underlying security types, called *holdings*, combine to form one mutual fund, also called a *portfolio* . . . baskets of investments." http://mutualfunds.about.com)

NASDAQ: National Association of Securities Dealers Automatic Quotation System: an electronic quotation system that provides quotations to market participants about the more actively traded common stock issues in the over-the-counter market. About 4,000 stock issues are included in the Nasdaq system (www.nasdaq.com).

Russell Indexes: U.S. equity index widely used by pension and mutual fund investors that are weighted by market capitalization and published by the Frank Russell

Company of Tacoma, Washington. For example, the Russell 3000 includes the 3,000 U.S. companies according to market capitalization (www.nasdaq.com).

Security: A security is "a tradable financial asset (for example, bonds and stocks). It is commonly used to mean any form of financial instrument, but the legal definition of a "security" varies by legal and regulatory jurisdiction (www.wikipedia.org).

Standard & Poor's Indices: S&P Dow Jones Indices is the world's largest, global resource for index-based concepts, data, and research. Home to iconic financial market indicators, such as the S&P 500 and the Dow Jones Industrial Average, S&P Dow Jones Indices has over 115 years of experience constructing innovative and transparent solutions that fulfill the needs of institutional and retail investors (http://www.standardandpoors.com/en_US/web/guest/home).

Stock: A kind of financial security granting rights of ownership in a corporation, such as a claim to a portion of the assets and earnings of the corporation and the right to vote for the board of directors. Stock is issued and traded in units called *shares* (www.thefreedictionary.com).

Stock Market: The aggregation of buyers and sellers (a loose network of economic transactions, not a physical facility or discrete entity) of stocks also called shares. These may include securities on a stock exchange as those only traded privately (www.wikipedia.org).

Value Fund: A mutual fund that invests in companies that it determines to be underpriced by fundamental measures (www.investorwords.com).

Retirement Plan Choices

There are basically three types of retirement plans: individual retirement plans, company-sponsored retirement plans, and self-employed retirement plans. This discussion will cover only the ones you will most likely consider in each category. Not every plan will be mentioned.

1. *Individual traditional IRA:* A tax-favored account that allows anyone under the age of 70 1/2 years, with earned income, to contribute annually. A nonworking spouse may do the same thing. Earnings are tax-deferred and contributions *may* be tax-deductible. Be aware of the income limits.
2. *Individual Roth IRA:* Contributions are not tax-deductible, earnings grow tax-free, and no taxes are due when you withdraw the money. Income limits apply here too, but no age limits apply.
3. *401(k):* Allows employees of "for profit" companies to make pretax contributions through payroll deductions. Employers may contribute to the employee accounts, and that contribution would be a tax write-off for the company.
4. *SIMPLE IRA:* Businesses with 100 or fewer eligible employees can establish this plan. It resembles the 401(k), but with less testing and lower administrative costs. The maximum contribution an employee can make is much lower than the 401(k) allows. Employer contributions are mandatory up to 3.5%.
5. *Profit-sharing plan:* This offers companies considerable flexibility, allowing them to decide each year whether a contribution will be made and how much, up to 25% of each participant's pay. These plans can include provisions for loans and vesting schedules, like the 401(k). It does have a maximum dollar contribution limit.

6. *Money purchase plan:* This is similar to a profit-sharing plan. Contribution limits are the same, but the plan is not as flexible. A fixed percentage of pay must be contributed each year. That percentage is determined when the plan is established.

7. *Defined benefit plan:* Once your dental practice is established and your income is much higher, we recommend you switch to this type of retirement plan. It is like the old pension plans. In the other plans mentioned, the contribution is determined, but you have no idea how much money you will have in the future. This plan allows you to determine the benefit you want in the future, and an actuary calculates each year how much you will need to contribute to stay on track to achieve that benefit. *Remember:* A high income is needed to qualify for this plan.

8. *Simplified employee pension (SEP) plan:* This allows self-employed people and small business owners to make tax-deductible contributions of up to 25% of W-2 income or 20% of form 1099 income, up to a maximum dollar amount. It is very easy to administer; however, employers must contribute the same percentage of income to their employees' accounts as they do for their own account.

We cannot encourage you enough to seek professional help when deciding which plan is best for you and your employees. In most cases, the fees you pay to a good financial planner will be more than offset by the improved tax-deferred growth and tax savings.

College Funding Investment Programs

Should all parents put away something to help finance their children's college education? Some people would say "yes." Should they use one of the government's designed savings vehicles for that purpose? Some people should not. There are two main programs to save for college:

1. *The Coverdell Education Savings Account:* A nondeductible cash contribution of up to $2,000 may be contributed each year, per child. The earnings grow tax-free. In certain circumstances, the account can be used to pay for elementary and secondary education as well. However, modified adjusted income limits may restrict your contributions.

2. *529 plans:* These plans give you the ability to front 5 years of the annual gift exclusion per donor to each child ($14,000 per year, as of 2015). It is not a tax deduction, but the earnings grow tax-free if the money is used for higher education. This cannot be used for elementary and secondary education expenses. No income limits apply. The wealthier use this program to remove money from their estate to save on "end of life taxes" that their beneficiaries may be exposed too.

These are good plans for the right situation, but they are not for everyone. For example, the American Opportunity Credit and the Lifetime Learning Credit may not be claimed for the same expenses paid for by money withdrawn from these plans. For some people these credits are more valuable than the tax-free growth. Salespeople love to sell these plans because most people want to help their children save. Talk to a tax professional who does not sell these plans. He or she can give you an unbiased opinion on which is the best way for you to save for college.

There are many ways parents can fund college costs, which include student loans and borrowing against your house. Do not rule out any options until you have thoroughly discussed all options with a competent financial planner. However, remember: you can always borrow for education expenses, but you cannot borrow for retirement. Take care of your retirement first.

The Need for a Budget

A budget should be the money plan that determines your spending. A budget is the most effective financial management tool available, allowing us to control our financial resources, set and accomplish goals, and plan how our money will work for us. The purpose of a budget is to save money up front for known and unexpected expenses. The benefits of a budget are numerous and include but are not limited to the following:

1. A budget allows you to control your money rather than your money controlling you.
2. A budget organizes your funds into categories of expenses and savings, automatically providing records of all your transactions.
3. A budget helps you live within your means.
4. A budget can get you out of debt and keep you out of debt.
5. A budget enhances family communication by setting common goals.
6. A budget helps meet savings goals.
7. A budget assists in planning for unexpected expenditures and emergencies.
8. A budget creates extra money.
9. A budget shows areas of excessive spending, which allows you to refocus on your most important goals.
10. A budget that is followed allows you to rest better at night because you do not have to worry about how you will pay your bills.

Not all people are able to make budgets work the first time they attempt to establish financial order in their lives. The following are the main reasons why people fail to make budgets work:

- Not understanding what a budget is and what a budget can do
- Setting unrealistic goals
- Giving up on the budget process

It is important to understand that the process of establishing financial order in your life is much like getting into and maintaining a physical exercise program. In a physical exercise program, you adjust the amount of exercise to accommodate to your physical condition and goals. You can expect to adjust your budget. You will have expenditures before all the money has been allocated for the expenditure (e.g., the clothes dryer breaks before enough money has been saved for a replacement). There will be times you or a family member purchase(s) an item on impulse. If you tell yourself you are in a learning process, the unexpected will happen and then you can get back to living on the budget. You can avoid the negative mindset and/or self-talks that lead to people giving up on the budgeting process by studying these sites: www.betterbudgeting.com/budgetformsfree.htm, www.soyouwanna.com/site/syws/budget/budget.html, www.youneedabudget.com.

Goal Setting

Just as you had to set goals and develop and maintain positive self-talks to graduate from dental school, you will need to develop life goals and maintain positive self-talks through your life. A good way to prepare yourself to tackle life goals is to ask yourself the following questions:

1. What do I want to be said about me at the end of my days?
2. What do I want to accomplish before I die?
3. Where do I want to visit or live before I die?

You may want to add, modify, or remove one of the three questions. It is the process that is important. Once you answer your questions, you are ready to start on your life goals. Life goals are dynamic and if tended too are alive and will need updating from time to time. Life goals need to center around your mission, vision, and values. Many people think of mission, vision, and values as something you do for your practice, not what you do for yourself or your family; however, if you don't know where you are going, it makes it harder to create mission, vision, and values statements for your practice. If you go to http://www.liquidplanner.com/blog/create-mission-vision-statement-year/ you will find How to Create a Personal Mission and Vision Statement for the Year. The same process that they identify can be used to develop your life mission and vision statement. When it comes to your values statement, answer the following question: What are the basic beliefs that guide how you do what you do? Another way to ask the question is what really matters to me?

To help get you started on developing your life goals, the following outline is presented for your consideration. You may want to add or drop a category. Also, the following website provides more elaboration and provides helpful suggestions for developing goals: http://www.mindtools.com/page6.html.

1. *Spiritual*: Do you or do you not believe in God and how does it look in your life mission trips, reduced fees for people in need or do not want this as a life goal?
2. *Personal Goals*: How do you take care of yourself so that you can care for your family, practice, and others. This includes your exercise, hobbies, free time, and so on. This may overlap with other life goals. Also this could be where you put your bucket list.
3. *Family Goals:* Include values you want your children to learn, time with spouse, time with each child, vacations, and so on. Some people put family goals before personal goals. Remember the airline admonishment to put your oxygen mask on before helping others. Implication is if I am not in good condition, it makes it harder to help/be there for others.
4. *Practice/Business:* This can include daily huddles with staff, C. E. courses to take, production goals for you and others in the practice, better ways to bring in patients, and others.
5. *Hobbies:* How much time and money do I (we) set aside for hobbies.
6. *Financial:* See below.

Your financial goals should reflect your values. For example, if it is important to financially help others, whether through your faith-based organizations or through nonprofit organizations that provide services for people in need, you should have a budget item for giving. If educating your children is important, you need a budget item for college. Professional money managers say that they can tell a person's priorities in life by looking at his or her checkbook and/or credit card bills. People spend on and save for things that are important to them.

It is a good idea to list your short- and long-term financial goals after analyzing your spending patterns and before establishing your budget. Keep in mind that goals are what you wish to achieve at the completion of your budget. You need to be prepared to adjust your goals, if necessary, to meet your financial target. See the following website for more information on setting financial goals: http;//genxfinance.com/setting-your-financial-goals-with-a-goal-worksheet.

Budgeting Process

Step 1: Setting Up Categories and Calculating Expenditures

How you start the budgeting process can set you up for success or disappointment. To maximize your success, keep all your receipts, or if married all your family receipts, for at least 2 months, preferably 3 months. Sort them by category as you accumulate them. At the end of the appointed time period, total each category. Now you have an idea of how much to budget for food, utilities, gas, lunches, coffee out, fishing, and so forth.

For periodic reoccurring bills such as car insurance and house insurance, consult your checkbook or credit card statements and budget monthly. Budget books are available at office supply stores, or you can purchase software that allows you to record your purchases and assists you with creation of your budget. Some personal computers come with software such as Microsoft Money. You can purchase other software programs such as Quicken or Microsoft Excel. Be sure to customize any budget worksheet you use. Add or delete categories to reflect your spending.

The important thing is to find a method that works for you and then use that method to record your expenditures. Table 26.1 provides an example of a personal/family budget. Two websites that can help you find/develop a budget work sheet are http://www.betterbudgeting.com/budgetformsfree.htm and http://www.soyouwanna.com/site/syws/budget/budget.html

Step 2: Matching Income to Expenses

The next step to successful budgeting is to take the summary of your 2- or 3-month spending patterns and compare the total monthly outflow with your monthly net (after taxes and deductions) income. If expenses run higher than income, you will need to make spending adjustments. The spending adjustments need to be severe enough to leave you with a surplus at the end of the month. Remember, the unexpected can and will happen, so put aside for the unexpected (see "Step 4: Setting up an Emergency Fund"). Savings should be a part of your budget. Savings should focus on your goals for retirement, investments, and vacations.

Step 3: Refining Your Budget

Look for ways to increase your buying power. You can increase your buying power by reducing expenses, increasing income, and taking advantage of unique opportunities.

Table 26.1   Personal/family monthly budget.

Estimated take-home monthly income: _____This assumes an emergency fund has already been funded. If not, fully fund this to last 3–6 months

	Monthly Amount
Automobiles (could do some through business)	
Gasoline	_____
Repairs/tires	_____
Taxes/insurance	_____
Leasing/loan payment	_____
Car replacement savings fund	_____
Clothing/shoes	_____
Food	_____
Nonfood (household cleaning supplies, shampoo, etc.)	_____
Gifts and stamps/postage	_____
Personal debt (credit cards, department stores, etc.)	_____
School debt	_____
Child care	_____
House/apartment	_____
Phone (local, long-distance	_____
service, cell phone)	_____
Water	_____
Electricity	_____
Natural gas/propane	_____
Garbage (service provided via city taxes in some cases)	_____
House maintenance (repairs, etc.)	_____
Mortgage/loan payment	_____
Escrow for insurance/taxes	_____
Cable/internet	_____
Replacement funds (furnace, roof, carpet, furniture, computer, etc.)	_____
Other insurance (life, liability, disability); could do through business but not recommended that you do so for disability insurance because of tax implications)	_____
Entertainment (movies, eating out, etc)	_____
Allowances	_____
Vacation fund	_____
Giving	_____
Health insurance, prescriptions, glasses, etc. (could do this through business depending on business entity and benefits offered)	_____
Savings/retirement (beyond retirement plans through your business)	_____
Pets	_____
Miscellaneous (newspaper, magazines, haircuts, sports for children, children's school expenses, etc.)	_____
Total Monthly Budget	_____

Reducing expenses can range from cutting back on purchases, delaying purchases, or eliminating some purchases. On the positive side, reducing expenses can include buying in bulk items that you will need or timing sales (purchase next winter's coat in the spring). Many books and online sites are available to give good ideas on how to reduce expenses.

Increasing income can be accomplished without you or a family member seeking additional employment. Consolidating loans or paying off loans early can increase income without substantially increasing taxes. Again, both your library and online sites have many useful resources to help you find ways to increase income.

Use credit cards (only if you can pay them off each month) to take advantage of money-saving offers such as free airline miles, discounts on gas, and points toward purchases. Make some of your necessary purchases online (only from reputable businesses with low or no handling charges). The cost of mailing may offset any reduced sales tax or gas required to purchase the same item locally. Again, many books and websites can help you find the bargains that best help you achieve your goals. Google Cut Costs: Guides on Bargains & Money Management.

Step 4: Setting Up an Emergency Fund

With some or all of the cash you free up when you establish and live on your budget, you need to create an emergency fund. The purpose of an emergency fund is to sock away, in a safe, out-of-sight, out-of-mind account, 3–6 months of living expenses. An emergency fund not only can support you and your family in the interim between injury and disability insurance payments or the interim between changing practices but can also fund unexpected expenses such as the broken dryer or an expensive car repair. Emergency funds are an absolute necessity for financial security because they give you funds to fall back on. Without an emergency fund, you may be forced to incur credit card debt that could take you many years to pay off. You never want to be in the position where you have to buy daily necessities like food and transportation on credit.

If you do not have dependents, a 3-month emergency fund may be adequate. If you have dependents, you should set your goal for 6 months of emergency funds. The more the people you support, the more likely you will be to have unplanned or unexpected costs.

It is best to keep your emergency fund separate from investment accounts used for vacations or cars. Keeping it separate makes it easier to leave alone. While you would not keep your retirement funds in savings accounts, money market accounts, certificates of deposit, or short-term bonds, these are good places to stash cash you may need on short notice. These are the most liquid investments.

If you determine you need $6,000 in your emergency fund and you can afford $100 a month, pay yourself, put it away, and let it grow. Once you have reached your goal, keep investing the money but put it in a nonretirement brokerage account and watch your savings grow.

If you have your emergency fund money transferred from your paycheck to your emergency fund account, your temptation to spend it will be reduced. Remember, financial security comes over time. Do not get discouraged. Refer to Why You Need an Emergency Fund (http://financialplan.about.com/od/savingmoney/a/emergencyfund.html).

Step 5: Passing on What You Have Learned

All the people affected by a budget should be involved in the budget as soon as they are old enough to understand the concept of money. Family budget meetings are excellent teaching opportunities for children and a good way to get the family working together on a goal or goals.

You will find many examples of budgets that give you a percentile range for how much you should be spending on housing, food, and so forth. The percentile ranges are based on average incomes. Consequently, if your income is lower or higher than average, the ranges will not be reflective of your spending patterns.

Remember that budgeting is a process that requires realistic goals and adjustments: adjustments to your goals, adjustments for unexpected expenses, adjustments in income, and so on. The more you scrutinize and understand your budget, the better the likelihood of achieving your financial goals. Stick to your budget and do not give up.

Exit Strategies

For Your Business

Should you structure your dental practice as a sole proprietorship, partnership, or limited partnership? What about a C corporation, S corporation, or limited liability company (LLC)? Chapter 10 addresses these organizational options in greater detail. We cannot advise you strongly enough to seek the help of a competent attorney-accountant team to help you decide which is best for you. Many times the decision is made based on which one offers the best tax situation or which best limits your exposure to a potential lawsuit. Sometimes the determination is made based on which has the least administrative costs. It is appropriate to consider all of these things. However, remember to consider something else. How will the structure I choose affect me when it is time to sell the practice? When first starting your practice, how it will be sold is probably one of the least important things on your mind. Even though this event is years away, give it some thought at the start.

For Yourself

You will die some day, a sobering thought for all mortals. How will you pass along your assets to your loved ones? Basically, it can be done in one of three ways:

1. Attach a beneficiary or transfer on death statement to everything you own. If you near the end of life with few assets, this may be all you need.
2. Use a will: Upon your death the executor will distribute your assets per your instructions. Probate court may be involved in some states and therefore the proceedings would be made public. The cost to probate a will can be substantial.
3. Use a trust: If you have considerable assets, a trust is probably best for you. It can shelter your loved ones from paying taxes needlessly. One need not die for the trust to be activated. A trust can actually start benefiting you while you are still alive. Since the trust does not go through a probate court, there are no proceedings to be made public. Your financial situation remains private. It costs more to prepare, fund, and manage a trust, but then you save by avoiding probate costs if all assets were held by the trust.

Make an appointment with a competent estate planning attorney. Professional guidance is very important.

Long-Term Care Planning

As we live longer, funding our care near the end of our lives is becoming a bigger concern. There are four ways to fund your long-term care expenses:

1. *Long-term care insurance:* It can be expensive and you will be paying regular premiums with no assurance you will ever use it. It is only as good as the company you buy it from. When the aging population starts making demands on these insurance companies, will they have enough money to meet these expenses? If not, the company goes bankrupt and you will not receive the benefits you were promised.

2. *Medicare and Medicaid:* Medicare is a federal program. Medicaid is a state program and therefore varies from state to state. Having federal and/or state programs pay for your longer-term care is designed for those who cannot afford to pay for it themselves. However, both programs cover very little long-term care costs. There are attorneys who specialize in designing programs to "give away" your assets so that you qualify for this support. More and more of these loopholes are being closed so that the wealthy cannot "beat the system." However, if you decide to pursue this, do not try to do it yourself. Hire a competent attorney who specializes in this area to handle the details. The process is very detailed and one minor misstep can derail your program.

3. *Self-insured:* Many people assume that only the very wealthy can afford to do this. Not so fast. Let us assume that the average cost of a long-term care facility in your area is $75,000 per year. If the average stay is 3 years, then one would need $225,000 to pay for it. Many dentists will have that much left in their retirement plans when they get to the last 3 years of their lives. Take the time to do the computations before you rule out this alternative.

4. *Relatives:* Most people assume that this means financial support from a relative. That is one possibility. But what if you have a son, daughter, niece, or nephew who is a doctor or nurse? Can one of them take care of you and in return you leave that person some or all of your assets when you die?

So, how do you determine which of the four is best for you? First, decide whether or not you want to protect your assets for your children or loved ones. Some people plan to spend every dollar they have saved and enjoy life. These individuals are interested in protecting their assets for their spouse, but not for anyone else. We have heard many times, "I've told my kids the last check I write before I die will bounce." If this is your philosophy, you will make different choices when it comes to paying for your long-term care than someone who wants to make sure his or her children inherit something. Keep in mind the reason you have saved your entire working life is to take care of you and your spouse in your final years. That is what the money is for. You did not save it to pass it along to the kids. However, some people want to protect it for that purpose. So, first decide whether or not you wish to pass along some of your assets to your children, then decide which way you will fund your long-term care to best achieve that goal.

Second, should you decide to purchase a long-term care insurance policy, be aware that not all insurance companies have strong enough balance sheets to have enough money to pay you when the baby boomers hit those peak years near the end of their lives. The drain on the assets of most insurance companies at that time will be enormous. Too many long-term care sales people focus only on the benefits of the policy they sell, which is important. But do not forget to explore the financial strength of the insurance company that issues the policy. This is best done by meeting with a competent professional who knows how to read profit and loss statements, balance sheets, and annual reports. Insurance companies are also rated by organizations. This information may also be helpful in evaluating companies.

Summary

If you decide to make financial independence and building and maintaining wealth a part of your way of life, then you will need to make a commitment as well as the necessary changes in attitude and behavior to achieve your goals. The changes in attitude and behavior will not be as difficult as your first year of dental school. In fact, if most people maintained their dental school lifestyle for a couple of years after graduation, they would make significant progress toward financial independence and building wealth. This assumes the money saved by not spending is wisely invested and/or used to pay-off "bad" debt.

The people who have achieved financial independence and accumulated wealth have left a trail to follow. All you need to do is to follow the signs and do as they did:

- Develop an accurate philosophy about money.
- Establish and be committed to financial goals.
- Save buying power.
- Make decisions on the revenue side.
- Make informed investment choices.
- Plan for the future (college, retirement).
- Develop and maintain a budget.
- Develop exit strategies early in life.

As a final reminder, it is imperative that your business and personal assets be protected with proper insurance coverages as discussed in detail in Chapter 25.

References and Additional Resources

Books

Chidester, Jane E. and Macko, John L. 1997. *BudgetYes!: 21st Century Solutions for Taking Control of Your Money Now*. Powell, OH: Tulip Tree Press.

Dahle, James M. 2014. *The White Coat Investor: A Doctor's Guide to Personal Finance and Investing*. The White Coat Investor LLC.

Graham, Benjamin. 1973. *The Intelligent Investor: A Book of Practical Counsel*, 4th ed. New York: Harper & Row.

Lawrence, Judy. 2004. *The Budget Kit: The Common Cents Money Management Workbook*. Chicago: Dearborn Trade Publishing.

Sander, Peter, and Sander Basye, Jennifer. 1999. *The Pocket Idiot's Guide to Living on a Budget*. New York: Macmillan.

Shiller, Robert J. 2015. *Irrational Exuberance*, 3rd ed. Princeton, NJ: Princeton University Press.

Websites

http://www.investmentterms.net
http://financialplan.about.com/cs/personalfinance/a/EmergencyFunds.htm.
www.betterbudgeting.com/budgetformsfree.htm.
www.genxfinance.com/setting-your-financial-goals-with-a-goal-worksheet
www.soyouwanna.com/site/syws/budget/budget.html.
www.youneedabudget.com.
www.frugalliving.about.com/od/moneymanagement/u/cut_costs.htm

Learning Exercises

1. Write out your philosophy on money.
2. Read at least two books on budgeting and develop your monthly budget.
3. Develop your life goals.
4. Identify your financial goals for the next 5 years.

Index

Dental Practice Transition: A Practical Guide to Management, Second Edition.
Edited by David G. Dunning and Brian M. Lange.
© 2016 John Wiley & Sons, Inc. Published 2016 by John Wiley & Sons, Inc.
Companion Website: www.wiley.com/go/dunning/transition